the
MediterrAsian
Way

the
MediterrAsian
Way

A Cookbook and Guide to Health, Weight Loss,
and Longevity, Combining the Best Features of
Mediterranean and Asian Diets

Ric Watson & Trudy Thelander

ISBN: 978-0-473-45376-3

Bedford House
P R E S S

CONTENTS

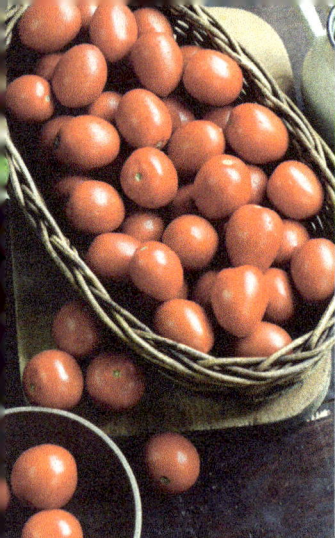

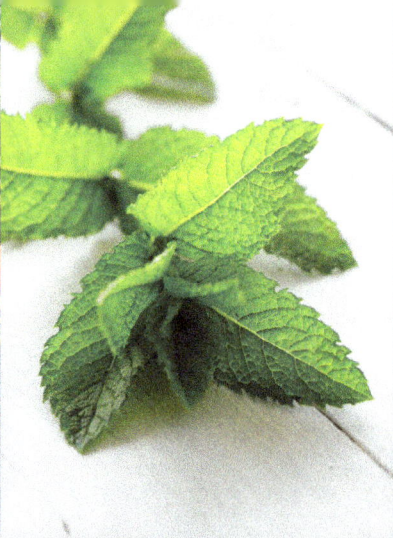

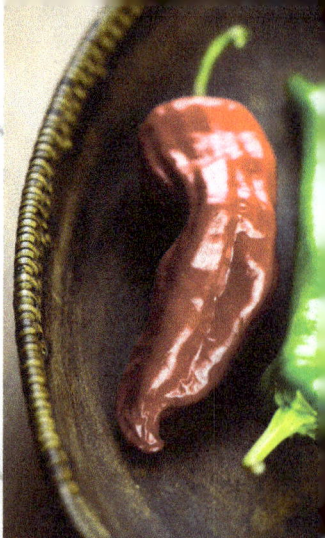

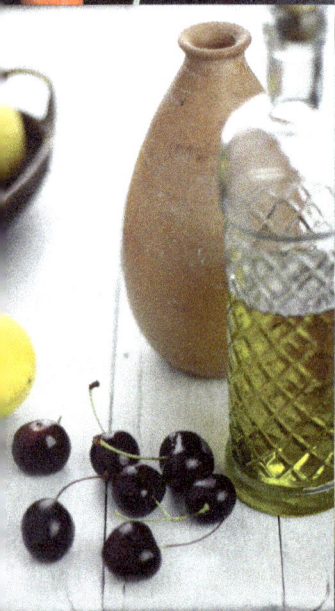

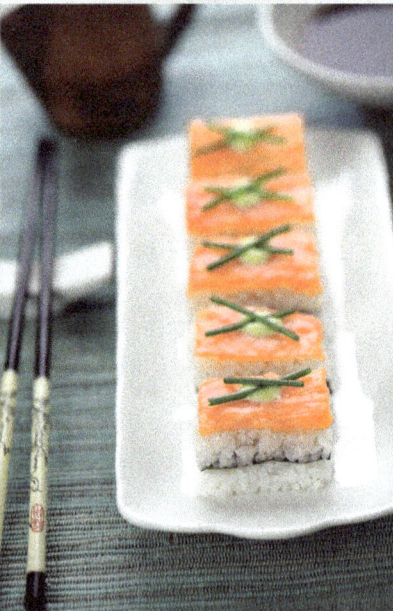

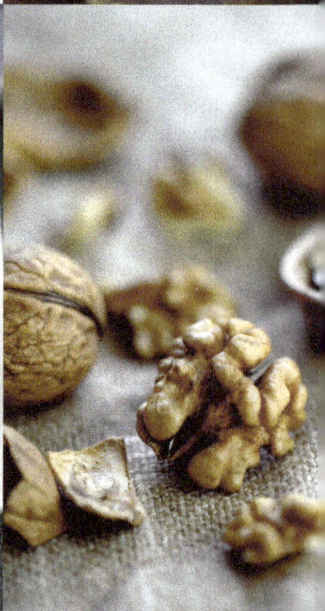

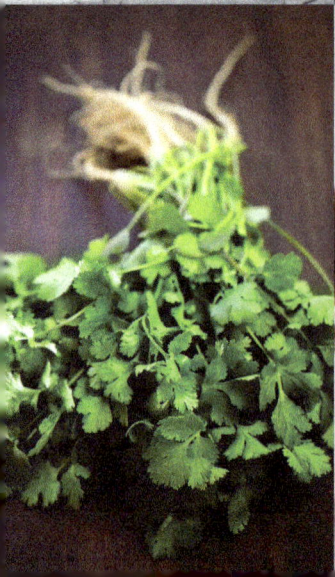

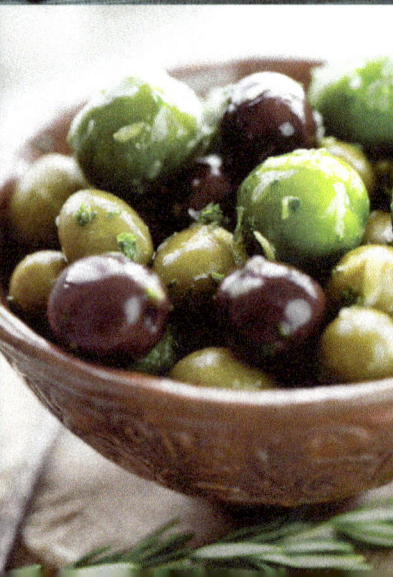

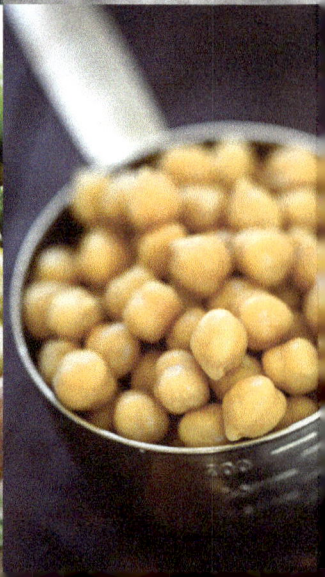

Discovering the MediterrAsian way

I believe that by following traditional Mediterranean and Asian dietary and lifestyle practices you can change your health, and your life, for the better. And I don't make that statement lightly. I know firsthand the benefits of this way of living, because it's had a very dramatic impact on my life. So, before describing this lifestyle in detail and how it can change your life, I'd like to tell you a little bit about myself and how a MediterrAsian lifestyle has changed my own life.

LIFE LESSONS

I was born to English parents in the beautiful Pacific Island nation of New Zealand. My parents had migrated to New Zealand because my dad, who was serving in the British Royal Airforce, had received a transfer there. And from as far back as I can remember, I'd dreamed of following in his footsteps by joining the military. But unlike my dad, who served in the airforce, I planned on becoming an officer in the army.

When I was a child, everything seemed to be heading in the right direction. I was very physically active when I was young and loved sports. I was lucky enough in my schooldays to be selected to play representative rugby for my city. One year I also set a school record in the 200-meter sprint. So, as far as I was concerned, I was well prepared for a physically demanding career as a soldier.

But, as the old saying goes, *the best-laid plans often go astray*.

First, when I was a teenager, I was called out of art class at school to the principal's office. My mother greeted me in tears and told me that my dad, who suffered from bouts of severe depression, had taken his own life.

Then, less than a year later—and while I was still grieving my dad's death—I was involved in a high-speed collision with a car while I was riding my motorcycle to a friend's house. My unprotected body slammed into the hard metal chassis with so much force that I broke most of the major bones on the left side my body. My left kneecap was shattered into several pieces, I sustained multiple lacerations, I severely bruised my liver and kidneys, and I lost a great deal of blood.

After being laid up for two months in the hospital, I was left with what my orthopedic surgeon described as "a permanent left-sided disability." And he told me that I might even need to use a walking stick for the rest of my life. He also told me flatly, but honestly, that I had "very little chance" of ever becoming a soldier.

These two horrible events, particularly one coming so soon after the other, took a toll on me, both physically and emotionally. But I'd already learned from my dad's death that you can't dwell on a crisis. You somehow have to see a positive (no matter how small that positive may be) and move on, or else it will just eat you up.

I started to look for positives, and thought about how my surgeon had given me very little chance of becoming a soldier, but he hadn't said no chance at all. As far as I was concerned, even if there was less than a 1 percent chance, I was still willing to give it a go. I knew I had nothing to lose.

A SEARCH FOR ANSWERS

So I decided to look for ways to regain my health and become fit and strong again. As Napoleon Bonaparte once said, "There are two ways to move men—interest and fear," and I certainly had both! Unfortunately, what I didn't have was any idea how to regain my health once it had been lost. I came to the conclusion that I needed to learn all I could about diet, health, and fitness if I was ever going to have a chance of reclaiming my future.

The first places I turned to for answers were bookstores and libraries. I was pleasantly surprised to find the shelves virtually overflowing with books promising a fast route to good health. However, on closer inspection, I noticed that most of these books offered different solutions from one another. In a lot of cases, one expert would totally contradict what another equally well-qualified expert said. I was staggered by the number of mixed messages I found.

In desperation I was forced to try a lot of different ways to regain my health. I found most of them were very restrictive and the results were mostly disappointing. But I persevered, because I realized that my entire future was on the line.

Eventually, after more than a year of *hard* work, I'd reached a point where I felt I could give the army a go. My knee was still causing me a lot of pain, and I knew I certainly wasn't back to 100 percent health, but I figured that army life would somehow "whip me into shape." In the end, I knew it was going to be a struggle but I was determined to grit my teeth and face the challenge.

However, although I was mentally prepared, physically my body certainly wasn't. By the end of the first day of training my knee started to swell and became increasingly painful. By the end of the week my knee was the size of a small balloon, and the pain was almost unbearable. I begged the army physician to let me stay to see if it improved, but he realized there was just no chance. So, after only eight days, I was honorably discharged from the army.

I returned home feeling like a failure. I couldn't believe that more than a year of struggle and sacrifice had amounted to absolutely nothing. But I knew I'd come too far to quit. I was still positive that the answer to regaining my health was out there somewhere, and at this stage I was more determined than ever to find it.

Again, I went back to the books and tried a number of other "miracle breakthroughs." Eventually, after four months of resolute effort, I felt I could give the army another go. It took a great deal of work to convince the army physician that I was fit and strong enough to reenlist, but after fervently pleading my case, he gave the go-ahead. I was over the moon. I couldn't believe I'd been given a second chance.

But my happiness quickly turned to despair when, after only a day of training, the swelling and pain in my knee started to increase. I tried lots of ways of covering up the pain and inflammation, but when my pants wouldn't fit over my knee anymore, I knew I was fighting a losing battle. So, after a little over a week back in the army, I received my second honorable discharge.

I returned home in a worse state than ever—both physically and emotionally. My orthopedic surgeon's report from the time highlights the poor state of my physical health:

"The wrist is painful . . . his left leg is troublesome and in particular the knee. Strenuous activity causes pain, standing causes the knee to ache and swell, he can jog for a mile but then has considerable pain which is quite persistent. He cannot run, cannot kneel, has difficulty getting up and down stairs . . . and the knee causes quite severe episodic pain."

The report finished on a high note: *"The situation is unlikely to change."*

I was devastated. And at this point I was well and truly fed up with what life had thrown at me: my dad's suicide, my accident, going in and out of the army twice, and trying everything in my power to regain my health, yet being in a worse state of health and in more pain than ever. As far as I was concerned, I was just destined to be a shell of my former self—one of life's "unlucky" people.

The outlook for my future seemed very bleak indeed. However, just as I was hitting rock bottom, something unexpected happened. I discovered that an accident compensation claim I'd filed many months earlier had been settled, and I'd received a lump sum payment.

But at first I wasn't quite sure what to do with it. Like most young guys, thoughts of fast cars, new clothes, and expanding my music collection all came to mind. But I knew there was a much deeper significance to getting this money. I knew it was the only ray of hope I had left for improving my future, and I was determined to use it very wisely.

One thing I knew for certain, I needed a break—a *big* break. My stress levels were going through the roof, and the severe pain in my left knee was really getting me down. I was also out of shape because my knee prevented me from being very physically active. I knew a long vacation would help me recuperate.

It didn't take me long to decide on the south coast of England as my vacation destination. Not just because of the peacefulness of this area, but because my uncle Tony lived there. And in many ways, Tony was the last hope I had for regaining my health.

THE VACATION THAT CHANGED MY LIFE

Tony, like my father, had served in the British Royal Airforce. But, instead of transferring to New Zealand, Tony had been stationed in the Middle East (where they traditionally eat a Mediterranean-style diet). It was there that Tony became a middleweight boxing champion for the airforce. When Tony returned to England he left the airforce became a sports coach and opened his own gymnasium.

When I arrived in England Tony and his wife, Muriel, were living in a quiet country village near the sea where they were running their own health spa. At the time Tony was in his late forties, but I was taken aback when I first saw him—he was in extraordinary physical condition and didn't look a day over thirty-five. Even more surprising was Aunt Muriel, who was nearly ten years older than Tony and approaching sixty. I could only describe her as radiant, and I would have sworn she wouldn't be blowing out more than forty candles on her next birthday. It was immediately clear that these people knew more than a few secrets about getting and staying fit and healthy, and I was determined to pick their brains!

One of my biggest surprises was when I discovered just how much good food Tony and Muriel ate. It turned out that the time Tony had spent stationed overseas had had a big influence on him, and there were no carrot sticks or cottage cheese anywhere in sight. Instead, I found delicious and hearty pasta, bean, vegetable, and rice dishes; a wide range of breads and cheeses; eggs; nuts; olive oil; seasonal and tropical fruits; and wonderful desserts.

Tony also told me that he and Muriel hadn't eaten red meat for years. He said that small amounts of red meat were fine, but that I should preferably eat chicken, or better still, fish and shellfish, which he said contained special health-giving oils. Tony also explained that eating the correct balance of these foods was just as important as the food itself.

At first it seemed almost too good to be true that by eating these sorts of delicious foods I could get healthy and in shape. But as soon as I started eating the correct balance of the foods Tony recommended, I could feel my body absorb the

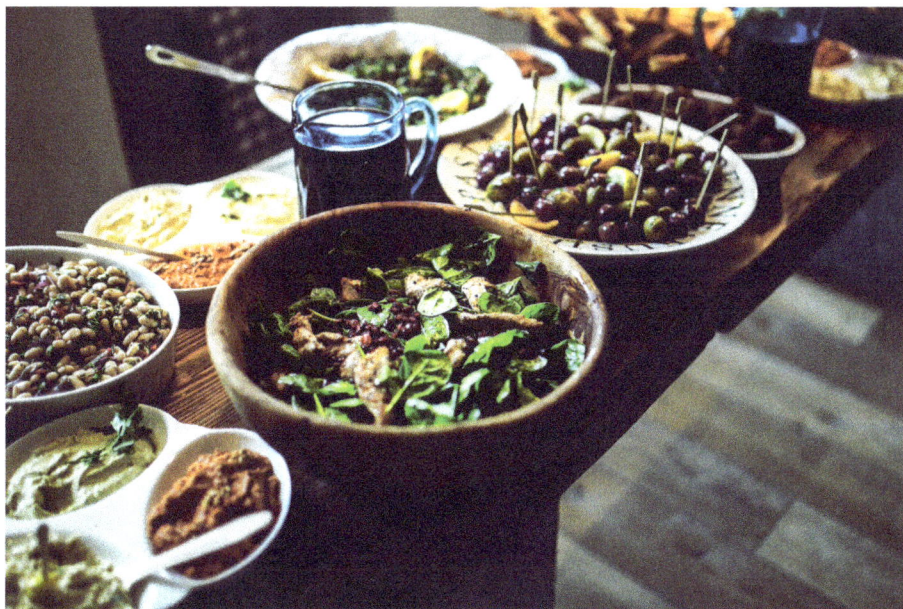

concentrated nourishment like a dry sponge soaking up water. Within days my energy level had increased substantially. Within weeks the pain and inflammation around my knee had started to improve noticeably. Even the excess weight I'd gained from my lack of movement started dropping off. And to my delight I discovered there was another positive side effect. Since I was six years old I'd suffered from migraine headaches almost weekly. My parents had taken me to a number of medical specialists in search of a cure, without success. But these nausea inducing headaches that had plagued me most of my life simply disappeared.

I'd heard that "you are what you eat," but I was amazed that something as simple as making the right food choices could have such a dramatic effect on my health. In fact, within six months my strength and energy had improved so much that I was even able to run for long distances, with only a minimum of discomfort.

After so much time fruitlessly struggling to regain my health, I could hardly believe the remarkable improvement in my health, fitness, and energy in such a short amount of time. A few months earlier I could barely walk up a flight of stairs, and running for any distance caused almost unbearable pain. Yet here I was, running for miles at a time with virtually no pain. My energy levels were at an all-time high, I was free of migraine headaches, and I was more than twenty pounds lighter. As far as I was concerned, it was nothing short of a miracle!

MOVING ON

With such a positive outcome, my vacation to England, which I'd originally planned to last no longer than two months, ended up turning into a working vacation lasting more than a year. But eventually I realized that although I'd sorted out my health, I was still single and without a career. I knew it was time to move on.

Instead of immediately returning home to New Zealand, I decided to visit my mother, who had remarried and moved to Australia. As it turned out, this was one of the most fateful decisions I've ever made, because it was in Australia that I met and fell in love with the co-author of this book, Trudy.

PERFECT MATCH

When I first met Trudy I couldn't believe how much we had in common. Like me, she was very interested in looking after her health (I found out that this was because she was the daughter of two practicing medical doctors). She also loved traveling (so much so that she was an international travel agent), and just like me she loved good food, good wine, and good conversation. With such an incentive to stay in Australia, I decided to indefinitely postpone my return to New Zealand, and Trudy and I moved in together.

With our common passion for good food, it wasn't long before we found ourselves naturally gravitating toward the kitchen. I was particularly keen to introduce Trudy to all the wonderful and healthy Mediterranean-style dishes I'd learned to cook in England. And I discovered that Trudy was equally keen to introduce me to her favorite style of food: Asian. It turned out that Trudy's sister-in-law was Chinese-Malaysian and had introduced her to authentic Asian cooking years earlier; Trudy had been hooked ever since. And as soon as I tasted my first mouthful of the authentic Asian seafood stir-fry that Trudy whipped up, I was well and truly hooked too!

At first I was worried about deviating too much from the Mediterranean style of eating I'd been following. I thought that if I ate too much Asian-inspired food, the pain in my knee could flare up, and my migraine headaches might return. Yet the more I looked into it the more I realized that, apart from basic differences in herbs and flavorings, the diets of the Mediterranean and Asia were actually remarkably similar.

For example, grain foods are a traditional dietary staple in both Mediterranean and Asian cultures. In Asia it's rice and noodles, and in the Mediterranean it's pasta, rice, bread, and other grain foods such as couscous and bulgur. And red meats don't feature prominently in either cuisine; instead fish, shellfish, poultry, and plant foods such as beans and nuts form the main sources of protein. Asian and Mediterranean peoples also traditionally eat lots of fresh vegetables and fruits, and even the type of fat they use is similar, favoring healthy plant-based fats such as olive or peanut oil over animal fats. Finally, the consumption of moderate amounts of alcohol, particularly over a meal, has been practiced by Mediterranean and Asian cultures for centuries. So, although each type of cuisine is unique, the nutrients found in both a Mediterranean and an Asian-style diet are almost identical. This delighted me because it opened up a whole new world of tastes and textures without compromising my hard-won good health. In fact, this way of eating made so much sense that it wasn't long before Trudy and I were living on an almost exclusive diet of what we called "MediterrAsian" food—literally, a fusion of Mediterranean and Asian cuisines.

GOOD FOOD THAT'S GOOD FOR YOU

As we experimented more and more with a MediterrAsian style of eating, we were delighted to discover that, in addition to all the health benefits, there were countless other bonuses too. For one, it never ceased to amaze us that foods this healthful were also the most delicious we'd ever tasted. And, as we began to experiment more with fresh Mediterranean and Asian ingredients, we found that the healthiest way to cook them was often the simplest, which meant less work for the cook! Best of all, this way of eating offered us such an endless variety of unique tastes, intriguing textures, vibrant colors, and tantalizing aromas that we were never bored. In fact, far from restricting our choice, we discovered a world of diverse foods and flavors.

To our delight, we also discovered that most of our favorite restaurant and takeout food was based on the cuisines of the Mediterranean and Asia. Italian, Greek, Chinese, Japanese, Thai, Vietnamese, Turkish, Spanish, and Moroccan were just some of the ethnic delights we could choose from.

With our love for this type of food we also became enthusiastic collectors of Mediterranean and Asian recipes. Our search for new and interesting dishes was helped immeasurably by Trudy's job as a travel agent. One of the perks of her job was traveling the world inspecting the facilities of international hotels. She used these overseas trips to such places as Indonesia and Hong Kong as the perfect opportunity to add to our growing collection of recipes. She would always return home with a notebook full of hastily scribbled recipes she had picked up from street vendors or in traditional back-street eateries—food that was so simple, yet so utterly glorious.

DISCOVERING MORE THAN FOOD

Over the years our love of Mediterranean and Asian food became a true passion. But it went a lot deeper than just food. We also became fascinated by the culture and rich history of these areas. And as we'd reaped so many positive rewards simply by adopting this style of eating, we started to wonder whether we could learn other lifestyle lessons from these cultures too.

Our first thoughts turned to our least favorite activity in life: exercising. At this stage, the main form of exercise in our lives was exercise sessions at our local fitness center. We both found this type of exercise extremely boring and a lot of hard work. Including the cost of yearly membership and parking, it was also very expensive. But we were under the impression that it was a necessary evil we just had to put up with if we wanted to stay fit. Then it dawned on us: For the past few thousand years Mediterranean and Asian peoples had never worked out on Stairmasters or Butt-Blasters or jumped around in aerobics classes to stay in shape. They kept fit by simply moving naturally as part of their everyday lives, so why couldn't we do the same?

This thought encouraged us to start looking for ways we could move naturally as part of our everyday lives, instead of moving artificially at the fitness center. We soon discovered dozens of ways we could easily and effortlessly slip physical activity into our lives without formally exercising, and all of them were a lot more fun than sweating away on a Stairmaster. Before long we decided to give up the fitness center and artificial exercise all together.

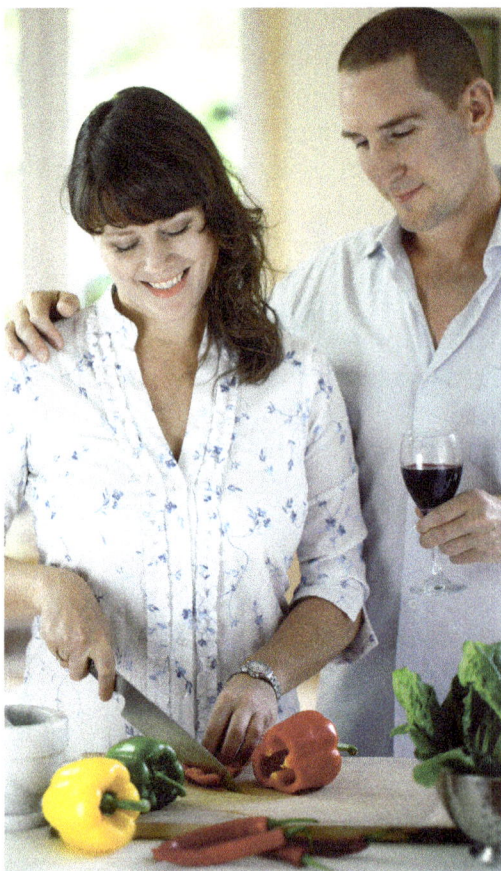

NOURISHING THE BODY AND THE SOUL

Between the healthy foods we were eating and the natural movement we were incorporating into our lives, we couldn't have been physically healthier. But as important as our physical well-being is, we also knew from personal experience that our emotional well-being is just as important.

By adopting a MediterrAsian style of eating, we had discovered how to enjoy lots of wonderful food while staying healthy and in shape, so this certainly went a long way toward providing us with a good sense of emotional wellbeing. But we knew that eating good food is only one of life's many pleasures. So we began to think of other ways we could achieve emotional well-being in our lives that didn't revolve around food. Through lots of fun experimentation we discovered plenty of ways to relax, rejuvenate, and achieve a sense emotional well-being in our lives, and none of them involved food. (This was good not only for our emotional well-being, but for the well-being of our waistlines too!)

We soon made it a rule that every day, no matter how busy we were, we each had to set aside time to do something relaxing and enjoyable. We found that one of the big benefits of setting aside relaxation time every day, apart from recharging our emotional and spiritual batteries, was that it also acts as a very effective stress-reliever.

PUTTING IT ALL TOGETHER

For us, incorporating relaxation time into our lives completed the foundations for achieving a healthy body and mind. And in many ways we had relied on the basic principles that Mediterranean and Asian peoples had instinctively been living for the past few thousand years: We were eating lots of good wholesome food; we were physically active as part of our everyday lives; and, by setting aside special time to relax every day, we were mimicking the relaxed, less stressful lifestyles that characterize people from these regions. With this simple three-pronged approach toward our physical and emotional health, not only did we feel empowered, but we ultimately felt we had achieved that most elusive of all states: *optimal health*.

SOLVING THE MYSTERY

Adopting a MediterrAsian way of living had made a profound difference to our health and vitality. Yet, although we knew that this lifestyle worked, we still didn't know exactly *why* it worked. This got us thinking: Was there a scientific explanation for the way we were feeling?

Yes, there certainly was a scientific explanation for the way we were feeling. We discovered that for over half a century some of the Western world's leading scientists and doctors had been thoroughly investigating the health-giving benefits of Mediterranean and Asian dietary and lifestyle practices.

Using the Internet we uncovered hundreds of interviews, reports, articles, and well-documented scientific studies confirming why this way of living was so beneficial. And as we investigated deeper we discovered dozens of remarkable stories of other Westerners, like us, who had adopted a similar lifestyle and were reaping incredible benefits. Among other things, we found that this type of lifestyle had been credited with the prevention of long-term crippling illnesses such as heart disease, many types of cancer, and arthritis.

SHARING OUR KNOWLEDGE

By now it was hard to believe how dramatically my life had turned around in the years since my accident. From thinking of myself as one of life's unlucky people, I now felt like one of the luckiest people in the world. I was healthier both physically and emotionally than ever before; I was sharing my life with someone I adored; and to top it off I'd even found a career I loved—I'd combined a lifelong passion for art with a computer and had started my own graphic design business.

But as happy and complete as my life seemed, I couldn't help thinking about how differently things could have turned out. I realized that if it wasn't for an extraordinary set of circumstances I never would have fully regained my health at all. This was reinforced to me every time I saw a new book or infomercial claiming to have finally discovered the "real answer" to getting healthy and fit. I knew most of these so-called answers were simply the same gimmicky personal theories that were around when I was struggling to regain my health years earlier, only with slick new packaging and flashy new marketing.

This made me feel incredibly frustrated because I knew we'd found a real answer: We'd discovered how someone living a busy Western lifestyle could successfully adopt the traditional dietary and lifestyle practices of the healthiest and longest-lived peoples on earth. And this answer wasn't based on someone's personal theory; it was based on dietary and lifestyle practices that had been successfully tried and tested for more than five thousand years, and was backed up by decades of scientific research.

We were positive there were lots of other people out there, like me, who had lost their health—either through accident, illness, or obesity—who would really appreciate knowing about this way of living. I certainly knew that if this sort of information had been available when I was fruitlessly searching for answers, it would have saved me a huge amount of frustration and emotional anxiety.

So we decided to become proactive. We made up our minds that we were going to share what we knew about this way of living with as many people as we could.

After a lot of deliberation, Trudy suggested that we record a phone message setting out the basic principles of a MediterrAsian way of living, and people could simply phone in and listen to it. This made a lot of sense to me because it seemed like the next best thing to actually speaking to people personally.

So we recorded our message, set up a special phone line that could handle multiple calls, and placed a small announcement in our local newspaper. At first there was just a trickle of calls. But as word of mouth spread, our phone line started to receive more and more calls. Within a short time we were getting dozens, then hundreds of calls a week. In a little over five months our phone line had received more than six thousand calls. We were blown away by the response!

We even started to receive letters from people who were putting our simple guidelines into practice and getting positive results. This gave us a warm glow of pride.

But we did notice one thing. Many of the letters would finish by asking for even more information, particularly written information. It soon became obvious to us that although our phone line was certainly helpful, it simply wasn't enough. People needed more. And most important, they needed written information they could refer back to.

So we worked hard in our spare time to achieve that goal, and for more than four years we compiled thousands of words about how to follow a MediterrAsian way of living.

We ended up condensing this information and presented it in a user-friendly format on the Internet. We called our site MediterrAsian.com and, thanks again to positive word of mouth, it's now grown to become one of the most popular ethnic diet websites on the Internet, and has shown millions of people how to incorporate traditional Mediterranean and Asian dietary and lifestyle practices into their own lives.

We see this book as an extension of our site, and we hope it gives you a good general understanding of the principles behind a MediterrAsian way of living. By following these principles, Trudy and I have profoundly changed our lives for the better. And we're confident that if you put these same simple principles into practice for yourself, your life will change for the better too.

–Ric Watson

CHAPTER 1

Introduction

I magine for a moment that every day you could indulge in a large variety of tasty and satisfying foods such as pasta dishes, stir-fries, pizzas, curries, risottos and sushi, all washed down with a glass of your favorite wine or beer. Imagine as well that you never had to formally exercise, and that you got to set aside special time every day to relax and unwind.

Now imagine that eating and living this way could help you stay lean and healthy; substantially reduce your risk of contracting heart disease, Type 2 diabetes, osteoporosis, and many types of cancer (including breast, prostate, and colon cancer); and increase your chances of living longer.

This way of living might sound like the impossible dream, but in reality people from Mediterranean and Asian cultures have been living like this, and reaping the rewards, for more than five thousand years.

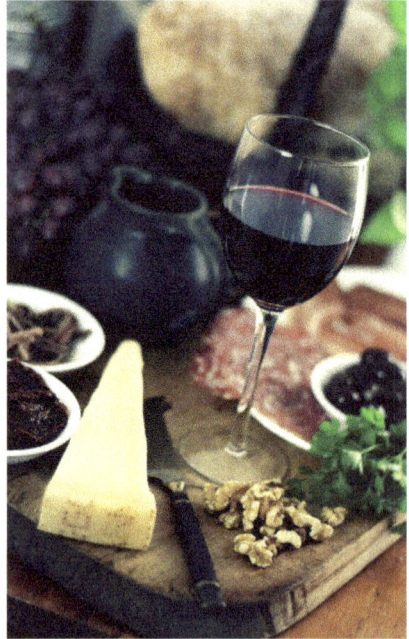

TRADITIONAL DIETARY AND LIFESTYLE PRACTICES

There's actually no such thing as a uniform Mediterranean or Asian diet and life-style. The Mediterranean region, for example, encompasses such diverse countries as Greece, Italy, Morocco, Turkey, Spain, and Tunisia. Not only do these countries share different ethnic, cultural, and religious backgrounds, but the dishes tra-ditionally eaten in these countries are equally diverse and use a wide range of different cooking techniques as well as different herbs, spices, and seasonings.

The cultural and culinary diversity seen throughout the Mediterranean is equally apparent in Asia, which includes such countries as Japan, China, Thailand, India, Vietnam, Indonesia, and Korea.

The Mediterranean Region

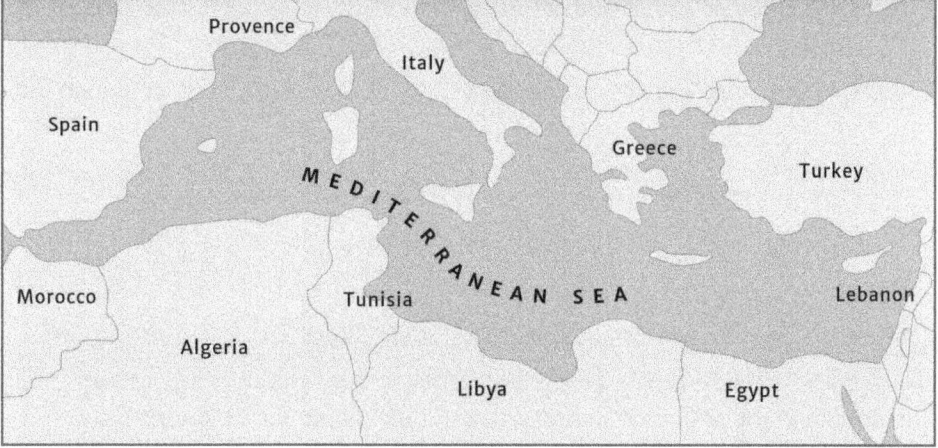

Provence
Italy
Spain
Greece
Turkey
M E D I T E R R A N E A N   S E A
Morocco
Tunisia
Lebanon
Algeria
Libya
Egypt

The Asian Region

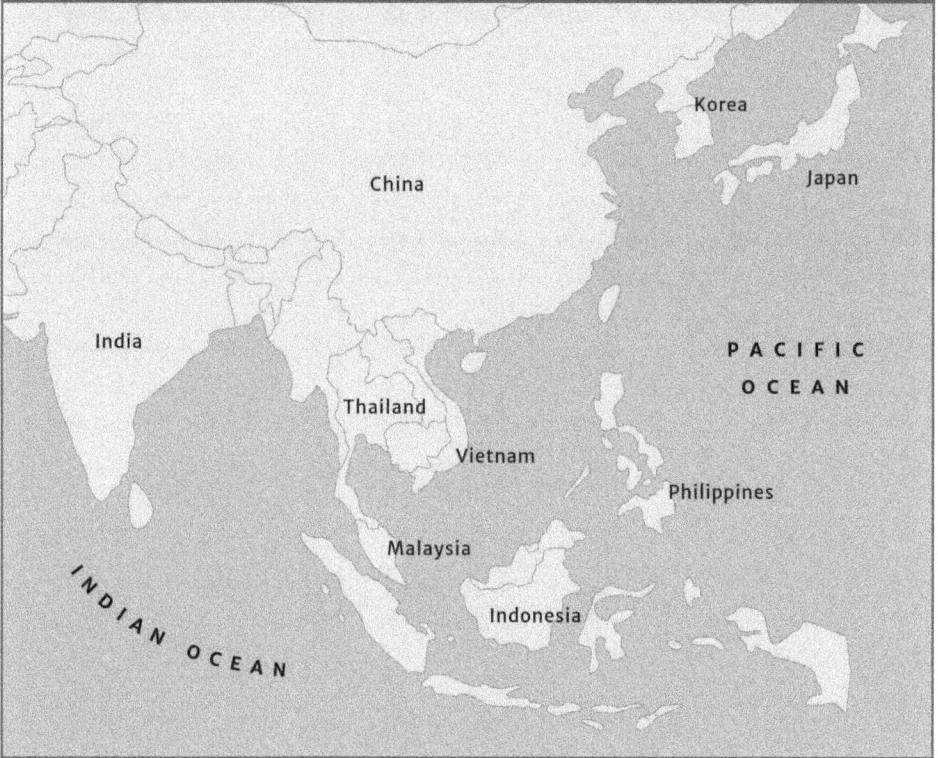

Korea
China
Japan
India
PACIFIC
OCEAN
Thailand
Vietnam
Philippines
Malaysia
INDIAN OCEAN
Indonesia

Yet, despite the differences, research over the last fifty years has shown that there are also many distinct similarities between the traditional dietary and lifestyle practices of Mediterranean and Asian cultures:

- Their diets include abundant amounts of plant foods such as vegetables, fruits, grains, legumes (beans, peas, and lentils), and nuts.
- They consume only small amounts of red meat.
- They consume fish regularly.
- Most of the fat they consume comes from plant and fish oils.
- They consume alcohol in moderation (usually with meals).
- They are physically active as part of their everyday lives.
- They tend to have an optimistic view of life, family ties are strong, and special time is usually set aside each day to relax the body and mind (such as the afternoon siesta common throughout the Mediterranean region, and tai chi and meditation, which are commonly practiced throughout Asia).

According to a large body of scientific research, these similar dietary and lifestyle practices help explain why Mediterranean and Asian peoples also share the same good health, low rates of chronic disease, and long life expectancy.

So how can a Westerner living in this fast-paced, high-stress modern world possibly adopt traditional Mediterranean and Asian dietary and lifestyle practices? If it sounds difficult, let us assure you that it's not. We both lead busy Western lives, and we've done it. In fact, for more than a decade we've been incorporating traditional Mediterranean and Asian dietary and lifestyle practices into our lives. Over that time, not only have we had lots of fun and discovered a world of wonderful tastes, we've also experienced a remarkable improvement in our physical health and emotional well-being. And through this book, we'd like to show you how to easily follow a "MediterrAsian" way of living too.

CHAPTER 2

Unlocking the secrets of the Mediterranean diet & Asian diet

O ne of the biggest benefits we've discovered through following a MediterrAsian way of living—along with how it makes us look and feel—is the peace of mind it gives us. With so many mixed messages out there, it's very comforting to know that a MediterrAsian lifestyle isn't based on unproven theories or current fads. It's based on what has worked for thousands of years.

And as well as being proven by the test of time, this type of lifestyle is also grounded in good science. In fact, for more than half a century some of the Western world's top scientists and doctors have been endeavoring to unlock the secrets behind the exceptional health, lack of chronic disease, and long life enjoyed by the peoples of the Mediterranean and Asia. What they have discovered—and are still discovering—is nothing short of remarkable.

THE GREAT CULTURAL DIVIDE

Scientists first started investigating the traditional dietary and lifestyle practices of Mediterranean and Asian cultures in the 1950s. They were looking for answers to why so many disorders common in Western society—such as coronary heart disease, breast cancer, diabetes, and obesity—were occurring frequently here, but very rarely there. What were these people doing that we weren't doing? Or was it simply a case of good genetics? The first person to attempt to answer that question was Ancel Keys, PhD, director of the Laboratory of Physiological Hygiene at the University of Minnesota School of Public Health.

Keys had already gained international notoriety in the 1940s for his research into the physiological effects of food and famine. Through his research he also developed a field survival ration for fighting troops, called the K Ration ("K" for

Keys), which became the official combat ration for U.S. troops during World War II. By the 1950s Keys's main focus was on preventing coronary heart disease, which was (and still is) the number one killer of both men and women in the Western world. He put forth a simple but powerful observation: "If some developed countries can do without heart attacks, why can't we?"

In the early 1950s Keys traveled to the Mediterranean region, where, working closely with local physicians, he conducted a series of studies. The first study involved a group of firemen from Naples, in southern Italy. Keys found that the firemen were still eating the same Mediterranean-style diet that had sustained their ancestors for thousands of years: plenty of plant foods (including grains, beans, fruits, and vegetables); fish and seafood eaten regularly; very little animal foods; and olive oil as the primary source of fat. When blood tests were taken, Keys found that the firemen had significantly lower blood cholesterol levels than the Western average. But at this stage it was still unclear how much of a role genetics played.

Next Keys traveled to another part of the Mediterranean, Spain, where he conducted a study on two different groups of people living in Madrid. One group lived in the poor quarter of Madrid; the other group was made up of fifty professional Madrid businessmen. Keys found that the Madrid poor, like the firemen from Naples, were still eating a traditional Mediterranean-style diet. But he found that most of the Madrid businessmen had abandoned their traditional diet and were eating a diet comparable to that in the West, complete with large amounts of red meat and dairy foods and only small amounts of plant foods.

In both groups the genetics were the same, but Keys discovered that blood cholesterol levels varied significantly. The Madrid poor had low levels, whereas the Madrid businessmen had much higher levels—and a correspondingly high rate of heart disease. Keys concluded that it was mainly the difference in diet that accounted for the greater incidence of heart disease among the businessmen.

To back-up this observation, Keys turned his attention to Asia, which, like the Mediterranean, had rates of heart disease far lower than that generally found in Western society. In 1956 he set up a long-range study of Japanese people living in Japan, Hawaii, and Los Angeles. Keys found that Japanese living in Japan had significantly lower blood cholesterol levels and far lower rates of heart disease than Japanese who had migrated to Hawaii or Los Angeles and adopted a Western diet. And he made another intriguing finding: The traditional diet that seemed to be protecting the Japanese in Japan was very similar to the traditional diet he had seen in the Mediterranean—high in plant-based foods, moderate in fish, and low in animal foods.

Keys's studies produced the first firm evidence that diet played a major role in the onset of heart disease. However, certain commercial interests—particularly the meat and dairy industries—still weren't convinced. But many others were, including the World Health Organization and President Eisenhower's heart specialist, Paul Dudley White. With their help Keys began planning one of the largest and most comprehensive studies ever conducted into the link between diet and heart disease, The Seven Countries Study.

A GROUNDBREAKING STUDY

The Seven Countries Study was launched in 1958. For more than a decade Professor Keys, with the help of an international team of specialists, studied the diet, lifestyle, and incidence of coronary heart disease among 12,763 randomly selected middle-aged men from seven countries: the United States, Japan, Italy, Greece, the Netherlands, Finland, and the former Yugoslavia. These areas were specifically chosen because of their differences in traditional diet. Another criterion was the availability of collaborators who understood the cultures and could provide logistical support and access to communities.

To make the research as thorough as possible, not only were extensive questionnaires recorded, Keys and his team collected actual foods eaten for a full week among randomly selected families and chemically analyzed their nutrient content. There were also repeat food collections in different seasons during different years to provide a valid estimate of the nutrients consumed.

When all the research was analyzed, a clear and predictable pattern emerged. In the Mediterranean and Asian regions of the world (Greece, Japan, and southern Italy)—where vegetables, grains, fruits, beans, and fish took center stage—heart disease was found to be rare. But in those countries where people filled their plates with red meat, cheese, and other foods high in saturated fat—such as in the United States and Finland—the rates of heart disease were found to be very high.

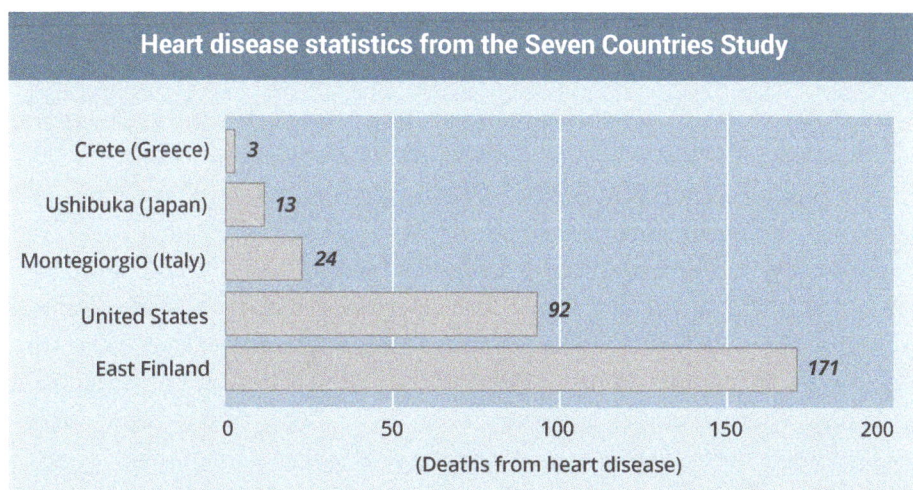

Heart disease statistics from the Seven Countries Study

Country	Deaths from heart disease
Crete (Greece)	3
Ushibuka (Japan)	13
Montegiorgio (Italy)	24
United States	92
East Finland	171

(Deaths from heart disease)

With hard figures from real populations, Keys was now certain that diet played the primary role in the onset of coronary heart disease. But, after so many years of research, he had come to realize that food might not be the only factor involved. Professor Keys also observed that Mediterranean and Asian peoples were physically active, family ties were strong, and the pace of life was leisurely. Keys concluded that although diet was the single most important factor, it was a combination of dietary and lifestyle factors that were responsible for the remarkably low rates of heart disease in Mediterranean and Asian regions.

The Seven Countries Study sparked a great deal of interest throughout the international scientific and medical communities. Dozens of studies on a molecular level followed in the 1970s and '80s, confirming Keys's findings. This led, in 1983, to the initiation of another large-scale population study. This time researchers concentrated their attention on Asia, and in particular on China.

THE CHINA STUDY

The China-Cornell-Oxford Project (also known as the China Study) was conducted by Cornell University in the United States, Oxford University in England, and the Chinese Academy of Preventative Medicine. Launched in 1983, the massive study focused on China and involved dozens of researchers, led by T. Colin Campbell, PhD, professor of nutritional biochemistry at Cornell University. Between 1983 and 1990 researchers traveled across the far reaches of China—from the southern coastal regions to the Gobi desert—studying the dietary practices and disease rates among 10,200 Chinese men and women.

To make the study as comprehensive and thorough as possible, Dr. Campbell and his colleagues collected every conceivable piece of information they could about their subjects. They found that a rural Chinese diet was the same diet that had been eaten in China for thousands of years. It was rich in plant-based foods such as rice and vegetables, low in animal foods, and contained around three times more fiber than an average Western diet. The rates of heart disease and breast cancer in these areas were also found to be many times lower than in Western society, as was prostate cancer and osteoporosis. Obesity was also very rare.

But further research conducted on Chinese populations living outside rural areas told a different story. It was found that the diet in many urban areas of China was a lot more Westernized, with far more animal food consumption at the expense of traditional dietary staples like rice and vegetables. The study also revealed that the urban Chinese who had abandoned their traditional diet had much higher rates of common Western ailments than their rural cousins, including heart disease, breast cancer, and prostate cancer. And obesity, which was rarely seen in rural Chinese populations, was found to be much more common among those Chinese eating a Westernized diet.

When the years of painstaking research were completed in 1990, the China Study had generated the largest database in the world on the multiple causes of disease. And the findings of the study were clear. "In the final analysis," reported Dr. Campbell, "we have strong evidence from this and other studies that nutrition becomes the controlling factor in the development of chronic degenerative diseases."

The China Study was hailed as a great success. The *New York Times* dubbed it the "Grand Prix of epidemiology," and went on to describe it as "the most comprehensive large study ever undertaken of the relationship between diet and the risk of developing disease . . . tantalizing findings."

The writing was now on the wall. It was clear that diet was the single most important factor in determining the onset of many chronic illnesses common in Western society. It was also clear that if people in the West wanted to live longer and reduce their risk of many chronic ailments, then the answer was to be found in adopting a traditional Mediterranean or Asian way of eating.

And two landmark studies have confirmed just how protective traditional Mediterranean and Asian diets can be for people who adopt them.

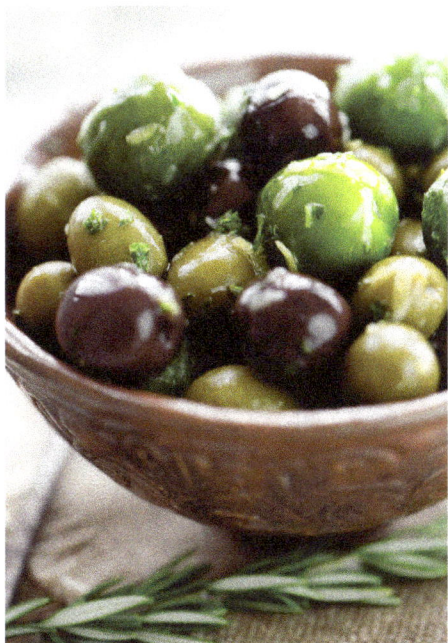

THE LYON DIET HEART STUDY

In 1988, researchers from the University of Saint-Etienne in France teamed up with researchers from the French National Center for Health Research to investigate the protective effects of a Mediterranean diet. In what became known as the Lyon Diet Heart Study, the researchers randomly divided 605 male and female heart attack survivors into two groups. One group was advised to eat the standard "prudent" low-fat diet suggested for heart patients. The other half were advised to eat a Mediterranean-style diet, complete with plenty of fresh vegetables and fruit, grains, olive oil, beans, small amounts of red meat, moderate amounts of fish and poultry, and wine with meals. Instead of butter they were advised to use a canola oil-based spread.

Although the study was originally scheduled to last for five years, after only two years researchers were so astounded by the differences in the two groups that the study was abruptly ended for ethical reasons. It was found that those following the Mediterranean-style diet had a 70 percent lower death rate compared to those following the prudent low-fat diet. In a follow-up report the researchers also discovered that cancer rates among the Mediterranean group were 61 percent lower than those of the other group.

"The results were spectacular and of unexpected magnitude," reported Serge Renaud, PhD, from the French National Center for Health Research, Bordeaux, who helped initiate the study. "The protective effects of the diet began to occur within two months of observation."

In fact, the results of the Lyon Diet Heart Study—results that hadn't been seen in any other diet, drug, or medical procedure—were deemed so important that they were published in three prestigious medical journals, the *American Journal of Clinical Nutrition*, the *Lancet*, and the *Journal of the American College of Cardiology*.

ASIAN-STYLE DIET ALSO SHOWS SIGNIFICANT BENEFITS

At the same time that French researchers were documenting the life-giving benefits of a Mediterranean-style diet, researchers in the United States were conducting a similar study into the role an Asian-style diet can play in reducing the risk of breast cancer in Western women.

In the study, conducted by a specialist team from the University of California, twenty-five breast cancer survivors were placed on an Asian-style diet and their progress was noted. Within only three months researchers saw biochemical changes in the breast in response to the change in the diet.

John Glaspy, MD, director of the University of California Oncology Center and lead author of the study reported, "My colleagues and I have shown that at least one aspect of human breast composition in American women can be altered to approximate the breast composition of women in certain Asian and European countries . . . in those countries, the incidence of breast cancer is much lower than it is here." Researchers also noted that the Asian diet promoted better cardiovascular health as well as weight loss.

THE GREAT PYRAMIDS

With decades of research confirming the health-giving benefits of traditional Mediterranean and Asian dietary and lifestyle practices, members of the scientific and medical communities decided the time had come to fully educate the Western public on the merits of this way of living.

In 1993, a group of experts from three highly respected organizations—Harvard School of Public Health, the World Health Organization, and Oldways Preservation and Exchange Trust—released the *Traditional Healthy Mediterranean Diet Pyramid*.

The aim of the pyramid was simple: to illustrate, in a graphical form, the traditional healthy dietary and lifestyle practices of Mediterranean cultures. It was based on a culmination of research dating back to Professor Ancel Keys's first studies in the 1950s.

The Traditional Healthy Mediterranean Diet Pyramid

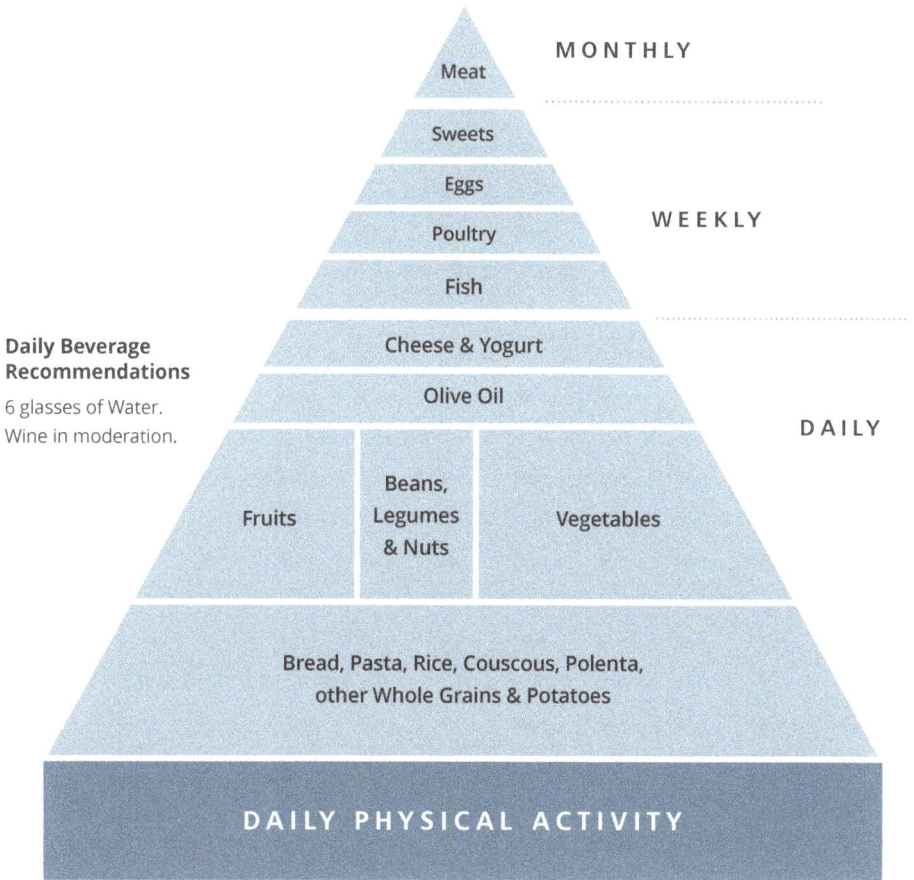

MONTHLY

Meat

Sweets

Eggs

WEEKLY

Poultry

Fish

Daily Beverage Recommendations

6 glasses of Water.
Wine in moderation.

Cheese & Yogurt

Olive Oil

DAILY

Fruits

Beans, Legumes & Nuts

Vegetables

Bread, Pasta, Rice, Couscous, Polenta, other Whole Grains & Potatoes

DAILY PHYSICAL ACTIVITY

www.oldwayspt.org

The Mediterranean diet pyramid was followed in 1995 by the *Traditional Healthy Asian Diet Pyramid*, which was developed by the same organizations as the Mediterranean pyramid, and also by senior scientists from Cornell University including Dr. T. Colin Campbell, director of the massive China Study.

The Traditional Healthy Asian Diet Pyramid

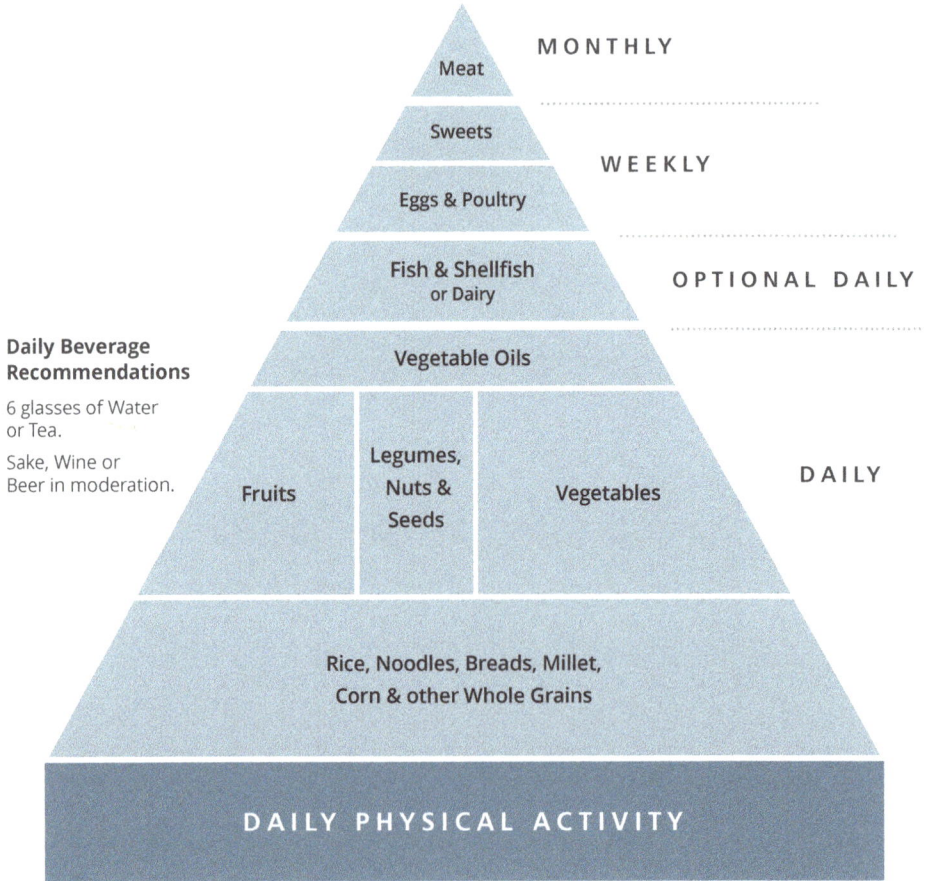

MONTHLY

Meat

Sweets

WEEKLY

Eggs & Poultry

Fish & Shellfish
or Dairy

OPTIONAL DAILY

Vegetable Oils

Daily Beverage Recommendations

6 glasses of Water or Tea.

Sake, Wine or Beer in moderation.

Fruits

Legumes, Nuts & Seeds

Vegetables

DAILY

Rice, Noodles, Breads, Millet, Corn & other Whole Grains

DAILY PHYSICAL ACTIVITY

© 2000 Oldways Preservation & Exchange Trust   www.oldwayspt.org

The Mediterranean and Asian pyramids are marvelous blue prints of the traditional dietary and lifestyle characteristics of people from these areas. They also highlight the remarkable similarities between traditional Mediterranean and traditional Asian dietary and lifestyle practices.

Many of us are now aware of the healthfulness of traditional Mediterranean and Asian dietary and lifestyle practices. In fact it seems like every week there's a new study touting the benefits of these traditional practices. But how do the

TRADITIONAL DIETARY & LIFESTYLE PRACTICES

MEDITERRANEAN	ASIAN
Grain foods such as bread, pasta, rice and couscous form a staple part of the daily diet	Grain foods such as rice, noodles and millet form a staple part of the daily diet
Fresh vegetables and fruits are eaten daily	Fresh vegetables and fruits are eaten daily
Plant oils and fish oils are the main sources of fat in the diet	Plant oils and fish oils are the main sources of fat in the diet
Red meat is eaten only a few times a month	Red meat is eaten only a few times a month
Fish is eaten regularly	Fish is eaten regularly
Legumes (beans, peas and lentils) and nuts are eaten regularly	Legumes (beans, peas and lentils) and nuts are eaten regularly
Alcohol such as red wine is consumed daily in moderation	Alcohol such as beer and rice wine is consumed daily in moderation
Moderate physical activity is a regular part of life	Moderate physical activity is a regular part of life

guidelines set out in the pyramids translate into real life for a Westerner living in this fast-paced modern world? That's what the rest of this book is all about. Over the coming pages we'll go through these guidelines in detail. I'll outline why each one is so important, and give you concrete, practical examples of how you can easily incorporate that guideline into your life. We'll also discuss one guideline that wasn't included in either the Mediterranean or Asian pyramid—the fact that Mediterranean and Asian cultures have known for centuries that emotional health is just as important as physical health. Indeed, more than two thousand years ago the Greek philosopher Aristotle defined the goal of all human endeavor as "happiness." We agree wholeheartedly! Then we'll put all these guidelines together into a plan. Not just a plan for a month or a year, but a plan for *life*.

Let's start by looking at one of the most misunderstood nutrients in the Western world: fat.

CHAPTER 3

Fat fundamentals

F at tastes great! It gives food a unique flavor and a feel in the mouth that's incomparable to any other type of food. And fat isn't only tasty, it's also an essential nutrient we need to survive.

Fat maintains cell membranes and blood vessels, it helps produce essential hormones that regulate numerous bodily functions, it provides your body with energy, and it helps maintain healthy skin and hair. Fat is also required in order to absorb the fat-soluble vitamins A, D, E, and K, which are essential for proper function of your eyes, immune system, and bones.

But when it comes to fat, it's not all good news. The crucial fact is that not all fats are created equal.

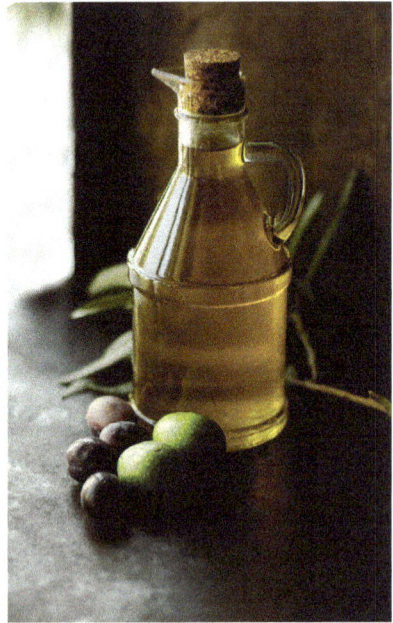

SOME FATS HARM, SOME FATS HEAL

One of the biggest conclusions drawn from over fifty years of research into eating patterns throughout the Mediterranean and Asia is that saturated fat (found in high amounts in red meat and dairy products) plays a pivotal role in the onset of many chronic diseases. At the same time, the weight of scientific evidence shows that unsaturated fat—found in high amounts in plant and fish oils—can actually help prevent disease.

Professor Ancel Keys saw firsthand how different types of fat can have vastly different effects on the chemistry of the body. During the 1950s Keys studied a group of woodchoppers in Finland, where heart disease rates were among the highest in the world.

Keys found that the diet of these men was very high in fat, particularly saturated fat from meat and dairy products. He even noted that many of the woodchoppers would butter their cheese. Keys found that a large percentage of these men were suffering from heart disease.

Later, during the Seven Countries Study, Keys conducted research on a group of villagers on the Greek island of Crete, where, along with Japan, heart disease rates were the lowest in the world.

Keys found that the Crete villagers, like the Finnish woodchoppers, also had a diet high in fat (up to 40 percent of their calories came from fat). But unlike the Finnish woodchoppers, who consumed lots of saturated fat from meat and dairy products, the fat in the Crete diets came primarily from olive oil and from the oil in the fish they ate. Both of these oils are made up primarily of unsaturated fat. Keys found that these villagers had low blood cholesterol levels, and heart disease amongst them was almost nonexistent.

So, what's the difference between saturated fat and unsaturated fat? And why do they behave so differently in the body? To really understand fat, it's important to learn a few basics first.

THE SKINNY ON FAT

Scientifically known as fatty acids, fats are divided into three main families: saturated fatty acids, polyunsaturated fatty acids, and monounsaturated fatty acids. The latter two are known collectively as unsaturated fats.

The major difference between these fatty acids lies in the type of molecules of which they're composed, and the degree to which these molecules are saturated with hydrogen atoms.

Every type of fat, whether it's from a plant source or an animal source, actually contains a mixture of all three of these fatty acids. But although all fats are made up of a mixture of saturated, polyunsaturated, and monounsaturated fatty acids, one type almost always predominates. And it's the fatty acid that predominates that classifies what type of fat it is.

For example, around 75 percent of the fatty acids in olive oil are monounsaturated, so scientists classify it as a monounsaturated fat. Safflower oil, on the other hand, contains around 75 percent of its fatty acids in the form of polyunsaturated fat, so it's known as a polyunsaturated fat. And animal fats, with between 50 and 70 percent of their fatty acids in the form of saturated fat are classified as—you guessed it—saturated fat.

In general, fat from animal sources is high in saturated fat, and fat from vegetable sources is high in unsaturated fat. Tropical vegetable oils (palm oil and coconut oil) are the exception to this rule and contain an amount of saturated fatty acids similar to that found in animal fat.

THE DANGERS OF A DIET HIGH IN SATURATED FAT

One of the first clues that saturated fat is vastly different from unsaturated fat is the visible fact that saturated fat (such as butter and lard) is solid at room temperature, whereas unsaturated fat (such as olive and safflower oil) is liquid.

The chemical structure of saturated fat also affects how your body metabolizes it. Controlled clinical studies, as well as large population studies, have repeatedly shown that consuming too much saturated fat can lead to elevated levels of potentially harmful LDL cholesterol in our blood.

Our bodies are ill equipped to deal with large amounts of LDL cholesterol in the blood, and the excess can accumulate on the walls of our arteries. This can lead to the formation of plaque and to a hardening and narrowing of the arteries, known as *atherosclerosis.*

What is Cholesterol?

Cholesterol (from the Greek words meaning "solid bile") is a soft, waxy substance that is found, to varying degrees, in everyone's body. We need cholesterol to survive, since it's used to form cell membranes and brain and nerve tissues. Cholesterol also helps the body produce hormones needed for body regulation, including processing food, and bile acids needed for digestion. Your liver actually produces all the cholesterol your body needs for these functions, so you don't need to consume any extra through your diet.

It used to be thought that eating dietary cholesterol was a major factor in raising potentially harmful LDL cholesterol levels in the blood, but in recent years studies have found that consuming dietary cholesterol has only a small effect. Consuming large amounts of bad fats (saturated and trans fats) has been identified as the main culprit.

Good and bad cholesterol

You may have heard about "bad" versus "good" cholesterol. Here's a simple explanation. Having high levels of LDL (low-density lipoprotein) cholesterol in your blood is considered bad because it can lead to a buildup of plaque inside your arteries, which can block the flow of blood to vital organs. HDL (high-density lipoprotein) cholesterol is considered good because it helps carry LDL cholesterol from the blood to the liver, where it can be naturally eliminated. An easy way to remember the difference is to think "H" for healthy and "L" for life-threatening.

Atherosclerosis displays no symptoms as it gradually restricts blood flow. Eventually this can end up causing a clot (thrombus), completely blocking an artery that feeds blood to a vital organ. Ultimately this can lead to a heart attack if a coronary artery is blocked, to stroke if an artery to the brain is blocked, or to kidney failure if an artery to the kidney is blocked.

Red Meat and Saturated Fat

The main source of saturated fat in a typical Western diet comes from red meat (beef, pork, and lamb). And red meat, in one form or another, usually takes center stage on most of our plates. Some typical examples include burgers, hot dogs, steak, meatloaf, bacon, spare ribs, roasts, meat pies, and sausages.

The opposite is true throughout Asia and the Mediterranean, where, for thousands of years, red meat has traditionally been reserved for special feast days, or eaten more as a flavor-enhancer than a main course. Instead, the peoples of Asia and the Mediterranean have traditionally gotten their protein from highly unsaturated foods such as fish, shellfish, and plant foods, including beans and nuts.

This way of eating certainly makes sense because numerous studies have shown that red meat, and the high amounts of saturated fat it contains, elevates LDL cholesterol levels and therefore raises the risk of arterial blockage.

The Hidden Fat in Red Meat

Many of us are unaware of exactly how much fat red meat contains. The simple fact is that a large amount of the fat in red meat is hidden in tiny pockets within the flesh, so it's hard to gauge how much you are really eating. Here are some examples:

- An 8-ounce T-bone has over 30 grams of fat
- An 8-ounce burger patty has almost 35 grams of fat
- An 8-ounce sirloin contains almost 40 grams

This hidden fat isn't just bad for health; it can also affect how you look. Quite simply, hidden fat equals hidden calories, and red meat contains lots of calories. An 8-ounce sirloin steak, for example, contains more than 400 calories. This compares to an 8-ounce tuna steak, which contains only around 240 calories.

Researchers at the University of Michigan in Ann Arbor believe the high calorie content of red meat could be one of the key reasons that many of us in the West are overweight. Several years ago they surveyed a group of obese men about what foods they liked the most; steaks and roasts topped the list.

Saturated Fat Confusion

Decades of research has shown the dangers of consuming excess saturated fat. But in 2014 a meta-analysis (a study of studies) headed by a recent graduate of the University of Cambridge, Rajiv Chowdhury, was published in the *Annals of Internal Medicine* which claimed that saturated fat wasn't linked to heart disease after all.

Because the meta-analysis was published in a respected scientific journal, it created headlines all over the world. But not long after the meta-analysis was published it was found to contain multiple errors and omissions, and Chowdhury had to make numerous corrections.

Dr. Walter Willett (Chair of the Department of Nutrition at Harvard School of Public Health at the time) had this to say about the study: *"Chowdhury's analysis was deeply flawed due to omission of important studies, extraction of incorrect data from some studies, incorrect interpretation of their own findings, and failure to mention results of other, superior analyses...Thus, the conclusions of Chowdhury et al. regarding the type of fat being unimportant are seriously misleading and should be disregarded."*

Unfortunately there was very little press coverage about the numerous errors in the meta-analysis, and the myth that saturated fat had been exonerated continued to spread—even causing worldwide butter shortages. This led in 2017 to the American Heart Association publishing a comprehensive review of the scientific evidence on saturated fat. The review, compiled by a group of 12 leading experts in the field of nutrition and health, showed that numerous well-conducted studies had found that replacing saturated fat with unsaturated fat reduced heart disease risk by at least 30 percent (as much as special cholesterol-lowering drugs called statins).

In 2018 The World Health Organization also reviewed the most up to date science on saturated fat. They found that the overwhelming weight of scientific evidence shows that when saturated fat is replaced with unsaturated fats from plant or fish oils, "bad" LDL cholesterol goes down and so does the risk of heart disease. Their latest, updated guidelines recommended that 10 percent or less of your calories should come from saturated fat, and that unsaturated fats should make up the majority of the fat you eat (which is very much in line with traditional Mediterranean and Asian dietary practices).

But high cholesterol, atherosclerosis, and weight gain aren't the only problems caused by overconsumption of red meat. In recent years a number of major international studies have confirmed that eating large amounts of red meat can also increase your risk of contracting certain types of cancer, particularly breast, colon, and prostate cancer.

THE CANCER CONNECTION

In late 1997 the World Cancer Research Fund and the American Institute for Cancer Research released the most comprehensive report of its kind into the link between diet and cancer. The report involved distinguished researchers from the United States, Britain, Japan, China, India, and Latin America, who reviewed over 4,500 studies to come up with their detailed analysis, which was titled "Food, Nutrition and the Prevention of Cancer: A Global Perspective."

The report found that people who lived in areas like the Mediterranean and Asia, where red meat consumption is generally low and plant-food consumption is high, had the lowest rates of cancer in the world.

It was also found that when these healthy people moved to industrialized Western nations like the United States and Great Britain, where meat consumption is high and plant-food consumption low, their rate of cancers soon matched that of their adopted country. These population studies, plus strong evidence from thousands of clinical studies, led the researchers to conclude that diet plays a vital role in preventing the onset of cancer.

The expert panel who prepared the report went on to recommend that if red meat is eaten at all, it should be limited to no more than 3 ounces per day, about the size of a deck of cards. Instead, it suggested eating fish and poultry.

Other large-scale studies have also shown a direct link between red meat consumption and increased risk of certain cancers. For example, Harvard scientists who have been conducting an ongoing study involving more than 80,000 women since 1980 found that women who had beef, lamb, or pork as a daily main dish had two and a half times the risk of developing colon cancer as those who ate the meats less than once a month.

Prostate Cancer Linked to High Red Meat Consumption

Prostate cancer is a leading cause of death for men in the Western world. Scientists have now identified red meat as a key risk factor. In one study, a group of researchers led by Dr. James Herbert of the University of Massachusetts Medical School reviewed a survey of prostate cancer deaths in fifty-nine countries. They found what a number of other studies have found: that prostate cancer deaths are much lower in countries where red meat is eaten rarely.

The researchers noted that the lowest death rates from prostate cancer are in countries such as Japan, where people traditionally eat a great deal of fish and very little red meat. "Animal energy was positively associated with prostate cancer mortality," commented Dr. Herbert. "On the other hand, intakes of cereals, soybeans, other nuts and oilseeds and fish were negatively associated with prostate cancer mortality."

The study concluded, "On the basis of the results of this study and other studies, it appears that the Western diet may contribute to the risk for prostate cancer mortality."

GRIM REPERCUSSIONS

As I mentioned earlier, Asians and Mediterraneans have traditionally eaten very little red meat in their diets. Unfortunately, in recent years many Asians and Mediterraneans, particularly those living in urban areas, have started to abandon their traditional diets in favor of a Western diet high in red meat and low in plant foods. The results have been dramatic.

For example, since the 1970s the Japanese diet has rapidly Westernized, and burgers, steaks, and processed foods have become increasingly popular, at the expense of the traditional Japanese staples of fish, vegetables, and rice. (Studies show that rice consumption in Japan has dropped by more than 50 percent in the last forty years.) As this change in diet has occurred, there has also been a corresponding rise in obesity and rates of heart disease and cancers of the colon, prostate, and breast. In fact breast cancer, which used to be rare in Japan, rose by a dramatic 58 percent between 1975 and 1985, and is still increasing at an alarming rate. Japanese researchers are convinced they know the reason why. In a *Time* magazine article, Dr. Akira Eboshida, chief deputy director of the Japanese Health and Welfare Ministry's Disease Control Division said, "The largest factor behind the sharp rise is the Westernization of our eating habits. We are eating more animal fat and less fiber."

The traditional Mediterranean diet that has sustained Greeks for thousands of years has also started to Westernize since the 1970s, and the outcome has been identical to that seen in Japan. Professor Antonia Trichopoulou from the Greek National School of Public Health has been monitoring the changes. In the 1990s she published a study showing that a dramatic twenty-year rise in rates of heart disease and cancers of the breast and colon corresponded with a large increase in consumption of animal fats and a large decline in plant-food consumption.

The governments of Greece and Japan are now enthusiastically urging their citizens to return to the culinary traditions that have sustained their ancestors for thousands of years, the same culinary traditions presented in this book.

THE UNSATURATED FAT STORY

Monounsaturated and polyunsaturated fatty acids, which are collectively known as unsaturated fats, act in ways vastly different than saturated fat. For a start, instead of raising potentially dangerous LDL cholesterol in the blood, decades of research has shown they do just the opposite, and actually help lower it.

Unsaturated fats are also a rich source of vitamin E. This vitamin, as well as being an essential nutrient needed for a number of body regulating functions, is also a powerful antioxidant, and antioxidants in their own right are thought to help prevent the buildup of cholesterol on artery walls. (See chapter 5, "Plant Power," for information about antioxidants.)

Polyunsaturated Fat

Polyunsaturated fat is actually divided into two groups: omega-6 polyunsaturated fatty acids (omega-6 fat) and omega-3 polyunsaturated fatty acids (omega-3s). Omega-6 fat is the primary fat in sunflower oil, corn oil, and safflower oil. It's also present in nuts and seeds, whole grains, and other plant foods. Omega-3s are found in fish and shellfish, particularly salmon, tuna, mackerel, sardines, and anchovies. It's also present in smaller amounts in dark green vegetables, walnuts, pecans, and flaxseeds.

You probably already know that vitamins are essential for good health, but did you know that polyunsaturated fats are just as essential? In fact, omega-3 and omega-6 fats are known scientifically as essential fatty acids, or EFAs. They're considered essential because they're not produced by the body and they are necessary for a wide range of functions, including cell membrane formation, brain development, good eyesight, and the production of hormone-like compounds that regulate inflammation, blood pressure, heart rate, and immune response.

Monounsaturated Fat

Although monounsaturated and polyunsaturated fats both lower your blood cholesterol levels, monounsaturated fat has been shown to do this more effectively. Omega-6 polyunsaturated fat lowers potentially harmful LDL cholesterol, but it tends to also slightly lower good HDL cholesterol. Studies have shown that monounsaturated fat, on the other hand, lowers LDL without affecting heart-protective HDL levels. In one study, researchers from the Pennsylvania State University and the University of Rochester in New York found that when twenty-two subjects consumed a diet rich in monounsaturated fat from olive oil, peanuts, and peanut oil, their LDL cholesterol levels dropped by an average of 14 percent in four weeks. At the same time, there was no change in heart protective HDL cholesterol levels. "These results show that eating more monounsaturated fat can reduce your heart-disease risk by 25 percent," reported Penny Kris-Etherton, the study author and a professor in the Pennsylvania State University's Department of Nutrition.

Recent research has also shown that monounsaturated fat has many other health-giving benefits. A study published in the *Archives of Internal Medicine*, for example, showed that olive oil can lower blood pressure and make blood pressure-lowering medications less necessary.

The study involved twenty-three people on medication to control high blood pressure, who were divided into two groups. Both groups ate a nutritionally balanced diet that was identical, except for the type of oil used.

During the first six months of the study, one group used olive oil (a highly monounsaturated fat), while the other group used sunflower oil (which is made up primarily of omega-6 polyunsaturated fat). During the last six months of the study, the two groups switched the type of oil they used. It was found that when the participants used olive oil, their systolic (top number) and diastolic (bottom number) blood pressure fell by an average of seven points; but sunflower oil had no effect. As blood pressure decreased, researchers adjusted the participants' medication regimen. Olive oil was so effective at reducing blood pressure that many patients reduced their drug dosage by half, and eight went off blood pressure drugs entirely.

Another study suggests that monounsaturated fat can also help maintain brainpower into old age. This time researchers from the University of Bari in Italy, led by Dr. Antonio Capurso, studied a group of 278 senior citizens. Those who consumed diets high in monounsaturated fat were found to be less likely to experience age-related cognitive decline compared with people who ate less monounsaturated fat.

Dr. Capurso concluded, "It appears that high monounsaturated fatty acid intakes, mostly present in vegetable oils and particularly in extra virgin olive oil, the main fat of the Mediterranean diet, protect from age-related cognitive decline."

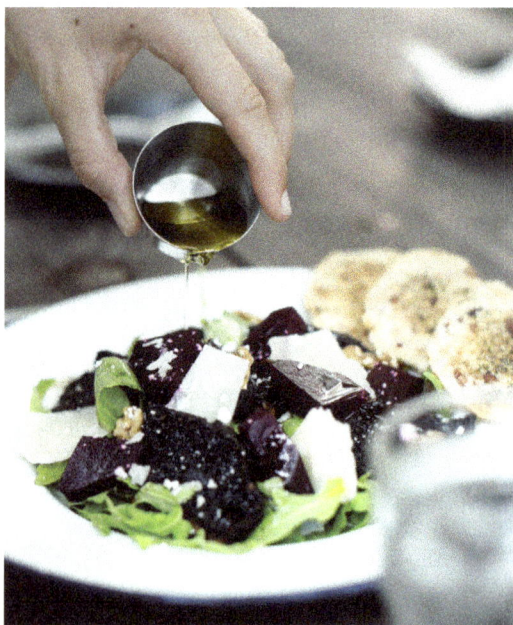

The Weight Loss Bonus

Monounsaturated fat may even help you lose weight and maintain that loss, according to a study by researchers at Brigham and Women's Hospital and Harvard Medical School.

In the study sixty-one overweight men and women consumed one of two diets: a standard low-fat diet or a Mediterranean-style diet with regular moderate consumption of healthy monounsaturated fat from olive oil, olives, nuts, and nut products (such as nut oils and peanut butter). Both groups were instructed to consume the same number of calories.

After six months both groups had experienced roughly the same amount of weight loss, but the big difference came at the end of the study, twelve months later. It was found that a large number of the Mediterranean diet group had stuck with the diet and maintained their weight loss. However, many of those on the low-fat diet couldn't stick with it and had not only regained their lost weight, but weighed more than they did before the study began. "In our study, three times as many people trying to lose weight were able to stick to a Mediterranean-style diet versus the low-fat diet," reported the lead author of the study, Kathy McManus, RD, director of nutrition at Brigham and Women's Hospital. She noted, "Patients loved this diet because they could include favorite foods if they carefully watched portion sizes."

The researchers concluded, "Motivation and adherence are very hard to sustain in any weight loss programs, but the results from this study suggest that the tastier the food, the greater overall success of the diet plan—even if it does include moderate amounts of fat."

Fats & Figures

"It's fat that makes you fat," proclaim the low-fat diet gurus. "No, you're quite wrong," say the low-carbohydrate gurus, "it's carbohydrates that make you fat." Meanwhile, we're stuck in the middle trying to figure out who's right.

Well, the truth is, they're both partly right. Yes, fat can make you fat; but so can carbohydrates—and in fact, so can protein. Here's how it works.

All foods are made up of macronutrients. The three primary macronutrients are fat, protein, and carbohydrates. All three of these macronutrients contain stored energy, which scientists call kilocalories, or calories for short. (Vitamins

continues on next page

and minerals, which are called micronutrients, contain no calories). The three primary macronutrients are used in various ways by the body:

PROTEIN is used primarily for building, repairing, and maintaining muscles, making blood cells and synthesizing hormones and enzymes.

CARBOHYDRATES are broken down into glucose (blood sugar) in the body. Glucose fuels your muscles and gives them energy to work; it's also the primary fuel for the brain and the central nervous system.

FAT is used for energy and is also an essential building block for the body's cells and is required in order to absorb fat-soluble vitamins.

If you eat more macronutrients than your body needs for these purposes and you don't burn them off through physical activity, those excess calories are converted into fat and stored on your body.

"Whether you store fat or don't store fat has to do with caloric balance," explains Alice Lichtenstein, DSc, a scientist at the Jean Mayer USDA Human Nutrition Research Center on Aging at Tufts University. "If you eat too many extra calories as protein, you'll store them as body fat, just as you would too many calories from carbohydrate."

Proof that calories are the only thing that matters in weight control was shown in a 1996 study where two groups of obese people were fed diets equally low in calories but different in their fat and carbohydrate content. One group received a diet with 15 percent carbohydrates and 53 percent fat; the other group got 45 percent carbohydrates and 26 percent fat. The researchers found there was no difference in weight loss between the two groups, and they concluded that it was the number of calories eaten, not the proportion of calories from carbohydrates or fat, that determined weight loss.

Calories count, but don't count calories

So, when it comes to maintaining a healthy weight, it's calories that count. But that certainly doesn't mean you have to count calories to stay in shape. Remember, for thousands of years Mediterraneans and Asians have kept lean and trim, yet they had absolutely no idea what a calorie was (this is a modern scientific term). They simply ate food that tasted good, and made them feel good.

Coincidentally the majority of this food also happens to be bulky, filling, and satisfying, but only moderate in calories. The great benefit about this way of eating is that it means you'll feel full and satisfied long before the calories can do any damage. Later in the book we'll show you just how easily this principle works in real life (see page 95).

NEW FAT ON THE BLOCK

We've looked at the different roles of saturated, polyunsaturated, and monounsaturated fat, but there's also a "synthetic" fat that's important to mention.

Early in the twentieth century scientists discovered they could create a new kind of fat by injecting hydrogen molecules into vegetable oil. This made the oil, which was normally liquid at room temperature, into a solid type of fat. The more hydrogen added to the oil, the harder the resulting fat. This process, called hydrogenation, is used to turn vegetable oil into margarine and vegetable shortening.

Although hydrogenated fats have some advantages over normal vegetable oils—namely, they have a longer shelf life and can be heated to higher temperatures—studies have shown that these fats are actually worse for your health than saturated fat.

The trouble lies in the fact that when liquid oils are turned solid through the process of hydrogenation, this changes the building blocks of the fat and creates what are called trans fatty acids, or trans fats for short. Research has shown that trans fat raises levels of bad cholesterol, lowers good cholesterol, and raises triglycerides (blood fats)—all of which are known risk factors for heart disease.

A typical Western diet is high in trans fat because hydrogenated vegetable oil is used in everything from margarine, cookies, crackers and pastries, to fried snack foods like potato chips, and foods fried in fast-food outlets. However, with the dangers of trans fat being scientifically recognized, many governments around the world are starting to heavily regulate or ban foods that contain more than trace amounts of trans fat.

OIL CHANGE: HOW TO EAT LESS BAD FAT, MORE GOOD FAT

Following are the five most effective ways of replacing bad fats in your diet with good fats.

1. Instead of making red meat the main source of protein in your diet, opt for fish, shellfish, poultry, legumes, and nuts. Because red meat is the main source of saturated fat in a typical Western diet, the ideal first step in any plan to lower saturated fat intake is to reduce your intake of red meat. But at the same time it's important to remember that red meat only becomes a health hazard when you eat too much of it. Learning from the traditions of Asia and the Mediterranean, it would seem that the key word is *moderation* not *elimination*.

A steak, some bacon, or a hamburger once in a while won't do you any harm. It's only when you start eating too much of these types of food—which is easy to do in our "meat loving" culture—that the problems can start arising.

Of course, the thought of cutting back on red meat usually leads to the inevitable question: "Where am I going to get my protein?" Our answer: from *fish, shellfish, poultry, legumes (beans, peas, and lentils) nuts, and seeds.* This is where Mediterranean and Asian cultures have gotten their protein from for the last few thousand years. Like red meat these foods are packed with protein, but unlike red meat, which is typically loaded with saturated fat, these foods contain mostly heart-healthy unsaturated fats.

But all this doesn't mean much if these foods don't taste good. The great news is, over the centuries the humble home cooks of Asia and the Mediterranean

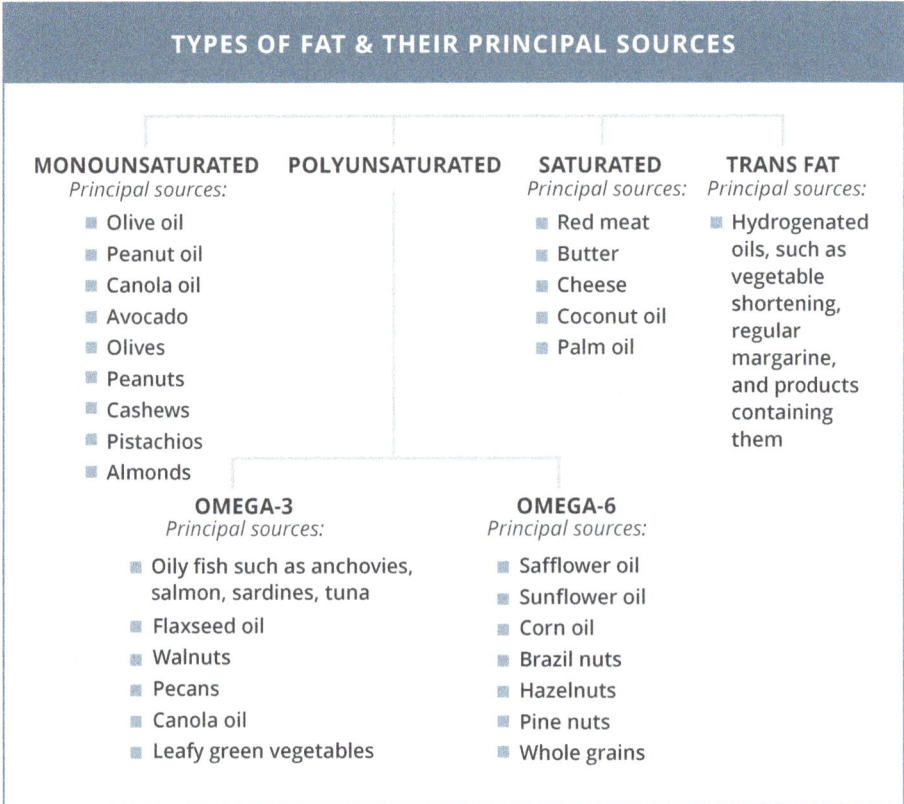

TYPES OF FAT & THEIR PRINCIPAL SOURCES

MONOUNSATURATED
Principal sources:
- Olive oil
- Peanut oil
- Canola oil
- Avocado
- Olives
- Peanuts
- Cashews
- Pistachios
- Almonds

POLYUNSATURATED

SATURATED
Principal sources:
- Red meat
- Butter
- Cheese
- Coconut oil
- Palm oil

TRANS FAT
Principal sources:
- Hydrogenated oils, such as vegetable shortening, regular margarine, and products containing them

OMEGA-3
Principal sources:
- Oily fish such as anchovies, salmon, sardines, tuna
- Flaxseed oil
- Walnuts
- Pecans
- Canola oil
- Leafy green vegetables

OMEGA-6
Principal sources:
- Safflower oil
- Sunflower oil
- Corn oil
- Brazil nuts
- Hazelnuts
- Pine nuts
- Whole grains

have discovered a myriad of ways to turn fish, shellfish, poultry, beans, and nuts into delicious, sometimes extraordinary dishes. The recipe section of this book will give you a good idea of what I mean.

2. Make olive and peanut oils your main cooking fats. These are traditionally the main cooking oils used throughout the Mediterranean and Asia. These oils are also made up primarily of monounsaturated fat, which lowers LDL cholesterol without affecting good HDL cholesterol.

Throughout the Mediterranean, olive oil has been revered as one of the basic staffs of life for thousands of years. The most commonly used olive oil throughout the Mediterranean is extra virgin olive oil, which is made from the first "cold pressing" (which means the oil is extracted with pressure, and no chemicals are involved) of the highest-quality olives. It has a greenish tinge and has a wonderfully rich aromatic taste. Extra virgin olive oil has a moderate smoking point, so is fine for lightly frying and sautéing, but it's unsuitable for cooking at very high temperatures. Another good use for extra virgin olive oil is to add it to food near the end of the cooking process as a texture and flavor enhancer. It goes particularly well with pasta dishes, grilled fish or vegetables, and stews, sauces, and soups. It's also delicious in salad dressings, marinades, or simply drizzled over a piece of fresh crusty bread.

Peanut oil has been used in Asian cooking for generations. It's mild in flavor and has a high smoking point, so it's good for general-purpose use (it's a particularly good stir-fry oil).

3. Instead of spreading bread with butter or margarine, use avocado, hummus, natural peanut butter, or trans fat-free margarine.

When studies started showing the dangers of a diet high in saturated fat, many of us switched from butter to margarine to save our arteries from becoming clogged. But now scientists are telling us margarine isn't such a healthy alternative after all because of the potentially dangerous trans fats it contains. (It can really start to seem like a case of damned if you do, damned if you don't!)

So what's the best solution? We believe it comes down to being a bit creative, and finding ways of substituting bad fats for good fats. For example, instead of using butter or margarine on your sandwich, try mashed avocado instead. The fat in avocados is mostly monounsaturated, so you get all the creaminess of butter or margarine without the guilt. Hummus (a Middle Eastern chickpea and sesame seed dip and spread) is another good alternative because it's also creamy but it contains mostly unsaturated fat.

If you're having a sweeter sandwich you could use peanut butter as the spread, because the fat in peanuts is mostly monounsaturated. But a word of warning: Use *natural* peanut butter with no added vegetable oil. The vegetable oil in many peanut butters is hydrogenated vegetable oil, which is high in trans fat.

If you're having bread or rolls at the side of your meal, instead of serving it with butter or margarine, do what Mediterraneans traditionally do and serve it with a small dish of extra virgin olive oil for dipping or drizzling. You can also use olive oil instead of butter or margarine to make garlic bread.

If you've still got a hankering for something that tastes like and resembles butter, you're in luck. In response to the highly publicized side effects caused by trans fat, many manufacturers now offer trans fat-free margarine in tubs. These are a great alternative to butter or normal margarine; especially if you select a brand that uses a monounsaturated fat like olive oil as its base.

4. Consume dairy products in moderation. After red meat, the second largest source of saturated fat in a typical Western diet comes from dairy foods (milk, cheese, butter, cream, and yogurt).

Research shows that throughout most of Asia, dairy foods have traditionally played almost no role in the diet. A traditional Mediterranean diet, on the other hand, does include a moderate amount of dairy. But, unlike in Western society, Mediterraneans traditionally have consumed very little butter or milk (these foods quickly spoiled in the hot Mediterranean climate). Most of their dairy intake has been in the form of cheese or yogurt. Even then, this type of food has been seen as an accompaniment to meals, and was mostly used in small amounts to add texture and flavor to dishes. The cheese was often a strong cheese like Parmesan, which also meant a little went a long way.

Of course, one of the biggest concerns in the West about cutting down on dairy food intake is the belief that it will inevitably lead to osteoporosis, the bone thinning disease. I remember constantly being told as a kid, "If you don't drink your milk, you won't grow up with strong teeth and bones." But science is now discovering that's not quite the case.

There is no doubt that calcium is good for your bones, and there is no doubt that dairy products are a good source of calcium. The trouble is, dairy products aren't the ideal food source for delivering calcium to your body, because they are also high in animal protein. For over thirty years studies have shown that if we consume too much animal protein, it tends to leech calcium from our bones. So by consuming lots of dairy products, we are naturally also consuming lots of animal protein—and leeching out calcium almost as fast as we're receiving it.

A Harvard study involving more than 80,000 women found that increased calcium consumption through milk did not decrease osteoporosis risk at all. In fact, those who drank three glasses of milk a day had more hip and wrist fractures (a common measure of the extent of osteoporosis) than those who rarely drank milk. A similar study in Australia showed identical results.

And the facts speak for themselves. In countries where dairy consumption is high—such as in the United States, Britain, and Australia—osteoporosis rates are also high. But in parts of the world where dairy product consumption is much lower, such as in Asia and the Mediterranean, osteoporosis rates are also low.

In the massive China Study, for example, researchers from Cornell University found that rural Chinese people rarely consumed dairy products, yet their rates of osteoporosis were among the lowest in the world.

Dr. T. Colin Campbell, who led the study, points out, "Dairy calcium is not needed to prevent osteoporosis. Most Chinese consume no dairy products and, instead, get all their calcium from vegetables."

And this is by far the best way to get your calcium. Sure, you can still get some calcium through dairy foods. The trick is to eat dairy foods in moderation, as the Mediterraneans traditionally have. This ensures that your animal protein intake won't go overboard, and calcium won't be leeched out of your bones. At the same time, it also means you'll automatically be cutting down on saturated fat.

The best calcium-rich plant foods are dark green vegetables, beans (including tofu), nuts, and fruit. And as a bonus, fresh produce like this also contains high levels of magnesium and potassium, which are other important minerals that are needed for strong, healthy bones.

5. Eat less trans fat packed snacks like potato chips, cookies and pastries, and eat more nuts and seeds. Nuts and seeds are the perfect snack food because they are rich in healthy unsaturated fat instead of trans fat. Nuts and seeds are discussed in detail on page 62.

This chapter has explored the subject of fat in lots of detail. I hope you now have a good basic understanding of the different types of fats, and the vastly different effects they have on your body.

But there is one type of fat that I have touched on only briefly in this chapter: omega-3 fatty acids. This special fat has been the focus of a great deal of research in recent years, and because the richest source of omega-3s is fish and shellfish, I've saved most of the details about this extraordinary fat for the next chapter, which deals exclusively with seafood. And the great news—as you're about to find out—is that fish and shellfish aren't only a delicious source of healthy omega-3s, they also have many other remarkable health-giving benefits.

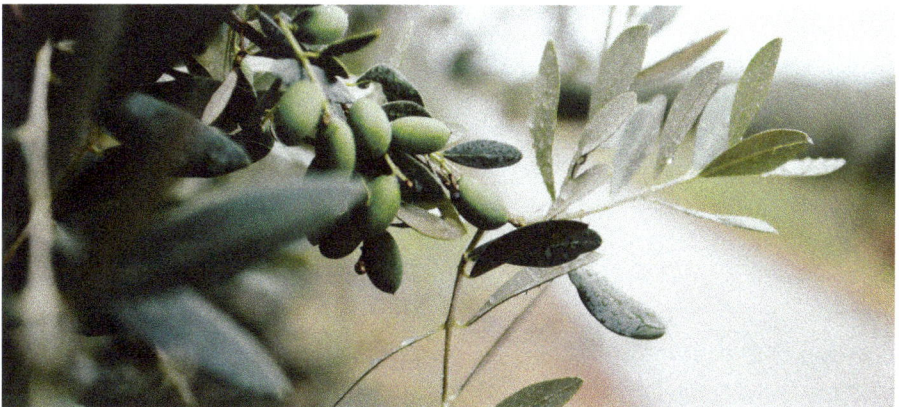

CHAPTER 4

A feast of health from the sea

For the past few thousand years the abundant waters of the Mediterranean Sea, Pacific Ocean, and Indian Ocean have provided the peoples of the Mediterranean and Asia with a treasure trove of edible delights. Some of the mouthwatering seafood plucked from these waters includes shrimp, salmon, crab, tuna, lobster, mussels, squid, oysters, and scallops.

And none of these delightful morsels go to waste either, because fish and shellfish are as popular throughout Asia and the Mediterranean as red meat is in the West. In Japan, for example, people consume an average of over 80 pounds of fish and shellfish per person each a year (this compares to only 15 pounds per person each year in the United States).

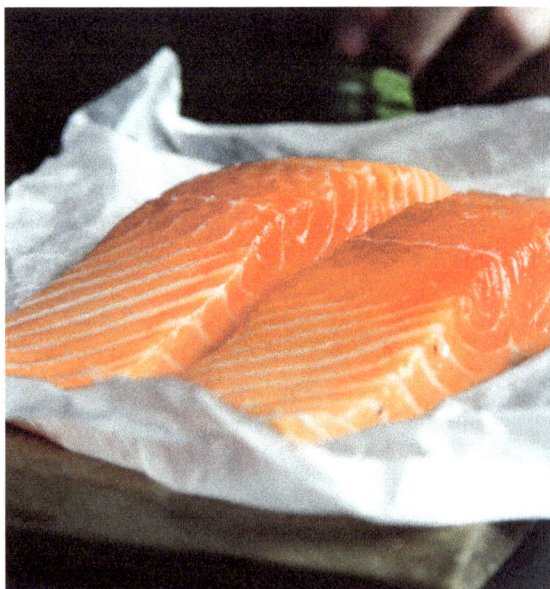

Researchers now believe this high consumption of fish and shellfish could partly help to explain why people in Mediterranean and Asian countries live longer, are leaner, and suffer from far less heart disease than we do.

So, what is the secret ingredient that makes fish and shellfish so healthy? Well, there are actually several reasons why these are among the most life-giving foods known to science, but a good place to start would be with the special fat found in fish and shellfish called *omega-3 fatty acids*, or omega-3s for short.

As you found out in the last chapter, we need to consume this special fat regularly to stay healthy. Research in recent years has also shown that omega-3s not

OMEGA-3 FATTY ACID CONTENT IN FISH & SHELLFISH

VERY GOOD SOURCE	GOOD SOURCE	MODERATE SOURCE
Anchovy	Cod, Pacific	Catfish
Herring	Flounder	Clams
Mackerel	Halibut	Cod, Atlantic
Salmon	Oysters	Crab
Sardines	Perch, ocean	Crayfish
Swordfish	Pollock	Haddock
Trout	Rockfish	Lobster
	Scallops	Shrimp
	Tuna, fresh	Snapper
	Tuna, white, canned	Tuna, light, canned
	Whiting	

only promote good health, but can also help prevent a wide range of illnesses common in Western society. An area of particular interest has been the ability of omega-3s to lower the risk of heart disease.

OMEGA-3 AND HEART DISEASE

For hundreds of years it has been known that people who consume fish regularly show striking patterns of good health. But it wasn't until research in the 1960s and '70s that omega-3 fatty acids were first isolated as being one of the primary health-giving components of fish. Studies during that time showed that Japanese fishermen who consumed fish regularly had very low rates of heart disease. Tests revealed that the fishermen had high amounts of omega-3s in their blood. Further research found that omega-3s helped thin the blood and inhibit the onset of atherosclerosis (clogged arteries). Researchers concluded that regularly eating fish rich in omega-3s could help reduce the risk of heart disease.

This research was widely publicized in the media and is now familiar to many of us. But the research on omega-3s certainly didn't stop there. Dozens of clinical trials and population studies have now been conducted showing that not only Japanese, but Mediterraneans, Dutch, and Americans who eat fish frequently also have less risk of heart disease.

In one study—involving 827 people matched for age, sex, weight, and family history of heart disease—researchers at the University of Washington, Seattle, found that the intake of just one portion of fatty fish a week (fatty fish is the best source of omega-3s) equaled a 50 percent lower risk of heart attack.

How Omega-3 Helps Prevent Heart Disease

Scientists believe there are several reasons omega-3s are so heart healthy. First, omega-3s have been shown to significantly reduce blood platelet cell stickiness (platelets are one of the components in the blood that causes clotting). Research has also shown that omega-3s can slow down the buildup of cholesterol in the arteries, which makes heart disease less likely.

It appears that omega-3s can even change the chemistry in the heart affecting heartbeat, the flow of blood, and chemical reactions in the blood vessels. "Potentially what happens is that fish actually can quiet the heart cells that might be irritated in a heart attack or during a period where the heart is not getting enough blood supply due to blockages in the arteries," says Dr. Christine Albert, who was involved in an eleven-year Harvard University study involving more than 21,000 people, which showed that just one serving of omega-3 rich fish weekly equaled a 52 percent reduction in sudden heart attack death.

On top of this, omega-3 has also been shown to help reduce blood pressure and high triglyceride (blood fat) levels, both of which are known risk factors for heart disease.

When you combine all these elements together, it's easy to see why omega-3s are one of the most powerful natural defenses against heart disease known to science.

Omega-3 and Stroke

Since omega-3s help prevent the arteries of the heart from becoming blocked, not surprisingly the rate of thrombotic stroke (stroke caused by a blockage to the arteries leading to the brain) has also been found to be much lower among those people who eat fish regularly.

In a study involving over 80,000 women, researchers from Harvard School of Public Health found that women who ate five or more servings of fish a week had one-third the risk of a thrombotic stroke compared to women who ate fish once a month or less.

"I wasn't surprised by the direction of this study, but I was surprised by the magnitude," reported Dr. Meir Stampfer, professor of nutrition and epidemiology at the Harvard School of Public Health and a coauthor of the study. "I didn't expect the protective effect of fish to be that strong."

BRAIN FOOD

Remember how your grandmother told you fish was good brain food? Well, these classic words of wisdom are now being backed up by modern science.

The brain is actually made up of more than 50 percent fat, and research has found that the most abundant of these fats is a type of omega-3 fatty acid called *docosahexaenoic acid* (DHA). Studies have shown that DHA is a crucial building block of the brain that enhances brain cell communication and nerve signal transmission. Other research has shown that diets that don't contain enough DHA-rich omega-3s can lead to behavioral changes, learning difficulties, and a change in the biochemistry of the brain. This means that omega-3s have wide-ranging effects on the healthy functioning of your brain, including your susceptibility to depression.

Omega-3 and Depression

Researchers have found an interesting relationship between consumption of omega-3s and the incidence of depression. In countries where fish consumption is low, depression rates tend to be high. On the other hand, in countries where fish consumption is high, depression rates tend to be low. Studies have also found that people with depression often have low levels of omega-3 in their cells, and these people typically respond well to an increase in omega-3 in their diet.

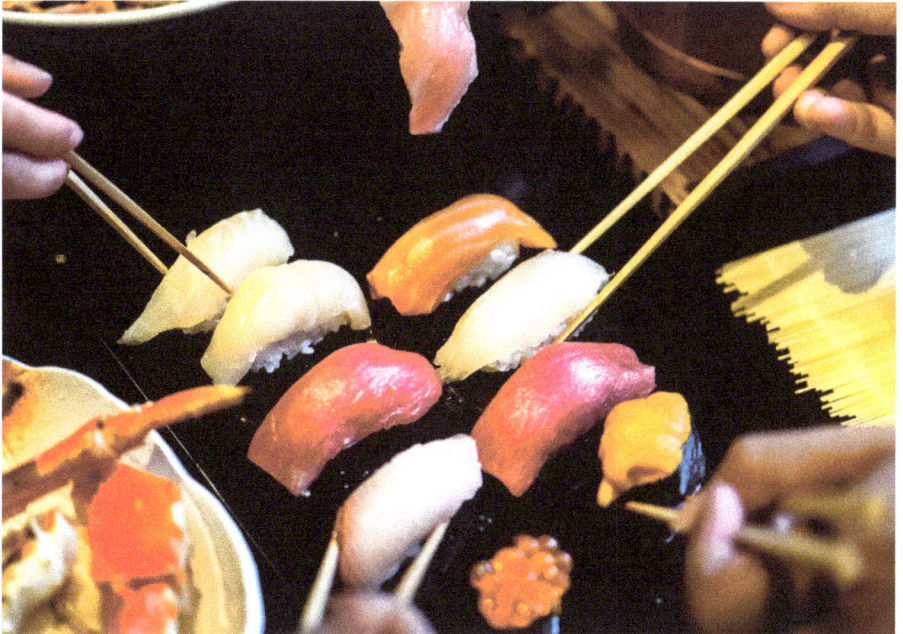

Omega-3 and Alzheimer's Disease

Because of the ability of omega-3s to improve brain function, it's not surprising that this remarkable fat has also been shown to be of benefit in reducing the risk of developing Alzheimer's disease. In one study of more than 1,000 people (average age seventy-five), those with high blood levels of omega-3s were found to be more than 40 percent less likely to develop Alzheimer's over a period of nine years than people with low omega-3 levels. Research by Danish scientists who compared the diets of 5,386 healthy older men and woman also found that the more fish in a person's diet, the lower his or her risk of developing Alzheimer's disease.

Omega-3 and Arthritis

Another area where omega-3s have shown great potential is with inflammatory illnesses such as arthritis and asthma.

In one study, by Dr. Jean A. Shapiro in association with Fred Hutchinson Cancer Research Institute, researchers used a food frequency questionnaire to compare 324 rheumatoid arthritis cases with 1,245 controls. They found that those who ate an average of just two servings a week of omega-3 rich fish were 57 percent less likely to develop rheumatoid arthritis as those who ate less than one.

Nearly two dozen studies have also shown that people with rheumatoid arthritis have less fatigue and joint stiffness and could lower their anti-inflammatory drugs when they increased their intake of omega-3s.

FISH: THE WEIGHT-LOSS SUPERFOOD

Fish is moderate in calories, yet filling and satisfying. In effect, this means that if you eat more fish, particularly in place of high-calorie red meat, losing weight should happen naturally. It certainly did for champion Australian weight lifter Dean Lukin. Dean won the gold medal for weight lifting in the super-heavyweight division at the 1984 Los Angeles Olympics. And Dean was certainly a super heavyweight himself, tipping the scales at over 300 pounds. But after his weight-lifting career ended, Dean was desperate to lose the pounds—not just to look better but to generally improve his health.

Dean decided to cut back on the highly processed foods and red meat that had made him fat. Instead he adopted a diet resembling that of previous generations of his family, who came from the Mediterranean region and ate a diet that included fish as their main source of protein. "My father grew up in a seaside village on the Dalmatian coast and he and his family basically lived off the sea," recalls Dean in his 1993 book *The Dean Lukin Diet*. "My great-grandfather lived until he was 96. My grandfather's brother is still going strong in his 90s, so I figure the stuff can't be all that bad for you!"

Dean came to the conclusion that a weight-loss program using fish as the main source of protein would be the commonsense way to go. And he soon discovered there was a big bonus to eating a diet that included lots of moderate-calorie fish: "I found that I can eat larger quantities of fish than most other foods without putting on weight—being a person who's big on volume I find it ideal."

So, what happened when Dean started eating like his Mediterranean relatives? He ended up losing an incredible 110 pounds of fat in less than a year, or as Dean puts it: "When I got to the stage of really ripping the blubber off, the rate of progress was quite startling." Just as incredible is the fact that, as I write, he has kept that weight off for well over two decades.

Of course, Dean doesn't put all his success down to eating more fish. He followed his Mediterranean relatives and also increased his consumption of highly nutritious vegetables, fruits, and grain-based foods such as pasta and rice. He also made sure he kept active. But Dean reckons that eating plenty of fish was a major contributing factor to his dramatic weight loss.

HIGH IN "QUALITY" PROTEIN

In the West we often base our meals around red meat such as beef, pork, or lamb. These foods all contain plenty of protein, which your body needs for growth and repair. Unfortunately, they also contain large amounts of saturated fat, which your body most certainly doesn't need.

Fish and shellfish, on the other hand, contain just as much protein as red meat, but instead of containing lots of bad fat they contain good fat. The protein found in all seafood is also identical to that found in red meat, and is a "complete" protein. This means it contains all the essential amino acids (the building blocks of protein) your body needs for repair and growth.

VITAMIN AND MINERAL RICH

As well as being a rich source of protein, fish and shellfish also contain high amounts of many important vitamins and minerals that are essential for optimal health including vitamin A, E and D, and also hard to get minerals such as selenium and zinc.

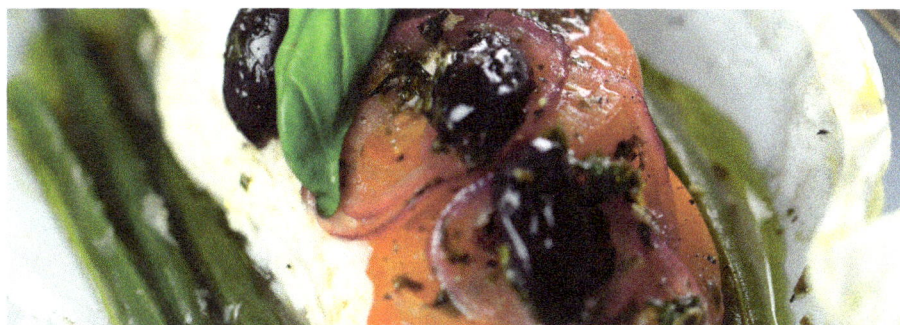

VITAMIN & MINERAL CONTENT OF FISH & SHELLFISH

NUTRIENT	BEST FISH & SHELLFISH SOURCES	MAIN ROLE
Vitamin A	Crab, halibut, salmon, sardines, swordfish, tuna, whitefish	Maintains healthy skin, bones, teeth and vision
Vitamin B12	Crab, herring, mackerel, oysters, salmon, trout	Needed for making red blood cells and maintaining the central nervous system
Vitamin E	Anchovies, haddock, herring, mackerel, salmon, sardines, tuna	An important antioxidant that protects body cells from free radical damage
Vitamin D	Anchovies, mackerel, salmon, sardines, tuna	Promotes strong bones and teeth and helps with the absorption of calcium and phosphorus
Calcium	Herring, oysters, salmon, sardines, shrimp	Builds bones and teeth, regulates blood clotting, is essential for normal functioning of muscles
Iron	Anchovies, abalone, clams, mackerel, mussels, oysters, perch, salmon, sardines, shrimp, tuna	Needed for making red blood cells and transporting oxygen in blood and muscles
Phosphorus	Cod, halibut, perch, salmon, scallops, snapper, trout, tuna	Needed for energy metabolism
Potassium	Cod, halibut, perch, salmon, scallops, snapper, trout, tuna	Helps transmit nerve impulses, controls muscle contractions, and regulates water balance in cells
Magnesium	Mackerel, oysters, salmon, shrimp	Regulates heart beat and promotes bone growth
Selenium	Cod, crab, lobster, oysters, scallops, shrimp	Helps to regulate blood pressure and protects cells from free radical damage
Zinc	Crab, lobster, oysters, halibut	Aids in wound healing, growth, and sexual development

THE MANY WAYS OF ENJOYING FISH AND SHELLFISH

There are countless ways to enjoy fish and shellfish—especially when you follow the example of people from Mediterranean and Asian cultures who have spent thousands of years developing tasty recipes with fish and shellfish in the starring role. And because fish and shellfish cook very quickly, this also means you'll end up spending less time in the kitchen than if you prepare a typical meat-based meal.

Here are some examples of different types of fish and shellfish and how you can easily incorporate them into your diet.

Anchovies. The salty flavor and oily texture of anchovies make them the classic complement for a wide variety of Mediterranean-style dishes. Sprinkle them over a pizza just before baking, add them to pasta sauces and risottos, and use them whole or finely chopped in Mediterranean-style salads. They also go wonderfully with a little chopped fresh basil as a topping for *bruschetta* (Italian garlic and olive oil toasts).

Clams. Clams add a delicious "taste of the sea" to pasta dishes, rice dishes, stews, and chowders. Canned clams can also be sprinkled on top of pizzas before baking.

Crab. Fresh crab is utterly delicious, but we regard it as "special occasion" food because it's expensive, and often hard to come by. More often than not we'll use surimi (imitation crab made from fish) instead. Whether you use real or imitation crab, either way you'll find plenty of uses for this versatile food. It can be added to stir-fries and noodle dishes; it tastes wonderful in risottos and pasta dishes, scattered in salads, or used as a filling in sushi, sandwiches, and rice paper rolls.

Oysters and mussels. Smoked oysters and mussels can be used as a pizza topping or as part of an Italian *antipasto* platter. Fresh mussels in the shell are also as an important element in the classic Spanish seafood paella (a saffron-infused rice and vegetable dish studded with a variety of seafood). Fresh mussels also taste wonderful in pasta dishes and risottos. Oysters served raw in the shell with a little lemon juice make a delicious appetizer, but be sure that the oysters are really fresh and come from a reputable source.

Salmon. Salmon isn't only one of the richest sources of healthy omega-3s; it's also one of the most versatile varieties of fish. Salmon steaks are particularly good cooked over a hot grill and served with salad and crusty bread, but be careful not to overcook the delicate flesh or else it will dry out. Fresh salmon fillets can be grilled, steamed, poached with fresh herbs, marinated and baked, or cut into cubes and added to pasta dishes and stir-fries. Thin slices of smoked salmon are delicious served with a bagel and a little avocado. Smoked salmon also makes a great pizza topping and sandwich or sushi filling, and goes wonderfully with scrambled eggs. Canned salmon is ideal served cold with salad and bread or in a sandwich or sub. It also works equally well on pizzas and in pasta dishes, bakes, and risottos and can be used to make burger patties. Choose canned Alaskan red salmon, since this is the best quality and is wild caught. Very fresh raw salmon can be eaten Japanese-style, in sushi or sliced and served as sashimi.

Sardines. Available fresh or canned. The canned variety can be mashed and used as a sandwich or toast spread, and the fresh variety goes well in pasta dishes or marinated and grilled.

Scallops. With their delicate milky flesh and clean flavor, scallops lend themselves to a wide variety of dishes including stir-fries, curries, pasta dishes, and bakes. Marinated and grilled scallops also make a delightful meal served with crusty bread and salad.

Shrimp. Shrimp happens to be one of our favorite foods. The possibilities with shrimp are virtually limitless: skewered with fresh vegetables, marinated, then cooked over a flaming grill; stir-fried with a colorful range of crunchy vegetables and served over rice or noodles; dotted throughout pasta dishes, risottos, pilafs, and paellas; as a filling for sandwiches and subs; or simply served as a classic shrimp cocktail with juicy tomatoes, crisp lettuce, tangy seafood sauce, and wedges of lemon. If you can't get your hands on fresh shrimp, frozen cooked shrimp is available in most supermarkets.

Squid. Squid goes well in Mediterranean-style dishes like pasta, risotto, and pizza. It goes equally well with Asian-style dishes such as stir-fries, noodles dishes, and Asian braises.

Swordfish. Swordfish is a delicious firm-fleshed fish with a mild flavor and a meaty texture. It's similar to fresh tuna and can be used in much the same way (see tuna below).

Tuna. Like salmon, tuna is a good source of omega-3s and is incredibly versatile. And even if you're not a big fan of fish you'll probably still enjoy tuna because its texture is more like chicken than fish. Fresh tuna steaks are ideal grilled or pan-fried and served with salad and crusty bread. Fresh tuna can also be cut into cubes and added to pasta dishes, stews, curries, and stir-fries. Another way to enjoy fresh tuna is served raw in sushi and sashimi. Canned tuna is a staple food in our pantry and can be used in a myriad of wonderful dishes including pastas, pizzas, risottos, and bakes. Of course, canned tuna is also the ideal sandwich filling with fresh crispy salad vegetables.

White fish. Firm white fish such as snapper, cod, and haddock can be cut into cubes and stir-fried, added to pasta dishes or grilled or pan-fried whole with a little olive oil and served with freshly ground pepper and lemon juice. White fish of any kind also tastes wonderful marinated and baked, or cooked in an Indian, Thai, or Malaysian curry until the flesh is soft and flaky.

Fish and shellfish are delicious, low in calories, easy to prepare, quick to cook, and incredibly versatile. And with all the wonderful health-giving benefits fish and other seafood have to offer, it's clear that including more in your diet (particularly in place of red meat) is a very sensible route to take. As Dr. Joyce A. Nettleton, a nutritionist and lecturer from Tufts University puts it, "The benefits of including fish at least every week is no longer doubted . . . helping ourselves to fish is helping ourselves to health."

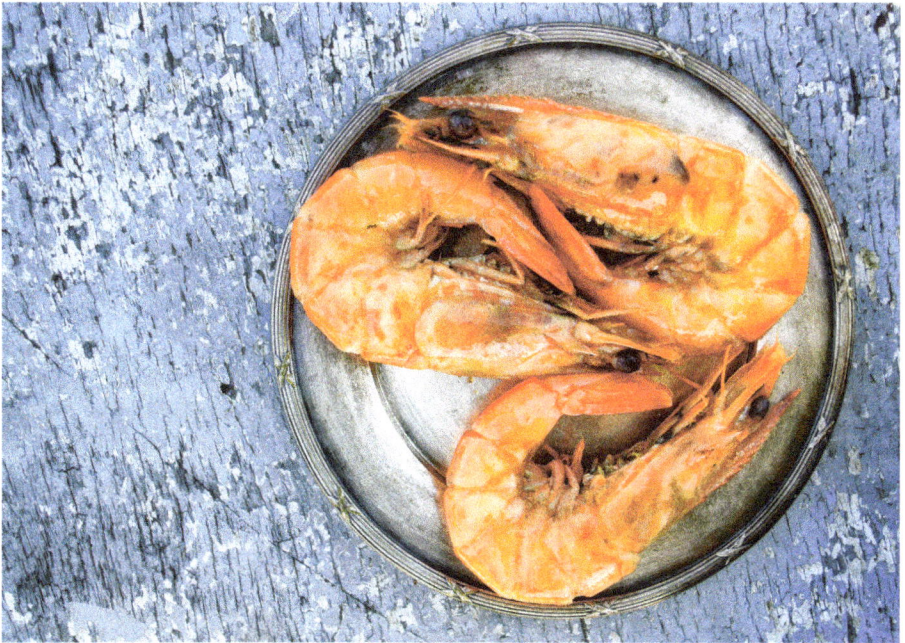

CHAPTER 5

Plant power

Plant-based foods form the backbone of traditional Mediterranean and Asian cuisines. One look at the Mediterranean and Asian Diet Pyramids (pages 10-11) and this fact becomes very obvious. The typical Western way of eating, on the other hand, generally includes lots of meat and highly processed foods but usually very little fresh or minimally processed plant foods.

As more and more scientific studies point to the role that plant foods play in the promotion of health and the reduction of disease, this situation is slowly starting to change. But unfortunately most of us in the West still fall short in our consumption of plant foods.

Yet incorporating more plant foods into your diet is actually very easy to do. This chapter will show you how, by following the example of Mediterranean and Asian cultures, eating more plant foods can actually be a highly pleasurable experience! This chapter will also identify the key reasons why you need to eat plant foods regularly if you want to give yourself the best chance of living a long and healthy life. I've divided this chapter into four main sections. Each of these different types of plant foods has distinctive health-giving qualities, which I'll cover in detail:

- Grain foods
- Vegetables and fruits
- Legumes
- Nuts and seeds

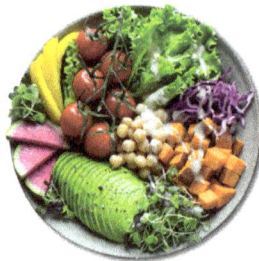

GRAIN FOODS

For thousands of years, grain-based foods such as rice, bread, pasta, noodles, couscous and bulgur have held a revered and sacred status throughout the Mediterranean and Asia. And it's not surprising that grains are so highly regarded by the peoples of these regions, because they really are an extraordinary food. They're inexpensive, filling and satisfying, and moderate in calories, and they can be used as a base for an almost endless variety of meals.

Grain foods are also highly nutritious. Wheat, for example, contains twenty-two different vitamins and minerals including vitamin E and B1, niacin, folate, iron, zinc, selenium, potassium, and magnesium. Grain foods are also a good source of antioxidants and phytochemicals, which help promote good health and prevent

---

COMMON TYPES OF GRAINS

- Wheat (used to make bread, pasta, noodles, couscous, and bulgur)
- Rice (comes in many different varieties and is eaten as a grain by itself or ground into rice flour to make various types of rice noodles)
- Oats

- Corn
- Rye
- Barley
- Millet
- Buckwheat (not botanically a grain but has a similar nutrient profile and is used in the same way)

---

disease. (I'll talk more about these incredible substances later in this chapter.) And like all plant foods, grains—particularly whole grains—are a good source of health-promoting dietary fiber (see "Dietary Fiber and its Benefits," page 41).

Studies have even found that whole grains can protect against heart disease and cancer. In one study, researchers from the University of Minnesota studied nearly 34,000 people and found that those who ate the highest amount of whole grains had a 23 percent reduced risk of death from heart disease and a 21 percent reduced risk of death from cancer, compared with people who ate little or no whole grains.

To many people's surprise, grains are also a good source of protein. Most varieties of grain contain 10 to 15 percent protein. However, unlike fish, soybeans, and meat, this protein isn't "complete" because it's low in *lysine* (one of the amino acids, or building blocks, of protein). But this problem is easily overcome by mixing a grain food with a complementary protein that contains lysine, such as legumes (beans, peas, and lentils), nuts, or fish. Indeed, this is what Mediterraneans and Asians have instinctively been doing for centuries.

GRAINS AND CARBOHYDRATES

Ever wondered how Chinese peasants or Greek farmers can toil away in the fields for long hours every day, even well into old age? Part of the answer could lie in the energy-giving foods these people eat every day.

Dietary Fiber & its Benefits

Dietary fiber is a type of carbohydrate found only in plant foods. It's basically derived from the material that helps give plants their shape and structure. Fiber falls into two distinct categories: insoluble fiber and soluble fiber. Most plant foods contain a combination of both soluble and insoluble fiber in varying amounts.

Insoluble fiber, which is found in high amounts in whole grains as well as beans, fruits, and vegetables, is coarse in texture. Soluble fiber, on the other hand, has a soft and gummy texture and is found in high amounts in legumes (beans, peas, and lentils), fruits, vegetables, oats, and barley. Soluble and insoluble fiber work in different ways to promote health.

Insoluble Fiber

Insoluble fiber acts like a sponge and absorbs water as it's digested, so it adds bulk and softness to bowel movements. This not only prevents constipation, but also speeds the rate at which food passes through your system, leaving less time for certain foods to deposit impurities and cancer-promoting compounds on the intestinal wall. This may be one reason why diets high in fiber are associated with low rates of bowel and colon cancer. Recent results from one of the largest studies ever conducted into the link between diet and cancer—the EPIC (European Prospective Investigation of Cancer and Nutrition) Study—involving more than 500,000 people from ten countries found that the people eating the most fiber had a 40 percent lower risk of colon cancer than those people eating the least.

Soluble Fiber

Soluble fiber works differently from insoluble fiber because it's broken down by the action of bacteria in the digestive tract and some of the healthy by-products of this process are absorbed into the bloodstream. Once in the bloodstream, these healthy by-products have been found to bind with bile acids (compounds originally derived from cholesterol stores in the liver) and escort them out of the body. This draws cholesterol from the blood, and in turn lowers cholesterol levels. In one study of men with high cholesterol levels, adding half a cup of cooked dried beans (rich in soluble fiber) to their normal diet reduced their blood cholesterol levels by 13 percent in twenty-one days. Soluble fiber also slows the release of glucose into the bloodstream, which helps regulate blood sugar levels.

Both soluble and insoluble fiber have also been shown to protect against heart disease and breast cancer. A study of over 43,000 U.S. male health professionals conducted by Harvard University found that over a six-year period those who ate the most fiber had a 55 percent lower chance of coronary death than those who ate the least. And a recent study of more than 1000 Australian women (half had been diagnosed with breast cancer, half were free of the disease) found that those who ate more than 28 grams of fiber per day had the lowest risk of the disease, while those who ate less than 14 grams per day faced the highest risk.

The Weight Loss Bonus

Fiber not only promotes good health and keeps you regular, but it can also help control your weight. Here's why. First, fiber is nature's best appetite suppressant because it fills the stomach and satisfies your appetite much earlier than fiber-depleted foods. And fiber isn't only bulky and filling; it also can't be digested like normal foods (it basically passes right through you) so it adds virtually no calories to your diet.

The chewiness of high-fiber foods also prolongs eating time, which, in turn, gives your body time to tell your brain that your stomach is full.

And a high-fiber diet may actually cut the number of calories you ingest by blocking your body's ability to digest the fat and protein consumed along with it. In a recent study by the U.S. Department of Agriculture, researchers set a certain number of calories for subject groups and altered the fiber content. Results demonstrated that fewer calories were absorbed with increased fiber intake. It was found that people who consumed up to 36 grams of fiber a day absorbed 130 fewer daily calories. Over a year, that adds up to over 47,000 calories!

Are You Getting Enough?

The importance of fiber as part of a healthy diet is beyond question. Unfortunately, most people in Western countries like the United States, the United Kingdom, and Australia consume very little dietary fiber—only around 10 to 15 grams a day. While this is better than none, it's too little for any appreciable benefits. Throughout the Mediterranean and Asia, fiber intake is traditionally between 30 and 40 grams a day. This is the level to strive for. Luckily, by following a MediterrAsian style of eating—which includes lots of fiber-rich whole grains, fruits, vegetables, nuts, and legumes—you'll naturally be eating this level of fiber without even having to think about it.

Traditional Mediterranean and Asian diets are based on a foundation of grain foods like rice, bread, pasta, and noodles. These foods also happen to contain energy-giving carbohydrates. All plant foods, including beans, vegetables, and fruits, contain carbohydrates; however, grain foods are one of the richest sources.

The reason why carbohydrates are so good at boosting energy levels is simple: when they're digested, they're broken down in your body and converted into glucose, or what is commonly known as blood sugar. This glucose is then released into your bloodstream and it supplies your muscles with their favorite source of fuel. So, by regularly eating carbohydrate-rich grain foods, you'll always ensure your energy levels stay high.

Just think, the grain-rich diets of the Mediterranean and Asia are what helped fuel the conquering Roman legions, sustained the laborers as they built the Great Pyramids, and provided the energy for the workers to build the Great Wall of China. Imagine how this same type of diet can help power you through your day!

Brain Fuel

The glucose supplied by carbohydrates isn't the favorite source of fuel for only your muscles: Your brain runs almost exclusively on glucose. That's why, if your blood sugar levels get low, you not only feel low in energy but often moody and fuzzy-headed, and it becomes difficult to concentrate. And carbohydrates have another important effect on the brain—they naturally increase the production of *serotonin*, a special chemical in the brain that has a calming effect.

So, by eating plenty of carbohydrates, you'll be more mentally alert and focused throughout the day, and at the same time you should also feel calmer and less moody.

Regulating Blood Sugars

Carbohydrate-rich grain foods are great for supplying your muscles and brain with glucose. However, to ensure this glucose is delivered most effectively, it makes sense to mix grain foods with foods that contain fat and protein. This is because fat and protein help to slow down the release of glucose into your bloodstream, which in turn helps regulate your blood sugars. (Soluble fiber, found in high amounts in legumes, vegetables, and fruits, also slows down the release of glucose into the bloodstream.)

This slow and steady release of glucose ensures you'll have a constant supply of fuel for your muscles and brain, which ultimately means more energy for longer periods of time, better concentration, and fewer mood swings.

The great thing is that grain-based foods like pasta and rice taste much better with the addition of protein and fat anyway. In fact, Mediterranean and Asian peoples have traditionally been mixing grain foods with protein sources (such as fish, beans, and poultry) and fat (such as olive oil and peanut oil) for thousands of years. Later in the book we'll show you just how easy it is to mix your meals in the same way.

White or Whole Grain?

When it comes to buying grain-based foods, you'll find there are two distinct categories: white and whole grain (also known as wholemeal). White pasta or whole grain pasta; white rice or brown (whole grain) rice; and white bread or whole grain bread are some examples.

What's the difference between white and whole grain varieties? Well, whole grains are just that—the whole grain. An unrefined kernel of grain is actually made up of three layers: the germ (innermost layer), the endosperm (central core), and the bran (protective outer layer). Refined (white) grains, on the other hand, have had their bran and germ removed in the refining process. Although the germ and bran layers make up less than 20 percent of the actual volume of a kernel of grain, two-thirds of the fiber and many of the vitamins and minerals are located in these layers.

So nutritionally speaking, white grain products are inferior to whole grain products. But does this make white grain products unhealthy? Well, think about it this way. If you took an apple and peeled it, would the apple suddenly become unhealthy? Sure, a peeled apple won't be as good for you as an unpeeled apple because lots of fiber, vitamins and minerals are stored in the skin of the apple, but this doesn't make what's left unhealthy.

The same is true with grains. White grain foods may not be as healthy for you as whole grain foods, but they're certainly not an unhealthy food. What is left when the germ and bran has been removed is the endosperm, or central core of the grain, which contains energy-giving carbohydrates as well as protein and B vitamins. And the endosperm still contains a third of the health-promoting fiber found in a grain's kernel.

So, white grain products aren't bad for you (unless they're combined with sugar or bad fats or cooked with unhealthy ingredients) and can definitely have a place in your diet. In fact, in most parts of Asia and the Mediterranean white rice and pasta have been more popular than whole grain varieties for many generations.

At the same time, it's clear that whole grains are very important because of the valuable nutrients they provide. The solution? If you enjoy eating brown rice and whole grain pasta, then continue to do so. But if you don't, then enjoy regular pasta and rice (mixed with lean protein, good fats and fiber-rich beans and vegetables) and when it comes to breads and breakfast cereals, opt mostly for whole grain varieties. This way you'll ensure you get a rich mix of nutrients.

Fitting Grain Foods into Your Life

With all the benefits that grain foods have to offer, it's now a matter of incorporating more of them into your life so you can reap the rewards. Luckily this is easily accomplished because a MediterrAsian style of eating features grain foods in a prominent role (as you'll discover when you try the delicious recipes in this book). Here's a rundown of the most common types of grain foods you'll be eating as part of a MediterrAsian way of eating.

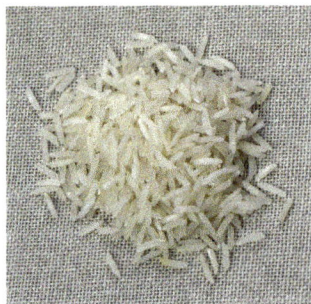

Rice. The Chinese eat the most rice in the world, at over four pounds (uncooked weight) per person each week. With this in mind, it's probably not surprising that the Chinese word for rice, *fan*, means "food." Rice is also a staple food in most other Asian countries including Japan, Thailand, Indonesia, Vietnam, and India.

But rice isn't popular only in Asia—for centuries it has also been widely enjoyed throughout the Mediterranean. The peoples of the Mediterranean have put their own flare into this versatile food and some of the delicious rice dishes popular in these regions include *risotto* from Italy, *paella* from Spain, and *pilaf* from Greece and the Middle East.

In recent years Western consumers have started to realize the benefits of this inexpensive and healthy grain. These days there are many varieties of rice available at your local supermarket. Some examples include fragrant Thai *jasmine*, Indian *basmati*, Spanish *valencia*, Japanese *koshihikari* (ideal for sushi), and Italian *arborio* (perfect for risottos).

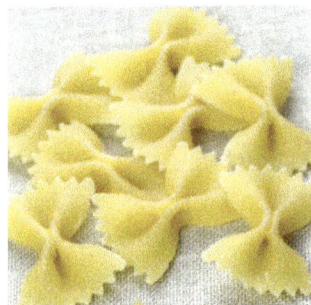

Pasta. Pasta has been a staple food in the Italian diet for centuries. As far back as 1300 the ships of Genoa had a "master of lasagna" on board to cook for the sailors. And there are so many reasons to love pasta: It's quick and easy to prepare, inexpensive, incredibly versatile, moderate in calories (a one-cup serving of cooked pasta contains only around 190 calories), and above all else it tastes delicious!

Pasta can be made from rice, corn, buckwheat, and other grains, but typically it's made from wheat, traditionally durum wheat (a special hard type of wheat that is digested slowly). You can buy pasta fresh, dried, and in high-fiber whole grain varieties.

Much of the appeal of pasta lies in its sheer versatility. Not only are the topping ideas limited only by your imagination, but the range of pasta shapes and sizes is enormous, with over four hundred different varieties. Some of our favorites include spaghetti, lasagna, fusilli (corkscrew shape), fettuccine (flat, ribbonlike), penne (tubular with ends cut on diagonal), farfalle (bow-tie shaped), cappellini (angel hair), and conchiglie (shells). One of the delights of eating a pasta dish is determining by experiment which kind of pasta best matches your favorite sauces.

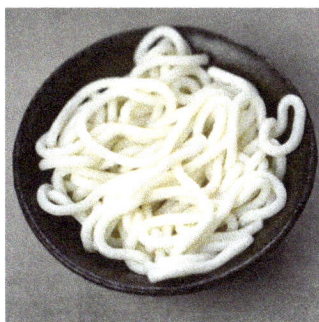

Noodles. Born in China around four thousand years ago, noodles are to Asians what pasta is to Italians. This endlessly versatile food can be boiled and served with sauces and toppings, simmered in soups and braises, or stir-fried with thinly sliced vegetables, seafood, and meats. Noodles are commonly made from wheat or rice flour, but other varieties are available made from buckwheat or bean starch. Depending on their shape and size, most noodles take only a few minutes to cook.

Although noodles are generally moderate in calories, some varieties like instant ramen noodles contain a fairly large amount of fat in the form of palm oil. Unfortunately, palm oil is as highly saturated as animal fat and so its use should be limited. Instead, look for noodles that contain just flour and water, since these are the healthiest option.

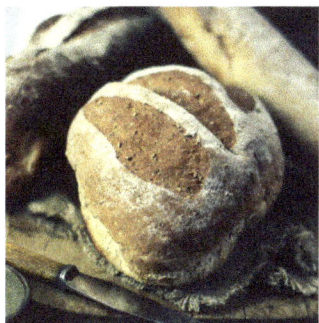

Bread. Bread, which has often been referred to as "the staff of life," is one of the most widely consumed foods in the world. In the Mediterranean region, where bread originated over four thousand years ago, it's a staple food that's eaten at most meals.

Bread is also a popular food in the West, but many of us tend to limit our choice of bread to sliced white. This is unfortunate because there is such a vast range of alternative breads available, offering a world of tastes and textures. Some examples include Italian ciabatta and focaccia bread, sourdough bread, baguettes, pita bread, whole grain peasant bread, Turkish pide bread, Middle Eastern lavash bread, Indian naan bread, as well as a large range of specialty loaves and rolls. Experiment with different breads to find your favorites.

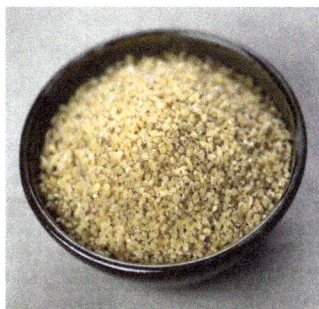

Couscous and bulgur. Both of these grain foods are actually made from wheat. Couscous is made from durum wheat (the same type of wheat used to make pasta), which is moistened with water, then rolled in small balls and steamed. It's a staple food in the north African countries that border the Mediterranean Sea, including Morocco and Tunisia, and is traditionally served in a big bowl and topped with various kinds of vegetable, fish, poultry, and bean stews. Couscous can also be added to salads, used to thicken soups, or mixed with fruit and other ingredients to make wonderful sweet desserts.

Bulgur is made from whole wheat that has been parboiled, dried, then sifted into particles. Bulgur is a common food in Greece and the countries of the Middle East, and like couscous it can be topped with various kinds of stews and sauces or used to thicken soups. It's also delicious used in pilafs and is an important ingredient in tabbouleh salad.

Breakfast cereals. Breakfast cereals fit in perfectly with a MediterrAsian way of eating because they're made from grains such as wheat, oats, and rice. With a little milk and topped with some fruit, breakfast cereals make an ideal high-energy start to the day.

Of course, all breakfast cereals aren't created equal, and many have a lot of added sugar and salt. The cereals to look out for are the whole grain varieties because these not only have more fiber but often contain little or no added nasties (oatmeal and untoasted muesli are ideal).

VEGETABLES AND FRUITS

More than two thousand years ago, the Greek physician Hippocrates proclaimed. "Let food be your medicine, and medicine be your food." Over the last few decades scientific research has proven just how true Hippocrates' words of wisdom are. Many types of foods are now known to contain nutrients that act like medicine and improve health, and also reduce the risk of becoming ill in the first place. Vegetables and fruits, more than any other types of food, contain the widest range of health-promoting compounds including antioxidants, phytochemicals, soluble and insoluble fiber, and a host of essential vitamins and minerals.

A large body of research in recent years has shown that these compounds can help your body resist cancer, heart disease, and other chronic health conditions. Vegetables and fruits are also generally very low in saturated fat and calories, are incredibly versatile, and when they're prepared correctly they taste great.

Notice how I say *when they're prepared correctly* they taste great. Because when vegetables and fruits—particularly vegetables—aren't prepared properly they can taste very unappetizing, to say the least. And that's probably one of the main reasons why vegetables aren't particularly popular in Western society—we really don't know how to prepare them properly.

Enjoying Vegetables

Remember the "eat your vegetables" routine at the dinner table? I certainly do; often followed by the threat that if I didn't, my dessert would instead be given to my older sister. And it's through similar threats and bribes that many of us were forced to eat vegetables as kids, and unfortunately a lot of us have grown up to hate vegetables as adults.

But compare this to people living in Mediterranean and Asian countries like Italy, Japan, Greece, or China; for thousands of years they've never had a problem eating and enjoying their vegetables. Why? because the traditional way Mediterranean and Asian peoples prepare and serve vegetables is very different from how we do it in the West, and vastly more appetizing.

In the West we often treat vegetables like a separate part of the meal and have them unflavored and pushed off into the corner of our plate. Throughout the Mediterranean and Asia, on the other hand, vegetables are rarely served in a pile by themselves. Vegetables are an integral part of the taste, texture, and color of most traditional Mediterranean and Asian dishes, and they're typically cut up and mixed in and cooked with the rest of the meal. And it's by combining vegetables with grain foods and protein-rich foods (like fish, shellfish, beans, and chicken), as well as sauces and flavorings, that vegetables taste their best.

Actually, we really already know this in the West, because a well-made sandwich is based on the same principle. If you munched away on plain lettuce or tomato you'd soon get bored; but when tomatoes and lettuce are combined with bread (grain food) and some tuna or chicken (protein-rich food) and some mustard or mayo (flavoring), you suddenly have a tasty sandwich. Indeed, the sandwich wouldn't taste as good without the crunchy lettuce and juicy tomatoes.

And that's the secret to enjoying vegetables: not having them plain and unflavored on the side of your plate, but using them as an integral part of your meal. Thankfully this is easy to do because generations of home cooks from the Mediterranean and Asia have developed countless mouthwatering dishes that use vegetables as a major component. Some good examples include stir-fries, curries, pizzas, pasta dishes, risottos, pilafs, and paellas.

Enjoying Fruit

Fruit also plays a very important role in traditional Mediterranean and Asian diets, and is typically eaten daily as a snack and dessert.

In Western society, although fruit is generally thought of in a more kindly way than vegetables are, again we don't eat nearly as much as we should. A recent study in the United States found that nearly half of all Americans eat no fruit on a given day, and there have been similar findings in the United Kingdom, Australia, New Zealand, and Canada.

There seem to be two major reasons why we don't eat very much fresh fruit in modern Western society. For a start, when was the last time you saw an advertisement for fresh fruit? Yet when was the last time you saw an advertisement for fruit's biggest rival, candy and processed desserts?

Not helping the situation is the fact that the Western way with fruits also tends to be rather unimaginative. For example, many of us limit our choice of fruit to apples, oranges, and a small handful of other fruits. But even though apples and oranges taste delicious, there are dozens of other equally delicious fruits to choose from. Let your imagination run wild when it comes to choosing fruit—mangoes, pineapple, kiwi fruit, berries (strawberries, raspberries, and so on), grapes, lychees, passion fruit, melons (watermelon, cantaloupe, and the like), papaya, persimmons, plums, figs, apricots, and cherries are just some delicious examples. And be adventurous with the way you eat fruits. As well as eating them by themselves, cut them up and mix different fruits together to create a varied range of fruit salads and fruit platters.

Fruit also makes a great base for lots of wonderful, healthy desserts and smoothies. Fresh or dried fruit can also add a sweet accent to savory salads and it makes a particularly good breakfast cereal topper.

Another way you can enjoy fruit is to lighten up a rich dessert. Instead of having a whole serving of rich dessert, have half a serving and mix it with pieces of fresh fruit of your choice. This will add wonderful color, texture, and taste to the dessert, as well as lower the overall calories. We enjoy putting this principle into practice regularly by having fresh fruit salad with a scoop of our favorite ice cream.

The Health-Giving Powers of Vegetables and Fruits

The examples above give you some good ideas of how to include more vegetables and fruits in your diet. And it's certainly not just your taste buds that will benefit. As I mentioned earlier, vegetables and fruits have extraordinary disease-fighting powers. An increasing body of scientific evidence dramatically highlights this protective effect.

The *Journal of the American Medical Association*, for example, recently reported on findings from a long-term study of more than 800 middle-aged men. The study found that the men who ate the most vegetables and fruits were the least likely to have had a stroke. For every three servings eaten a day, researchers found the risk of stroke dropped 22 percent. Two large-scale studies by researchers at Harvard School of Public Health and Brigham and Women's Hospital in Boston also found that eating plenty of vegetables and fruits offers protection against stroke. Both studies found that eating five servings of vegetables and fruits a day was associated with a 30 percent lower risk of stroke for men and women.

To date more than three hundred studies have also found that vegetables and fruits protect against different types of cancer. These include most of the cancers common in Western society, such as breast, prostate, colon, and lung cancer.

In a major study published in the *Journal of the American Dietetic Association*, researchers from the United States and Germany reviewed more than two hundred of these studies. They found consistent evidence that people who ate plenty of vegetables and fruits (five or more servings a day) had about half the risk of developing a broad range of cancers compared with people who ate few vegetables and fruits.

More than twenty studies have also shown that vegetables and fruits protect against heart disease. One study in Finland that tracked over 5000 Finnish men and women for fourteen years found a 34 percent reduction in the risk of a fatal heart attack in the third eating the most vegetables and fruit compared with the third eating the least.

Vegetables and fruits have even been found to offer protection against the bone-thinning disease osteoporosis. A study by researchers at Tufts University found that a high intake of vegetables and fruits helped determine the strength and density of bones in old age.

The lead investigator of the study, Katherine L. Tucker, PhD, associate professor of nutrition at Tufts University, reported, "This suggests that a good quality diet in adulthood is important to bone health beyond the better known contributions of calcium and vitamin D, and provides yet another reason to emphasize the intake of fruits and vegetables."

When you combine this sort of evidence with the fact that the vegetable- and fruit-loving peoples of the Mediterranean and Asia also have low rates of these same diseases, it becomes pretty clear that an apple a day really does keep the doctor away.

Nutrient Rich, Calorie Poor

Vegetables and fruits may be nutrient rich but they're also calorie poor. In other words, vegetables and fruits give you the biggest bang for the buck—lots of nutrients for the lowest amount of calories.

Did you know, for example, that two quarter-pound cheeseburgers contain the same number of calories as fifty carrots or seventy tomatoes?

Of course, I don't expect you to sit down to a plate of seventy tomatoes for lunch tomorrow, but this comparison gives you a good idea that when you add lots of different vegetables and fruits to your diet, you'll be adding lots of taste, texture, flavor, color, and nutrients but very few calories.

And the reason is quite simple: Vegetables and fruits generally have a very high water content. Because water contains no calories, vegetables and fruits, in turn, contain very few calories.

As an added bonus, the calories in vegetables and fruits generally come from carbohydrates, which are broken down into glucose in your body. Because glucose provides fuel for your muscles to work, it makes it much easier to incorporate more activity into your life, which in itself burns calories.

Vegetables and fruits are also a good source of dietary fiber. Fiber fills you up without filling you out, and because it can't be digested it adds virtually no calories to your diet.

However, not all vegetables and fruits are the same. When fresh vegetables or fruits are dried or turned into juice it changes their concentration of calories. In the case of fruit and vegetable juice, the calories become more concentrated because most of the fiber and bulk have been removed. Dried fruit, on the other hand, contains a much higher concentration of calories than fresh fruit because most of the water has been removed.

Removing the fiber or water from fruits and vegetables not only concentrates calories, but also makes them less bulky and not as filling and satisfying. This was clearly demonstrated in a study by Dr. Kenneth Heaton and colleagues at Bristol University, England. They gave ten volunteers either a whole apple or the same amount of apple made into puree or into juice. The volunteers took, on average, seventeen minutes to eat the apple, six minutes to eat the puree, and only one and a half minutes to drink the juice. Predictably, the volunteers said that the whole apples were more satisfying and kept them fuller for much longer.

Of course, juiced or dried vegetables and fruits are fine in moderation, but the most satisfying and certainly the healthiest way to eat vegetables and fruits is in their natural "whole" state.

LEGUMES

For centuries legumes have played a major role in the traditional diets enjoyed by Mediterranean and Asian peoples. In the Tuscany region of Italy, for example, there is such a wide variety of bean dishes that Tuscans are fondly known as the "bean eaters." Throughout India, legumes such as chickpeas, lentils, and green peas form a cornerstone of many Indian curries, such as dahl (lentil curry). In Greece and the countries of the Middle East, beans and lentils are traditionally eaten daily in soups and stews, or turned into sauces and pastes such as hummus. And in Asian countries such as Japan and China, the soybean in its many forms— such as tofu and soy sauce—is an essential ingredient in traditional cooking.

But legumes aren't only a delicious base for countless tasty meals. In recent years scientists have discovered that legumes are also nutritional powerhouses containing many essential nutrients we need for good health from the cradle to the grave. In addition to being a nutritious food source, studies have shown that legumes can also help lower LDL cholesterol levels, decrease the risk of certain cancers, help control Type 2 diabetes, relieve symptoms of menopause (such as hot flashes and night sweats), and assist in weight maintenance.

continues on page 57

Pick of the Crop: The Top Vegetable & Fruit Superfoods

All vegetables and fruits contain health-giving powers to a certain extent, but researchers have identified a number of vegetables and fruits that are particularly beneficial. Not surprisingly, all of these vegetables and fruits happen to be eaten extensively throughout Asia and the Mediterranean.

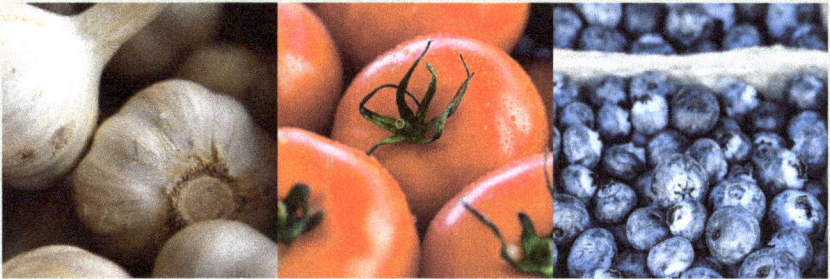

Garlic

A classic ingredient in traditional Mediterranean and Asian cooking, garlic has long been regarded as one of nature's most effective cure-alls. As long ago as 3000 BC, Egyptians were worshipping garlic and using it as a medicine (clay models of garlic were found inside Tutankhamen's tomb). Traditional Chinese medicine used garlic for the treatment of coughs, colds, bronchitis, tuberculosis, diarrhea, and many other infectious diseases. The ancient Greek physician Hippocrates used garlic to treat certain cancers. And it has been used throughout history to treat a host of other ailments including the plague in Europe and typhus and dysentery during World War I.

Since the 1950s dozens of scientific studies have evaluated the health and healing powers of garlic, and a number of other benefits have been discovered. Donald D. Hensrud, MD, a nutrition specialist at the Mayo Clinic in Minnesota notes, "Research is concentrating on several areas where garlic may have positive effects: cardiovascular health, immune function, antimicrobial action and anticancer activity."

In a recent study of 42,000 women in Iowa, for example, those who ate garlic more than once a week were half as likely to develop colon cancer as non-garlic eaters. Garlic has also been shown to lower LDL (bad) cholesterol and boost HDL

continues on next page

(good) cholesterol, which can decrease the incidence of heart attack and stroke.

So what makes garlic such a powerful superfood? Researchers have found that garlic is full of health-giving compounds, including vitamin C, potassium, phosphorus, selenium, and a number of amino acids. But one of the most important health-giving compounds found in garlic is *allicin*, a phytochemical compound formed when garlic is cut or crushed.

Garlic is enjoyed daily throughout the Mediterranean, and is used as a flavor enhancer in pasta dishes, paellas, risottos, pilafs, pizza, stews, soups, salad dressings, and sauces. Garlic is an equally essential ingredient in Asian cooking. "The pungent flavor of garlic is part of the fabric of Chinese cuisine," points out renowned Chinese American cook and author Ken Hom. "It would be inconceivable to cook without its distinctive, highly aromatic smell and unique taste."

Tomatoes

Tomatoes are a staple ingredient in Mediterranean cooking (they were brought back from the New World by Spanish explorers more than five hundred years ago), and are also popular in Indian and Southeast Asian cooking.

The unique flavor and texture of tomatoes complement a multitude of dishes, including hearty stews, robust pasta dishes, spicy curries, and mouthwatering soups (such as Italian minestrone and Spanish gazpacho). Many types of salad also rely on the juiciness, flavor, and color of tomatoes, including Greek salad, and Salade Niçoise. And, of course, pizza wouldn't be quite the same without a layer of luscious tomato sauce.

But tomatoes aren't renowned only for their taste and versatility; research in recent years has found that tomatoes also act as a potent medicine. And the characteristic deep red color of tomatoes is one of the reasons they're so healthy. It turns out that the pigment that gives tomatoes their color—called *lycopene*—has powerful antioxidant properties, and also protects against cancer. Research has shown that lycopene is particularly effective at reducing prostate cancer risk. In a large-scale study by Harvard researchers involving more than 48,000 men, it was found that those who ate ten or more servings of lycopene-rich tomato products a week had one-third the risk of developing prostate cancer than those eating two servings or fewer. A review of more than seventy studies published in the *Journal of the National Cancer Institute* also found strong evidence that lycopene is protective against prostate cancer, as well as lung and stomach cancers.

And lycopene doesn't only offer protection against cancer. A study involving 1,300 European men found that those consuming the most lycopene from foods had about half the risk of heart attack as men who consumed the least.

Along with lycopene, tomatoes are also rich in vitamin C and beta-carotene (both powerful antioxidants), and are a good source of health-promoting dietary fiber and potassium. To top it off, tomatoes are also very low in calories.

Berries

Berries are sweet and satisfying superfoods. Strawberries, cranberries, raspberries, and blackberries are all packed with powerful antioxidants and phytochemicals that can ward off disease and premature aging. Berries also supply your body with a host of other essential nutrients, including potassium, vitamin C, iron, B vitamins such as niacin (which releases energy from food and protects against heart disease), and folate.

Raspberries and strawberries are one of the richest food sources of a phytochemical compound called *ellagic acid*, which studies have shown to be a powerful cancer blocker. Cranberries and blueberries contain antibiotic-like compounds that help prevent bladder and urinary tract infection. And all berries contain high amounts of *pectin*, a soluble fiber that has been shown to be effective at lowering blood cholesterol levels by binding with LDL cholesterol and eliminating it from the body. There are plenty of ways to enjoy berries: sprinkled over cereals, added to fruit salads, whipped up in a smoothie, served with a small scoop of your favorite ice cream, or simply eaten by themselves as a sweet and juicy snack.

Avocados

Avocados are one of the few fruits that are high in fat. But unlike saturated fat, which can raise potentially harmful LDL cholesterol levels in your body, the fat in avocados is mostly made up of heart-healthy monounsaturated fat. Avocados also contain high amounts of special phytochemical compounds called *phytosterols*. Studies have shown that phytosterols can inhibit cholesterol absorption from the intestine, which results in lower levels of LDL cholesterol in the blood. In animal studies, phytosterols have also been shown to inhibit the growth of cancerous tumors.

In addition, avocados are a rich source of vitamin E, a powerful antioxidant that protects your cells from free radical damage. They also contain high amounts of folate, which has been shown to protect against heart disease as well as prevent birth defects. And they are one of the richest sources of the mineral potassium, which helps to maintain the stability of heart cells and the central nervous system.

But although avocados are very healthy, it's important to remember that they're also very high in calories (one medium-size avocado contains around 500 calories), so it makes sense not to go overboard when you eat them. Luckily, because they're so rich and creamy, a little avocado goes a long way. Use them diced into salads and sandwiches, blend them up with some lemon juice and salt for an instant guacamole dip, or try them Japanese-style in sushi rolls with smoked salmon or shrimp. A particularly good way to enjoy avocados is as a healthy alternative to butter. Simply mash some avocado in a cup or bowl and smear it onto your sandwich before you add the fillings.

continues on next page

Cruciferous Vegetables

I was put off the cruciferous family very early in life when my mother introduced me to Brussels sprouts. They were usually served overcooked and soggy and were always the last thing on my plate to get eaten. Thankfully I'm now on good terms with the cruciferous family because I've discovered that when they're cooked the right way (the MediterrAsian way, of course) they can taste absolutely delicious! Here are some choices from this vegetable group:

Bok choy	Cauliflower	Mustard greens
Broccoli	Chinese cabbage	Rutabaga
Brussels sprouts	Choy sum	Swiss chard
Cabbage	Gai lan	

Yet again the home cooks of the Mediterranean and Asia have come up with a delightful array of ways to use these vegetables to add flavor, depth, and texture to a wide range of wonderful dishes from soups, salads, and stir-fries to curries, stews, and pasta dishes.

And the cruciferous family isn't only a tasty addition to a myriad of dishes. These vegetables also happen to be one of the most powerful disease-fighting plant foods known to science.

About twenty years ago studies first indicated that a high consumption of cruciferous vegetables equaled a reduced risk of certain cancers. Then in the early 1990s a phytochemical called *sulforaphane* was identified in cruciferous vegetables that was found to guard against cancer by stimulating the production of protective enzymes that detoxify carcinogens (cancer-causing compounds). In addition, another compound was discovered called *indol-3-carbinol*, which was found to reduce breast cancer risk by preventing estrogen overproduction. A Harvard study even found that a high intake of cruciferous vegetables, such as broccoli and cabbage, could reduce bladder cancer risk in men.

Cruciferous vegetables are also a rich source of many other potent disease-fighting substances, including potassium, calcium, and dietary fiber. And broccoli and cabbage are a good source of immune-system-boosting, antioxidant-rich vitamin C. For example, one medium stalk of broccoli provides 200 percent of the daily recommended intake of vitamin C.

Carrots

Remember being told that carrots helped you see better in the dark? Well, they do. Carrots are rich in *beta-carotene*, which is converted by the body into vitamin A, a nutrient essential for the functioning of the retina of your eye.

Beta-carotene, which is a powerful antioxidant, has also been shown to improve immune function, inhibit the early stages of tumor development, and lower cholesterol levels. In one study, participants who ate seven carrots a day for three weeks dropped their cholesterol levels by 11 percent.

Carrots are also one of the best vegetable sources of health-giving dietary fiber, containing high amounts of both soluble and insoluble fiber.

Carrots make a colorful and crunchy addition to stir-fries and stews, and they taste wonderful finely chopped in pasta dishes, shredded on sandwiches, added to salads, or simply eaten raw as a snack.

Citrus Fruits

The citrus family includes oranges and lemons, which have been widely cultivated in the Mediterranean region since ancient Roman times; limes, which are native to India; and mandarins, which have been grown in China and Japan for thousands of years. Other citrus fruit include grapefruit, tangerines, and tangelos.

All citrus fruits are a good source of *flavonoids*—a special group of phytochemicals, which have been found to inhibit the growth of breast, prostate, and skin cancer cells. In addition oranges and tangelos are a rich source of a phytochemical called *5-desmethyl sinensetin*, which has been shown to effectively inhibit human lung cancer cells.

Citrus fruits, as we've always been told, are also a good source of vitamin C (one orange, for example, contains two times your daily requirement of vitamin C). Vitamin C not only works as a powerful free-radical-destroying antioxidant, but also makes blood less likely to clot, which reduces the risk of heart attack and stroke.

Citrus fruits can be enjoyed in dozens of different ways. Oranges, tangelos, and tangerines can be eaten by themselves or chopped and mixed in with other fruits to make a variety of fruit salads. Citrus fruits also go well as a sweet addition to savory salads. Lemon or lime juice and zest can be used as a flavor enhancer in a myriad of dishes such as curries, pasta dishes, and soups, and lemon juice or lime juice adds a delightful tang to salad dressings. Fresh lemon juice squeezed over fish and shellfish is also the perfect accompaniment.

Onions

Onions are related to garlic, and like garlic, onions are a staple in traditional Mediterranean and Asian cooking. Onions also share many of garlic's health-giving properties. They have been shown to boost good HDL cholesterol levels while lowering potentially harmful LDL cholesterol. They increase blood-clot-dissolving activity in the blood, which reduces the risk of heart attack and stroke. And studies have identified a phytochemical in onions called *quercetin*, which is a powerful antioxidant and cancer-preventing agent.

Sautéed chopped onions are used as the base for a wide variety of Mediterranean and Asian meals including risottos, curries, pasta dishes, pilafs, and paellas. Thinly sliced raw onion also adds a wonderful boost to salads, sandwiches, and burgers (red onions are particularly good because they're milder, sweeter, and more colorful than regular onions). And when whole onions are roasted they lose their potency and become sweet, delicate vegetables.

continues on next page

Bell Peppers

Bell peppers come in many colors—green, red, yellow, and even orange. Their color depends on the variety and their stage of ripeness.

Red peppers are particularly healthy because they are a rich source of the powerful antioxidants vitamin C and beta-carotene (red peppers contain around ten times more beta-carotene than green peppers). One 3½ ounce red pepper contains the recommended daily allowance of beta-carotene and more than 300 percent of the recommended daily allowance for vitamin C. And red peppers, like tomatoes, contain cancer-fighting lycopene.

Bell peppers can be enjoyed in many different of ways, such as cut into thin strips and lightly cooked in stir-fries, or cooked until melt-in-the-mouth tender in stews and pasta sauces. Roasted and marinated peppers also go wonderfully in an Italian antipasto platter or a Middle Eastern meze platter. And thinly sliced raw peppers make a crunchy and colorful addition to salads and sandwiches.

How to Easily Consume These Superfoods Regularly

When you eat the MediterrAsian way you'll find that most of your meals will contain at least one of the nine vegetables or fruits listed above, and often more. A stir-fry or pasta dish, for example, could easily contain garlic, onion, bell pepper, broccoli, and carrots. If you finish with a fresh fruit salad that includes berries and oranges, you've eaten seven different types in one sitting!

A Health Jackpot

There are so many reasons why legumes are such a health-giving food. First, they are a valuable source of both carbohydrates and protein. Carbohydrates are your muscles' and brain's favorite fuel source, and protein is used by your body for growth and repair, so both of these nutrients are vital for good health. Legumes also contain high amounts of soluble fiber, which helps slow the rate at which glucose (blood sugar) enters your bloodstream—so you'll have more energy and better concentration for longer periods of time. The soluble fiber in legumes has also been shown to help lower blood cholesterol levels.

In addition to carbohydrates, protein, and fiber, beans and other legumes are also a good source of zinc, phosphorus, magnesium, and potassium. These minerals are important for maintaining healthy muscle tone, combating fatigue, and promoting energy and endurance. Legumes are also a good source of iron (which helps deliver oxygen to all your cells) and B vitamins (which are important for a number of bodily functions, including maintaining healthy nerve cells and strengthening your immune system).

Meat for Vegetarians

Legumes have often been called "meat for vegetarians," and for a very good reason. Beans, peas, and lentils contain more protein than any other plant food and they're also a good source of many vitamins and minerals that are commonly found in red meat, such as iron and B vitamins.

But that's where the similarities end, because as far as health is concerned, beans are a far wiser choice than red meat. For instance, unlike red meat, beans contain hardly any saturated fat. The fat they do contain is made up mostly of heart-healthy unsaturated fat. Another big difference is that legumes contain lots of cholesterol-lowering soluble fiber, whereas meat contains no fiber at all. At the same time, legumes are a good source of anticancer and heart-protecting phytochemicals, which, again, red meat contains none of.

If there is one drawback to replacing a red meat-based meal with a legume-based meal it is the question of protein. While the quality of protein in legumes is high, with the exception of soybeans, the quality isn't quite as high as the protein found in fish, shellfish, poultry, and meat. This is because legumes don't contain all the essential amino acids (the building blocks of protein) needed for growth and repair. Luckily this problem is easily overcome, because the amino acids missing from legumes are found in grain foods; and coincidentally, the amino acids missing from grain foods are found in legumes. So by mixing beans and grains together in one meal, you end up with a complete protein that is of the same quality as that found in fish, soybeans, and meat. Here are some good examples of legume and grain combinations that form a complete protein:

- Dahl (lentil curry) with rice or naan bread
- Beans with pasta
- Lentil or bean burger
- Bean risotto
- Tortilla bread with beans
- Bean salad and crusty bread
- Chickpea stew served over couscous
- Bean dip and baked corn chips
- Falafel kebab (gyro)
- Beans with rice
- Lentil or bean soup served with bread
- Hummus and pita bread

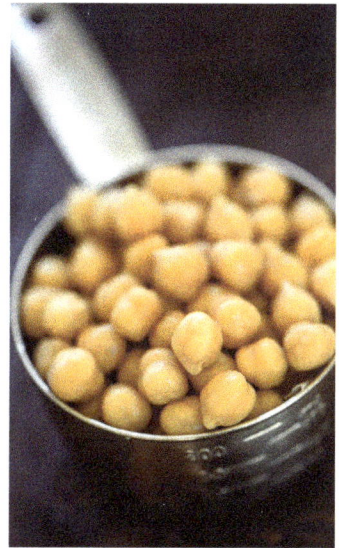

The Fat-Fighting Powers of Legumes

One of the most visible benefits associated with adding more legumes to your diet is weight maintenance. Legumes are ideal for maintaining a healthy body weight for a number of reasons. First, they are only moderate in calories, which means you have to eat a great deal of them before they can do any damage. And it's very hard to eat too many legumes for the simple fact that they're bulky and high in fiber, which is nature's best appetite suppressant. Legumes are also effective for shedding those extra pounds because they contain natural carbohydrates, which give your body lots of energy to be more active—activity in turn burns body fat.

THE HEALTH-GIVING BENEFITS OF SOY

Although all legumes have health-giving properties, one legume stands out as being the healthiest of all—the soybean.

Soybeans have played an integral part in Asian culture, both as a food and as a medicine, for many centuries. In fact, according to ancient Japanese mythology soybeans are a gift from the gods. And if recent scientific research is anything to go by, the humble soybean certainly lives up to this accolade.

Soy and Heart Disease

Can soybeans reduce your risk of heart disease? If soy protein is substituted for meat protein the answer is yes, according to a report published in the *New England Journal of Medicine*. In the report, researchers at the University of Kentucky, Lexington, reviewed thirty-eight separate clinical studies on soy and found that people who substituted soy protein for about half of the meat protein in their diet reduced their LDL cholesterol by 12.9 percent and triglycerides by 10.5 percent. According to the lead author of the report, Dr. James Anderson, the results suggest that a diet that regularly includes soy has the potential to reduce heart disease risk 25 to 30 percent.

Soy and Cancer

Rates of breast and prostate cancer are low in Asia, where soy is eaten regularly. Scientists believe they have now identified one of the main reasons why soy could offer protection. Soybeans contain special phytochemical compounds called *isoflavones*. Research has shown that these compounds can work as powerful cancer blockers.

For example, the isoflavones in soy have been shown to block the growth of new capillaries that supply tumors with blood. Without an adequate blood supply, a tumor can't grow. Isoflavones have also been shown to directly inhibit the growth of different types of cancer cells in test tube experiments.

And direct studies on soy consumption have shown just how powerful a cancer blocker it is. One study by researchers at Loma Linda University in California found that men who consumed soy milk at least once a day had a 70 percent lower risk of developing prostate cancer than those men who didn't. Another study by Dr. Wei Zheng of Vanderbilt University in Tennessee found that women in China who consumed the most soy had the lowest risk of breast cancer.

Soy and Women's Health

Legumes in general have many health benefits for women, but studies have shown that soybeans in particular offer the most benefits. Part of the reason could be that soybeans contain high amounts of natural phytochemical compounds called *phytoestrogens*. These compounds are similar to the human hormone estrogen, except they are much weaker. As weak estrogens, these compounds act as a substitute form of estrogen in the body, and actually compete with the more potent estrogens made by a woman's body. As a result, phytoestrogens can help to regulate estrogen levels. This is of great importance to women because high estrogen levels have been associated with a range of problems, including increased risk of breast cancer, fibroid tumors of the uterus, and PMS.

The phytoestrogens found in soybeans are helpful not only when estrogen levels are high, they're also helpful when estrogen levels are low—such as during menopause—because they can provide much needed hormonal support for the body. This is why many of the symptoms of menopause that are taken for granted in the West, like hot flashes and night sweats, are rarely seen in countries where soy is a staple food. In Japan, for example, where soy products are consumed regularly, there isn't even a term for "hot flashes."

In addition, studies have shown that soybeans can slow down the loss of bone mass, which causes the bone-weakening disease osteoporosis.

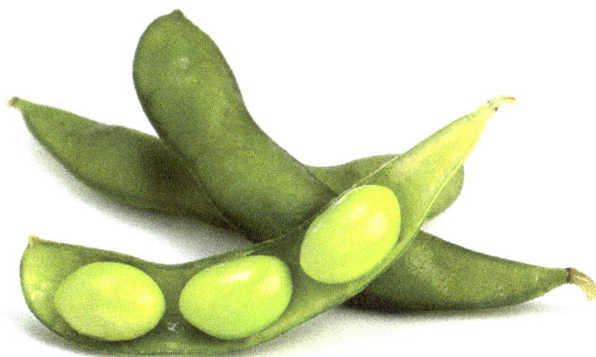

The Many Ways to Enjoy Soy

Are you wondering how you can fit this remarkable protein-rich bean into your diet? Here are some tasty and nutritious ways that you can enjoy soy:

Tofu (bean curd). Tofu is incredibly versatile because it has little taste of its own (but a delightful texture), which means that when you mix it with grains, vegetables, and seasonings, it soaks up their flavor. It comes in two main varieties: soft (silken) and firm. Firm tofu can be diced and sautéed in stir-fry dishes, and can replace meat or poultry in casseroles, soups, and stews. Soft tofu can be cut into cubes and added to asian-style soups. It also adds creaminess to smoothies, soups, sauces, dips, salad dressings, and desserts.

Baked pressed tofu. This form of seasoned, extra-firm tofu comes in several marinade-type flavors and is ready to use straight off the supermarket shelf. Slice it and use it to replace meat as a tasty sandwich filling; serve it over noodles or rice, in salads, or with stir-fried vegetables.

Dried soybeans. These can be used to replace any other variety of beans in dishes such as bean salad, homemade baked beans, or chili. The only drawback is that they take two to three hours to cook. Luckily you can now buy canned precooked soybeans, which you can heat and eat in only minutes.

Fresh soybeans. Called *edamame* in Japanese, fresh soy is harvested while green and sold as "sweet beans" in Asian grocery stores in the summer months. Steamed or boiled in salted water, these make a great appetizer or snack, or they can be added to stir-fries and salads.

Tempeh. This traditional Indonesian food is made from cooked and coagulated soybeans and is slightly higher in protein than tofu. It has a distinct flavor and a dense, chewy texture. Try it crumbled and used as a ground meat substitute; diced and sautéed, it can be tossed into rice, noodle, or vegetable dishes; and it can also be sliced and sautéed like cutlets and served with barbecue sauce.

Miso. Miso is a paste made from fermented soybeans, salt, and grains. It's delicious used as an all-purpose stock to flavor Asian dishes, casseroles, and soups. The only drawback is the high salt content, but this is offset somewhat by the fact that it is high in flavor, so you only need small amounts.

Soy milk. Soy milk has come a long way since its early bland-tasting days and is now more than satisfactory as a replacement for regular milk. Pour it over cereal, stir into hot drinks, or use in shakes, soups, or baking.

NUTS AND SEEDS

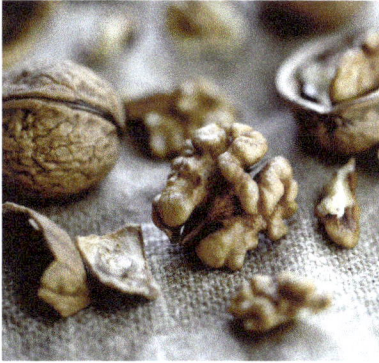

Because of the high fat content of nuts, people in the West were often told to avoid them in order to reduce blood cholesterol levels and prevent heart disease. But, as Dr. Frank Hu, a nutritional epidemiologist at Harvard School of Public Health points out, "In reality, nuts reduce your blood cholesterol and protect against heart disease because most of the fats in nuts are healthy fats—unsaturated fats, monounsaturated fats, polyunsaturated fats."

In fact, a study by Loma Linda University scientists on 34,000 people over six years found that those who consumed a handful of nuts four or more times a week had 50 percent fewer heart attacks than people who ate nuts less than once a week. A fourteen-year study at Harvard University involving more than 80,000 women showed similar results.

Nuts and seeds aren't only a rich source of good fats, they also contain many other health-enhancing substances. For example, they're a good source of protein, fiber, vitamin E (a powerful antioxidant), magnesium, and zinc. Nuts also contain high amounts of an essential amino acid called arginine. This special protein has been shown to help relax blood vessels and make blood less sticky, which, in turn, reduces the risk of heart attack and stroke. And certain nuts and seeds—particularly walnuts, pecans, and linseeds (flaxseeds)—are a good source of omega-3 fatty acids.

TYPES OF NUTS & SEEDS

- Almonds
- Brazil nuts
- Cashews
- Chestnuts
- Flaxseeds (Linseeds)
- Macadamia nuts

- Peanuts (actually a legume, not a nut, but has the same nutritional profile as nuts and used in the same way)
- Pecans
- Pine nuts
- Pistachios
- Sesame seeds
- Sunflower seeds
- Walnuts

The Perfect Snack Food

Nuts and seeds are high in fat; but most of the fat in nuts and seeds is made up of heart-healthy unsaturated fats. But it's also important to remember that nuts are still high in calories. An ounce, which is about a handful, provides between 165 to 200 calories (depending on the type of nut). So the idea isn't simply to add nuts to your diet, but to substitute them for other foods—especially less wholesome foods.

This works particularly effectively when you replace junk food with nuts, because calorie for calorie there is simply no comparison between the two. Snack foods are generally calorie-rich but nutrient poor. Nuts, on the other hand, are calorie rich, but also nutrient rich. The fiber, protein, essential fats, and other nutrients in nuts sustain and nourish your body, and satisfy your hunger for far longer than an equal number of calories from "empty calorie" snack foods.

A Tasty Addition to Meals

As well as being a great snack food, nuts and seeds also make a delicious and healthy addition to meals. You can even use them to replace animal protein in a dish. Here are a few ways you can incorporate nuts and seeds into your meals:

- Adding a handful of cashews or slivered almonds to an Asian-style stir-fry, braise, or noodle dish makes a wonderful crunchy addition.
- Nuts go well with many pasta and risotto dishes. Pesto, for example, is a delicious sauce that originates from Genoa in Italy. It's made up of a mix of fresh basil, nuts (usually pine nuts), Parmesan cheese, garlic, and extra virgin olive oil. It makes an incredibly delicious creamy sauce that can be tossed through pasta or spread on bread or toasts. Walnuts also make a rustic addition to pasta.
- Toasted sesame seeds sprinkled over a stir-fry add a wonderful flavor and texture.
- Crushed peanuts make a tasty and crunchy garnish for Thai, Indonesian, and Vietnamese dishes, and peanuts are one of the main ingredients in Indonesian satay sauce.
- Nuts add a flavor and texture boost to salads.
- Crushed nuts go perfectly sprinkled over cereal, oatmeal, yogurt, or fruit salad.
- Whole and crushed nuts and seeds can be added to your own homemade muesli.
- A handful of crushed almonds or pistachios is wonderful sprinkled over a Middle Eastern pilaf.

CHAPTER 6

Drink & be merry

For thousands of years alcohol has been enjoyed in Mediterranean and Asian cultures. The inclusion of moderate alcohol consumption in the Mediterranean and Asian pyramids reflects this fact. Researchers now believe that drinking alcohol in moderation isn't only an enjoyable social experience but it can also benefit your body, particularly your heart and arteries.

LIQUID ASSETS

Does a drink a day keep heart attacks away? Yes, according to no fewer than sixty scientific studies that have shown alcohol to be protective against heart disease. Indeed, as far back as 1981 researchers from Johns Hopkins University School of Medicine cited over a dozen studies in their article "The Beneficial Side of Moderate Alcohol Use" in describing alcohol's heart-protective benefits. "A number of well designed and executed case-control studies," wrote Thomas Turner, MD, and colleagues in the *Johns Hopkins Medical Journal*, "indicate that the risk of coronary heart disease, especially myocardial infarction (heart attack), is lower in persons who use alcohol moderately than in abstainers."

In a scientific review published recently in the *British Medical Journal*, Harvard researchers looked at forty-two studies and concluded that regularly consuming alcohol in moderation equaled a 24.7 percent reduction in heart-disease risk.

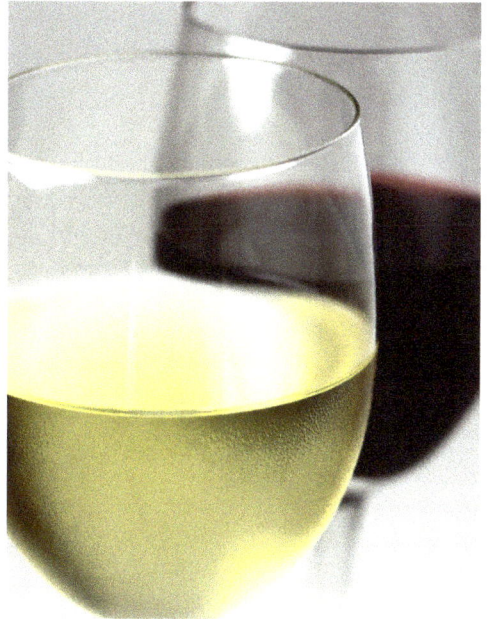

WHICH ALCOHOLIC BEVERAGE IS THE MOST HEART PROTECTIVE?

Research has found that *any* alcoholic drink (beer, wine, or spirits), when consumed in moderation, can raise your "good" HDL cholesterol levels, thus helping inhibit the onset of heart disease. However, red wine has been found to contain other health-giving compounds that make it especially good for your health.

Unlike other alcoholic drinks, red wine is a rich source of a special group of phytochemicals called *phenolic compounds*, which are found in grape juice and particularly grape skin. These compounds, which give grapes their color, have been shown to reduce the artery-clogging properties of LDL cholesterol, as well as to reduce the formation of blood clots and inhibit cancer tumor growth. And phenolic compounds have a duel role because they also work as powerful antioxidants—mopping up potentially dangerous free radicals that can destroy healthy cells, speed up the aging process, and increase your risk of heart disease and cancer.

This is why, out of all alcoholic beverages, red wine has been found to be the most protective. In one study, for example, Danish researchers followed more than 13,000 people over ten years and found that teetotalers had twice the risk of dying from heart disease as people who drank a moderate amount of red wine every day.

The Great Stress Reliever

The warm, relaxing feeling after a glass of wine or beer goes a long way toward relieving the tensions of the day.

Dr. David Benton, a psychologist at the University of Wales, has been studying the impact of food and drink on behavior for over fifteen years and says that, in moderation, alcohol acts as a mild sedative. "In the short term, alcohol is a relaxant," he says. "It may even improve performance that has been disrupted by stress."

When combined with good food and conversation at the dinner table, the stress-relieving benefits of alcohol become even more pronounced. Unfortunately, the stress-relieving benefits of alcohol soon diminish when it's consumed in excess, and alcohol can end up working as a depressant. So take it easy and drink only in moderation—you'll get the best stress-relieving benefits that way.

CONSUMING ALCOHOL WITH YOUR MEAL IS BEST

In the West, alcohol is often consumed before a meal or on its own. Throughout the Mediterranean and Asia, on the other hand, alcohol has traditionally been consumed at meal times. Recent research has shown that this interaction between food and alcohol could also help to explain some of the benefits associated with moderate alcohol consumption.

Dr. Maurizio Trevisan from the University of Buffalo has reported—based on results from the Risk Factor and Life Expectancy (RIFLE) Study of more than 70,000 men and women in Italy—that benefits with respect to heart disease and overall mortality were more pronounced when wine was consumed with meals. His research helps support the results of a 1994 study by health researchers with the Japanese government that reported that wine with meals prevents the modification of LDL cholesterol to a form that can increase heart disease risk.

The consumption of alcohol at meal times also limits its abuse, according to Italian researcher Amedeo Cottino. "This is precisely what is meant by the very common Italian saying, 'Never drink wine between meals.' This ensures that alcoholic beverages never fill an empty stomach, and it also controls the amount of drinking by relating it to eating times."

HOW MUCH IS TOO MUCH?

Although alcohol certainly has its advantages, experts point out that there's only a small window of opportunity for deriving positive effects; this means that *moderation* is the key word. Studies have shown that around two drinks a day for men and one drink a day for women are the maximum limit (one drink equals 12 ounces of beer, 4 ounces of wine, 1.5 ounces of 80-proof spirits, or 1 ounce of 100-proof spirits). More than that and the advantages of alcohol start turning into disadvantages such as these:

- **Liver disease.** If alcohol is consumed regularly in large amounts it can lead to a number of serious liver complaints such as cirrhosis of the liver, alcoholic hepatitis, and liver cancer.
- **Mouth and throat cancer.** High levels of alcohol consumption increase the risk of cancers of the mouth, throat, and tongue.
- **Heart disease.** Heavy drinkers are more susceptible to coronary heart disease and high blood pressure, and they are more likely to suffer a stroke.
- **Depression.** A high level of alcohol intake can result in depression, memory loss, and mental deterioration.
- **Digestive disorders.** Heavy drinkers may suffer from digestive tract diseases including gastritis, pancreatitis, and cancer of the upper digestive tract.

Another thing to remember is that alcohol is fairly high in calories, which means that if you consume too much alcohol you could easily gain weight.

Of course it's important to note that these down sides only come about when you consume *too much* alcohol. If you follow the example of people from Mediterranean and Asian cultures and consume no more than one to two drinks a day, preferably with meals, then you only have to look forward to the benefits.

But, with that said, one of these days you'll no doubt find yourself in a situation where it's going to be difficult to have only a couple of drinks—for example at holiday celebrations or at a party. So what's the best solution? Well, you basically have two options:

- Find creative ways to consume less alcohol (more about this shortly) *or*
- Drink whatever is served and resume your healthy moderate drinking habits immediately thereafter.

From a health point of view, you can choose option two without fear of ruining your well-being, as long as you limit this kind of activity to once in a blue moon. If you feel like taking option one by finding creative ways to consume less alcohol, here are some effective tips that you might find useful:

- Add some fresh fruit juice to champagne for a delicious champagne cocktail.
- Turn a glass of white wine into a spritzer by adding some soda water.
- Turn a glass of beer into a sweet refreshing shandy by adding some lemonade.
- Sip a nonalcoholic drink like a soft drink, cordial, soda, or mineral water (or just plain water) in between alcoholic drinks.

Remember that the first few drinks are usually used to quench your thirst. By quenching that thirst with a nonalcoholic drink first, you'll probably find you'll end up drinking less alcohol.

In short, consuming moderate amounts of alcohol (particularly red wine) is a simple and effective way to improve your health and relieve stress. The fact that it's also a highly pleasurable experience makes it all the more worthwhile. The cardinal rule is not to drink too much (no more than two drinks daily for men, and one drink daily for women), and to make sure that you usually drink with your meal. If you follow these simple guidelines, you can feel confident in raising your glass and toasting to your health!

CHAPTER 7

Stop exercising, start living!

These days it almost seems as if there's a conspiracy to stop us moving. Most of us now have sedentary jobs that involve very little movement. Devices such as washing machines, vacuum cleaners, and dishwashers have reduced how much physical labor is required of us. Our leisure time revolves around passive activities such as watching TV, playing video games, or surfing the Internet. To top it off, our main form of transportation is now our car instead of our legs.

As a society we've virtually stopped moving. And when you don't move much, you dramatically reduce the number of calories your body burns. This, in turn, leads to weight gain. At the same time, lack of movement leads to a loss of muscle tissue. Muscles are active tissues that increase your fat-burning metabolism. In simple terms this means the less muscle you have, the easier it is to get fat.

To make matters worse, by not moving much, your heart and other vital organs are not working as they should. This can increase the risk of heart disease, Type 2 diabetes, high blood pressure, osteoporosis, and dozens of other potentially debilitating conditions. That's why movement is so important—every bit as important as eating the right foods.

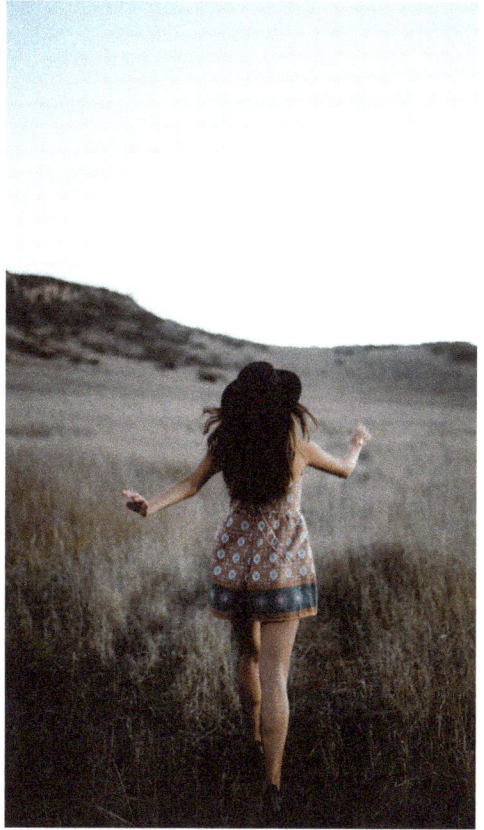

The great news is that by moving your body only a little each day, it won't degenerate. You'll keep all your fat-fighting muscle tissue, your health and fitness will improve measurably, and you'll look and feel great. But when I say moving, I don't mean exercising. The fact is, the best way to bring movement into your life is to stop exercising and start living!

INCORPORATING PHYSICAL ACTIVITY INTO YOUR LIFE

The Mediterranean and Asian pyramids both include a reference to the importance of regular physical activity for maintaining good health. But the way Mediterranean and Asian peoples have gotten their physical activity for the past few thousand years hasn't been through exercising. When Professor Ancel Keys studied Greeks, Japanese, and Italians in the 1950s and '60s, he noted that most of them kept physically active by walking to see friends, gathering crops, pumping water, and carrying out other general day-to-day tasks. In fact, this is how humans have always kept physically active. We've never formally set aside time to exercise—not ever before in history. We just went about our day and, lo and behold, we stayed fit and in shape. These days, because modern technology has forced us into laziness, we think the only way to compensate is to set aside special time, put on special clothes, and formally "exercise."

What sorts of thoughts usually go through someone's mind when they're exercising? Most people aren't thinking, "Oh great, this is fun!" It's more likely to be "How much longer to go?" or "C'mon, I've got to keep this up for my own good." Ultimately, most of us are exercising not because we want to, but because we think we have to.

But the simple fact is that we would all still be living in caves if our nature didn't dictate our need for diversity. Our senses crave stimulation to stay alert and engaged. For most of us, working out on the same exercise machine, jogging past the same sights, or just sticking to the same old exercise routine—no matter what it is—will eventually lead to boredom. And once boredom rears its head, it's only a matter of time before we give up altogether. Who can blame us!

NATURAL MOVEMENT

The revolutionary news is you don't have to stick to a grueling structured exercise plan to get health benefits. The latest research reveals what history has always shown us: You can attain a good level of fitness simply by being more physically active in your everyday life.

The idea is to take the focus off formal "exercise" and put the emphasis on *natural movement*. By natural movement I simply mean moving as part of your everyday life—just like Mediterranean and Asian peoples have traditionally done for thousands of years. Of course, you can't be expected to start gathering crops or pumping water, but it doesn't matter because there are lots of other ways you can slip movement unobtrusively into your hectic twenty-first-century lifestyle.

For example, instead of trying to find excuses not to exercise—like housework, shopping, and letters to write—why not make these tasks the regular exercise in your day? Think of everyday activities as an opportunity to kill two birds with one stone; in other words, to accomplish a task and at the same time collect some movement.

Don't think of it as "having to do the housework," but instead use the chance to do a ten-minute aerobic workout by turning housework into a cardio cleaning blitz. (You'll be amazed how vigorous vacuuming, dusting, and window cleaning can be!) Instead of circling to find a prime space, park at the far end of the lot and walk the rest of the way—adding another few minutes to your "activity bank." If you've got some shopping to do, use the opportunity to collect another five minutes and slip in a resistance workout by carrying your shopping bags to the car. And those letters you had to write—instead of mailing them by car on the way to use the treadmill at the gym, just walk to the mailbox instead (take the scenic route), and deposit another ten minutes into your activity bank so you can skip the gym altogether.

NO PAIN, ALL GAIN

Five minutes here, ten minutes there—without even thinking about it you've "exercised" for around half an hour today, just the right amount to the enjoy the benefits that a healthy level of fitness offers. Before you know it, depositing movement into your activity bank will become as natural as brushing your teeth. After a few short weeks you'll notice improvements in your body tone and energy levels; you'll look better, get fitter, and generally feel great.

Our days are filled with activities that provide us with the chance to bring extra movement into our lives. Walking the dog (both you and your dog benefit), using the stairs (forget the Stairmaster!), and pushing the stroller or carriage (choose the hilly way for extra intensity) are all ideal activities you can do that happen to get you moving at the same time. Even the most unlikely times and places can provide the perfect opportunity to slip in some form of activity. For example, the bedroom can be very conducive to working up a light sweat...I think you get the idea!

By using your imagination to slip activity unobtrusively into your busy life-style, you'll not only find you've exercised without even thinking about it, but you'll also have more time for yourself instead of spending it at the gym or fitness center.

Here are some other good examples of *natural movement*:

Clean your car by hand. Instead of taking your car through the gas station car wash, clean it at home by hand. Give it a good wash and polish with extra intensity. Washing your car by hand is also far gentler on your car's paintwork than taking it through a mechanical car wash.

Walk to your local store instead of driving. Walk to the local store for convenience items like milk and bread instead of taking the car or sending the kids. The physical benefits of brisk walking are many, including better endurance and an increase in your metabolic rate. Pop your small child in a shoulder carrier or push him or her in a stroller—the extra weight adds intensity and makes you work a little harder. Even subtle lifestyle changes like this are effective ways to add physical activity to your life and get you out into the fresh air and sunshine at the same time.

Park and walk. When you go to the mall, rather than circling the parking lot for the prime position closest to the entry, make a conscious decision to park as far away from the stores as possible and walk the extra distance instead. Although this may sound time-consuming, you'll probably find that you get inside the mall faster than if you circled around searching for a prime spot anyway.

Toil in the soil. Get out into the garden, get your hands dirty, and get your body moving. Mow the lawn, rake the leaves, weed the flower bed, dig holes, pot plants, and saw off overhanging tree limbs. All of these cardio-intensive activities contribute to the maintenance of your yard as well as of your body. Although it's become commonplace for the time-poor, cash-rich among us to have a gardening service perform these tasks, why not experience the pride and satisfaction of doing them yourself? What's more, it's free and it can be fun!

Clean out your attic, basement, or garage. Spring-cleaning is a great way to get rid of all those boxes of unwanted stuff, as well as to help shed unwanted pounds. You'll be amazed at how active you'll get, and astonished at how much junk you can clear in the process.

Walk to your local park for lunch. Instead of being stuck at home, at a desk, or in the office cafeteria, head to your local park or gardens instead. The fresh air is good for your lungs and the sunshine beats artificial lighting any day (vitamin D, which is essential for bone growth and maintenance, is also produced by the body when you're exposed to sunlight). A brisk walk and a change of scenery will do wonders for your physical and mental well-being. Even big cities have patches of green to use as a quiet respite from the hectic pace of modern life. Take off your shoes, loosen your tie, and close your eyes. Even after just a short time away, you'll return home or to work renewed and ready for the afternoon ahead.

Get to work on two wheels. Avoid traffic jams and cycle to and from work. Wear a helmet and have front and rear lights fitted to your bike if you plan to cycle at night. A word of caution: Long skirts and trouser cuffs tend to get caught in the bike chain, so wear more suitable clothing and change into your work clothes when you arrive—you'll be much fresher that way too!

Catch public transportation to work. Instead of driving to work, take the bus or train instead, which means walking to and from the bus stop or train station on both ends. Walking gives you a chance to plan the day ahead and arrive at work refreshed and alert. Likewise, a brisk walk after work gives you time to wind down and get some fresh air before arriving home. As well as the extra movement you're slipping into your life, you'll also save time and money (no more gasoline, parking fees, and traffic jams).

Shop and carry. One of the best ways to justify a shopping spree as a bona fide workout is to make a point of carrying your shopping bags on foot to the car or while you're window shopping. Just think—the more you buy, the better the workout! Similarly, cruise the supermarket aisles carrying a shopping basket instead of pushing a shopping cart around. The extra weight acts as resistance to give you an upper-body workout.

Park a few blocks from work. By walking the rest of the way, this burst of physical activity will give you a chance to stretch your legs and boost your metabolism before getting to the office. Alternatively, choose a parking space as far away from your building as possible and then walk the rest of the way at a brisk pace. Even the famous multimillionaire media mogul, William Randolph Hearst, had his limousine driver drop him off a few blocks from his mansion so he could walk the rest of the way home. It just goes to show that you're never too rich or too old to slip in some physical activity.

Work out at the office. If your job is sedentary and involves sitting at a desk in front of a computer screen for most of the day, use your initiative to incorporate movement in various ways. For instance, if you need to go and see colleagues on the fourth floor, take the stairs. Use the restroom that's most

The Benefits of Regular Movement

Helps control weight. In addition to burning calories while you're moving, physical activity also boosts your *basal metabolic rate*—the rate at which your body burns calories while at rest. In other words, when you're physically active, you continue to burn extra calories even after you stop moving.

Reduces the risk of heart disease. Heart disease is the Western world's leading cause of death. Physical activity helps prevent it by strengthening the heart, reducing blood pressure, boosting "good" HDL cholesterol, and combating obesity. A study by researchers from the University of Washington in Seattle and the University of Michigan in Ann Arbor found that people who walk for exercise can reduce the risk of having a first heart attack by 73 percent and those who garden can reduce the risk by 66 percent compared with people who are not regularly physically active. "When performed for more than sixty minutes a week, walking for exercise or gardening was associated with a similar risk reduction to that of high-intensity leisure-time physical activity," reported Dr. Rozenn N. Lemaitre, who helped conduct the study.

Reduces high blood pressure and the risk of stroke. High blood pressure is a key risk factor for stroke, and regular physical activity has been shown to help reduce it.

Helps you live longer. Physical activity strengthens your heart and immune system, and helps reduce the risk of atherosclerosis (clogged arteries), thus giving you a more robust age-fighting body. As Professor Ancel Keys noted while conducting the Seven Countries Study: "During the field work of this study it was not uncommon to see men [in Greece] of 80 to 100 years of age and more going off to work in the fields with a hoe."

Builds strength, flexibility, and stamina. When you move regularly your muscles become stronger, your joints become suppler, and you can remain active longer without tiring.

Helps preserve bone. Regular weight-bearing movement (walking, gardening, dancing, and the like) helps prevent the bone-thinning disease osteoporosis, which is a major health problem for many older women and men in the Western world.

Helps the body deal with stress. Regular movement strengthens your body's circulatory and immune systems. This in turn helps your body to better deal with the damaging effects of stress.

Improves love life. James White, PhD, director of the Human Performance Laboratory at the University of California in San Diego, recruited ninety-five healthy but sedentary men, average age forty-seven, into one of two exercise programs four days a week. One group engaged in low-intensity sixty-minute walks. The other participated in an hour of aerobics. After nine months, both groups reported increased sexual desire and pleasure, and more orgasms.

Improves sleep. When you move regularly throughout the day it helps your body wind down at night so you can sleep more deeply. This is why many sleep disorder experts recommend regular movement to treat insomnia.

distant from your work area; if it's up several flights of stairs, great! Don't ask someone to bring you something, like a file or coffee; instead, go and get it yourself. Post the daily mail on foot rather than taking the company car. Walk to the local sandwich shop to get your lunch; if it's a block or two away, all the better. Instead of sending an interoffice memo or email, deliver it personally. These activities all add up to keep you more active and give you short, regular breaks in your work routine.

Walk and talk the kids to school. Rather than chauffeuring the kids to and from school, walk with them. Both you and the kids will benefit from the exercise and it will give you the chance to have a good chat with them. Stop off on the way home from school at the playground or park and spend time with each other having fun. If your children catch public transportation, walk with them to and from the bus stop or train station instead of waving good-bye from the front door.

Make the most of vacations. Instead of using your vacation as an excuse to do nothing but eat too much and do as little as possible, use it as an opportunity to have fun and get moving at the same time. For instance, take a cycling tour through the countryside, go on a guided walking tour, go hiking in national parks, or go kayaking or white-water rafting.

A LESSON IN NATURAL MOVEMENT

If you think it's going to be tough to add natural movement into your life because you're just "too busy," think again. Even people with the busiest lifestyles can still slip moderate physical activity into their everyday lives. A classic example is that of busy executive Geoffrey Cannon, Director of Science for the World Cancer Research Fund.

Cannon lives and works in busy central London, and he decided that it didn't make sense for him to own a car. He now mostly cycles to work, which takes around fifteen minutes each way. Sometimes, instead of cycling to work he walks twenty minutes to an underground station and at the other end he walks up the escalator (instead of just standing on it like a dead weight). He also doesn't use the elevator at work, and walks up and down the stairs to see his work colleagues. As well, he regularly carries bags of food on foot or on his bicycle, and he walks to most of his appointments in central London.

This example clearly demonstrates that no matter how busy or hectic your life may be, there are always plenty of ways to slip in some natural movement.

FUN FITNESS

Slipping physical activity into your day-to-day tasks is a very effective way of getting lots of natural movement, but it certainly isn't the only way. Another good way of getting lots of natural movement is what Trudy and I call *fun fitness*.

As I mentioned earlier, exercising may keep your body active, but it usually fails to keep your mind active; more often than not, this means you eventually get bored and quit.

But what if an activity you do is fun and enjoyable, something that keeps your body and your mind active—surely you wouldn't be in such a hurry to give it up? For example, I love playing Frisbee. When I go out to play Frisbee, the last thing on my mind is exercising; I'm just having fun, doing an activity I enjoy. But without thinking about it I'm giving myself a full-body, cardio-intensive workout. Golf is another activity I enjoy doing that also happens to exercise my body at the same time. You can probably think of dozens of activities you enjoy that also happen to get you moving at the same time. To start you thinking, here are some more examples of *fun fitness*:

> **Go for a scenic walk.** It's easy, free, and enjoyable. Let your mind roam freely and absorb the beauty of nature around you. For added enjoyment, buddy up with friends, family, and coworkers, or join a walking group. Depending on your level of fitness, you may want to walk fast for short distances or you may prefer to walk at a slightly slower pace for longer distances. Instead of walking the same way every time, explore different routes. Venture out into

the countryside and hike along nature trails or go orienteering. Other good places to walk around include the zoo, art galleries, museums, and gardens.

Have a ball. Whether you opt for a football, soccer ball, baseball, softball, or basketball, throwing or kicking a ball around in your backyard or at the local park is great fun and provides excellent cardiovascular conditioning and coordination.

Dive in. Get fit in the water by heading to the local swimming pool for some aquatic activity. Most pools conduct classes such as aqua aerobics if you prefer a routine. But you don't need to join these structured programs to get the benefits of water exercise. If you get bored swimming up and down lanes, take a ball in with you and throw it around, or have a friendly game of water volleyball. As an added bonus, since water partially supports your weight and provides resistance to work against, gentle water exercises are excellent for people who suffer from back pain or other muscle or joint problems (including arthritis).

Go for a leisurely ride. Cycling is a great form of exercise, it's easy to fit into a busy schedule, and it's suitable for people of most ages and fitness levels. Choose pleasant scenic routes and cycle ways that bypass heavily congested main roads or rush-hour traffic. For company, contact a local cycling club and join one of their regular riding tours. If you're the adventurous type, buy or rent a mountain bike, gear up with helmet and protective clothing, and head to the country.

Dance to the beat. Put on your favorite upbeat music and have a dance around the house. If you have a partner, get him or her involved, or ask the kids to join in. Energetic dancing is a great way to condition your entire body. It uses all the major muscle groups and speeds up your metabolism. Who cares if you look a bit silly—unlike in a crowded aerobics class, no one is there to see you! If you're feeling social, why not head to a night club or dance club and enjoy a sweaty bop on the dance floor?

Go skating. Rollerblading and ice-skating help to build strong ankle and leg muscles and to develop balance. You'll get aerobic benefits if you push yourself hard and skate vigorously, using your arms to speed up, rather than gliding along with minimal effort. If you choose to skate outdoors, stay away from traffic and wear protective clothing. If the weather's inclement, head to the rink and, if you get bored skating around in circles, get involved in the games that are usually run.

Play with the kids. Encourage the kids to take a break from computer games for the old-fashioned excitement of real-life games in the open air: hide-and-seek, hopscotch, ball games in the yard, leapfrog, and jumping rope. All of these activities will get you and the kids outdoors for some physical activity and give you a chance to do something fun together.

Go to the beach. But don't just lie there like a beached whale. There are so many ways to give your body a fun seaside workout: go swimming or splash in the ocean, ride the waves on a surfboard, body board, or use your own body, play beach volleyball, fly a kite, paddle a kayak, or go paddleboarding or windsurfing. Alternatively, enjoy more leisurely pursuits like building a sandcastle or walking along the beach.

Join a dance class. With so many dance styles available, you're sure to find one that appeals to you. Line, tap, belly, ballroom, rock 'n' roll, African, Latin American, jazz—all are great for improving general fitness, flexibility, and well-being. Dancing to music is also a great way of improving your coordination, concentration, balance, and rhythm, and is a wonderful social activity. Don't worry if it's your first time; remember that everyone's a beginner at some stage, and there are usually classes especially designed with beginners in mind.

Go skiing. Whether you choose to ski on the snow or in the water, skiing is an exhilarating activity that strengthens muscles and burns calories.

Try martial arts. Even if you're not interested in developing "fists of fury," martial arts can be a wonderful form of exercise for anyone to learn self-defense, gain confidence, and develop physical control. It's also a good outlet for stress. Check your local telephone directory or the Internet to find a class that suits you, or learn at home from a book or video.

Play racquet sports. Tennis, badminton, squash, and table tennis are all fun ways to have an aerobic workout, build muscular strength and endurance, and improve balance and coordination. Book a tennis, squash, or racquetball court at your local sports center or buy your own gear and play at home. Even throwing a tennis ball against a brick or wooden wall is challenging and can be performed solo. Badminton sets (complete with net, racquets, and shuttlecocks) are cheap and can be set up in the backyard. Table tennis tables are relatively inexpensive new but are downright cheap purchased secondhand, and can be folded up and wheeled away when not in use. Get family and friends involved in fun tournaments, or join local club fixtures if you're of a more competitive nature.

Fly a kite. Find a large open space (such as a park or beach) and return to your childhood by flying a kite. Not only does flying a kite involve plenty of physical activity, but it also improves your hand-eye coordination.

Get competitive. It's amazing what a bit of friendly competition can do to up your fitness without you even thinking about it. Competitive sports (where you're playing against someone else) is one of the easiest ways to have a high-intensity workout without pain—in fact, quite the opposite. You're focused on the match, you're having fun and enjoying yourself, yet at the same time you're getting fit and healthy. Competitive sports like basketball, softball, baseball, or football are also good for relieving stress and are great for making new friends and expanding your social life.

The benefits of incorporating more activity into your life are overwhelming: a leaner body, more energy, less disease, and a longer life. And fitting physical activity into your life, as you've discovered, is a pretty straightforward affair. As a bonus, you no longer have to put yourself through sweaty workouts or boring, structured exercise routines in order to get fit. The key now is simply to incorporate some form of physical activity into your life on a regular basis. The rewards will speak for themselves.

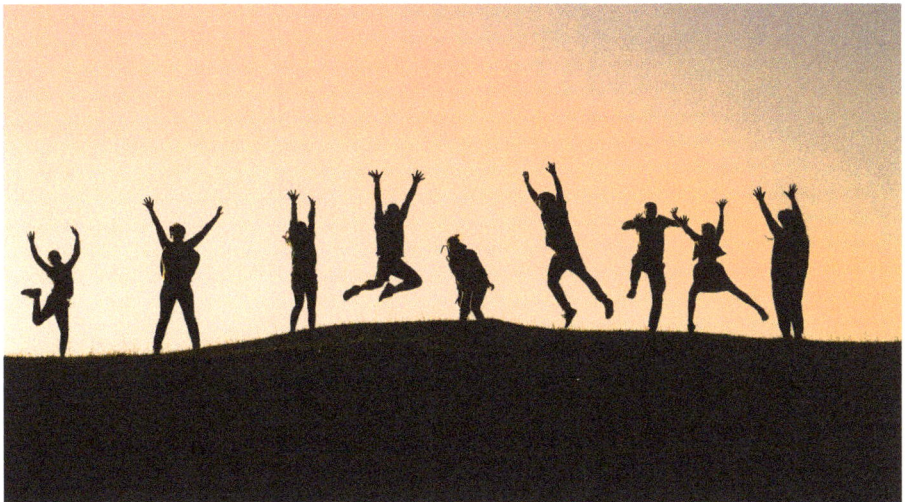

CHAPTER 8

A healthy mind in a healthy body

Achieving optimal health isn't just about looking good on the outside—it's also about feeling good on the inside. This has been known for thousands of years throughout Asia and the Mediterranean, and the ancient Romans even had a saying for it: *mens sana in corpore sana*, which literally means "a healthy mind in a healthy body."

But, although there are many effective ways that you can go about improving your physical health, exactly what steps can you take to directly improve your emotional health?

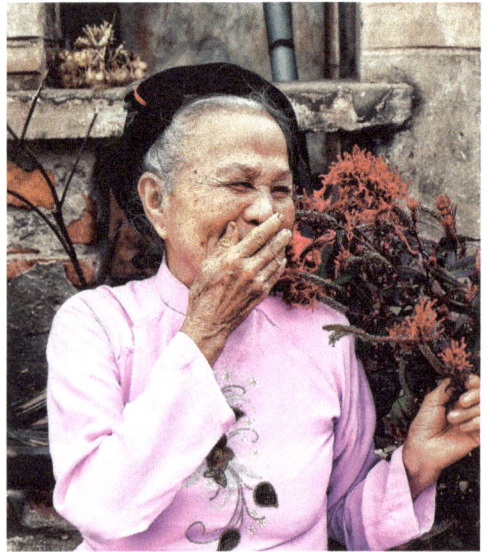

Learning from the traditional cultures of the Mediterranean and Asia, as well as from our own personal experiences, we believe there are five fundamental ways that you can substantially improve your emotional health and well-being:

1. **Enjoy good food and the rituals surrounding it**
2. **Have a more relaxed and optimistic attitude toward life**
3. **Truly appreciate the people and things around you**
4. **Pursue your passions**
5. **Set aside "calm time" each day**

Let's take a look at each of these steps in detail, starting with one of my favorite subjects: food!

ENJOY GOOD FOOD AND THE RITUALS SURROUNDING IT

There can be no doubt that the food you'll be eating as part of a MediterrAsian way of living is very good for your body in a physical sense. But so far we haven't touched much on the emotional aspect of food.

Food is not simply fuel, as some would like us to believe. Food is one of life's wonderful and glorious pleasures. Good food uplifts the emotions; provides comfort, satisfaction, and a sense of well-being; and can be spiritually fulfilling.

Think of all the senses that are involved when you enjoy good food: the smell, the sight, the texture, and the taste. You're smelling, seeing, feeling, as well as tasting—talk about hitting a lot of senses at the same time. Is it any wonder we love food so much!

Unfortunately, although the enjoyment of food should be one of the emotional highlights of our lives, in Western society good-tasting food is usually associated with food that's bad for you. This is very often true.

Many popular Western foods that taste good also happen to be loaded with calories, and at the same time they fall short in the nutrient department. Because of this, many of us have come to associate good-tasting food with food that's unhealthy and fattening.

But good-tasting food and food that's good for you certainly don't have to be mutually exclusive. Far from being unhealthy and fattening, traditional Mediterranean and Asian-style foods taste delicious, but they're typically packed with nutrients and contain only a moderate number of calories. This means that this food satisfies the stomach, the senses, and the soul—all without compromising your health.

The Emotional Pleasures of Food

So, by eating the MediterrAsian way you can start rejoicing over food, savoring it, getting full and satisfied, and all without guilt. This is how people from the Mediterranean and Asia have done it for centuries. They've always eaten lots of good-tasting food that made them feel good—physically *and* emotionally.

Indeed, the emotional aspect of food has always been a point to be celebrated in Mediterranean and Asian cultures. Traditionally mealtimes have been cherished—and the enjoyment of the food seen as paramount. In Italy, for example, they use the term *"Mangia!"* which means "to eat." But according to Italian-American food writer Anthony Del Plato, it means much more than that. To Italians, *mangia* means "eat and enjoy this food, relish all food, taste as much as you can, eat up life, eat and be well!"

This same fundamental philosophy is shared throughout the Mediterranean region and equally in Asia, where enjoyment of food has always been regarded as a deep-rooted part of the emotions and mealtimes are considered a blissful ritual.

More Than Just Food

The emotional fulfillment that eating provides doesn't just come from the enjoyment of the food—your surroundings can often be equally important.

In the Mediterranean and Asia mealtimes are traditionally seen not only as a time for eating wonderful food, but also as a time for relaxing, de-stressing, coming together with friends and family, and enjoying good conversation and a good laugh.

From our own personal experience, we have certainly found that sharing the pleasure of good food washed down with wine or cold beer is very conducive to relaxation, conversation, and laughter! And because of this, mealtimes (particularly dinnertime) have become one of the most emotionally and spiritually fulfilling times of the day for us.

We've also discovered something else quite extraordinary—the preparation and cooking of MediterrAsian-style meals can be a very fulfilling experience in its own right.

Unlike a typical Western meal, where the most exotic flavorings are usually salt, pepper, and ketchup, Mediterranean and Asian dishes contain a host of wonderful fragrant herbs, spices, and condiments. And instead of bland, colorless, lifeless ingredients to work with, there are lots of vegetables, fruits, fish, beans, nuts, and grains—in all sorts of shapes, colors, sizes, and textures. It's a true pleasure for the senses preparing and cooking these sorts of ingredients. And we still constantly marvel at how such simple ingredients can be transformed so quickly into such wonderful creations.

We also find that the time we spend in the kitchen preparing and cooking is a great bonding experience. Coming together and working to achieve something is a great way to catch up and get in touch with each other. And it really gives us a tremendous sense of achievement when we sit down to enjoy the meal knowing that it was created from the fruits of our own labor.

Of course, although we get a lot of emotional satisfaction from preparing and cooking meals at home, it certainly doesn't stop us from regularly eating out at Mediterranean and Asian-style restaurants. Greek, Italian, Chinese, Spanish, Japanese, Indian, Moroccan, Lebanese, Thai, and Vietnamese restaurants are some of our favorites.

Because these types of restaurants have a large number of dishes that fit within MediterrAsian eating guidelines, we get the emotional satisfaction of enjoying good-tasting food that's good for us, with the added bonus that we don't have to clean up afterward!

Eat to Your Heart's Content

Food is *not* a science experiment. It isn't something that should be counted, weighed and dissected—it should be savored and thoroughly enjoyed. And by eating the MediterrAsian way you really can enjoy the pleasures of eating to your heart's content—your emotional heart as well as your physical heart.

HAVE A MORE RELAXED AND OPTIMISTIC ATTITUDE TOWARD LIFE

Enjoying lots of delicious food throughout the day is great for improving your emotional well-being; but there's a lot more to life than just mealtimes. So how do you go about looking after your emotional well-being at other times of the day?

Again, we can learn a great deal from the traditional cultures of the Mediterranean and Asia. A common trait throughout these cultures is that people generally have a more relaxed and laid-back attitude to life. Simple celebrations of daily life are also common. And there's a general acceptance that life is fleeting and that time, as well as loved ones and friends, are precious commodities that can't be taken for granted.

We believe that having a similar sort of attitude in your own life is one of the key steps to dramatically improving your emotional well-being. But in this chaotic, high-stress twenty-first-century Western world, how can you possibly have the same laid-back, optimistic attitude to life as people from traditional Mediterranean and Asian cultures?

Well, there's no doubt that the twenty-first-century Western world can be a highly stressful environment to live in—stressful events seem to bombard us constantly. And this constant stress doesn't affect just our emotional health and well-being—it can also have a direct impact on our physical health. But it's very important to remember one simple point: your *attitude* determines your stress levels.

Stress and Perception

You may have noticed that some people are virtually immune to stress. No matter what comes up, they seem to be able to deal with it, often without batting an eyelid. Could it just be a case of enormous self-control? Perhaps. But part of the reason could lie in the fact that each of us has a different perception of what stressful is.

More than two thousand years ago the Greek philosopher Epictetus said that it's never the things that happen to us that upset us, it's our view of these things. In other words, it's your view of an event that makes it stressful and not the event itself.

As an example, in 1900 the polar explorer Sir Ernest Shackleton put the following advertisement in the *London Times*:

Men wanted for hazardous journey. Small wages, bitter cold, long months of complete darkness, constant danger, safe return doubtful. Honor and recognition in case of success.

You wouldn't really expect many people, if any, to reply to such an advertisement. But, surprisingly, there were hundreds of eager responses. This shows that what some people may find stressful, others may find desirable.

As another example, you've probably noticed that when some people get caught in a traffic jam they soon become frustrated and "stressed-out" and often shout at the cars ahead, or pound on the horn. Yet at the same time other people who are caught in the same traffic jam are quite calm. In the end, it's the same situation, but it leads to two completely different reactions.

Both of these examples demonstrate that stress is an emotional state—it's not the situation itself but your view of the situation that makes it stressful. Unfortunately the stress that starts in your mind can end up affecting your emotions, your body, and your spirit (see "The Stress Story").

How to Change Your View of a Stressful Situation

Inside each of us we have the power to control whether a situation becomes stressful or not. What it basically comes down to is changing your mindset when a situation arises that you would usually find stressful—for example, accidentally backing into the neighbor's fence, or having a stack of bills all arrive at the same time, or trying to meet an important deadline, or having your car break down, and so on.

Instead of seeing these events as stressful, change your perception and look at these events from a more optimistic viewpoint. And I don't mean "head in the clouds" optimistic; I'm talking about being a realistic optimist. Being a realistic optimist means that you're aware that life is inevitably going to throw you curveballs, but instead of seeing these curveballs as *problems*, you see them as *challenges*.

After my accident I spent a fair amount of time wallowing in self-pity, and it just got me more and more stressed and depressed. But when I changed my mindset and saw a challenge instead of a problem, it was like a switch had gone off in my head. It immediately made everything much easier to deal with, and I felt a lot happier and much more in control. This experience showed me that emotional

The Stress Story

There's nothing new about stress, nor is it an unnatural phenomenon. Stress is actually a kind of ancient survival mechanism, built into us by thousands of years of evolution. When our prehistoric ancestors were confronted with danger (like a hungry saber-toothed tiger), this set off an instant survival reaction that caused changes in body chemistry, including increased heart rate, higher blood pressure, and a release of large amounts of the hormones adrenaline and cortisol—all in preparation for either a physical showdown or a hasty retreat! After this "fight or flight" reaction, the body would eventually return to its normal, relaxed state. This biochemical reaction to external pressure is popularly known as stress.

Although stress is nothing new, the amount of stress we're now dealing with on a day-to-day basis is higher than ever before. These days we're constantly subjecting our stone-age bodies to space-age lifestyles—from traffic jams and noisy crowded cities, to juggling responsibilities and family arguments—all combined with our ongoing struggle to balance work, relationships, children, and finances.

The Dangers of Stress

What happens when you're constantly in a state of high stress? Instead of returning to the desirable, relaxed post-stress phase, the body adapts to the pressures, so in effect your body ends up being in a constant state of fight or flight. Constricted blood vessels, increased heart rate, and high blood pressure become permanent fixtures. Under these circumstances we begin to measurably harm our health.

In the end too much stress can lead to a range of problems, including neck, shoulder, and back pain; frequent headaches; attacks of arthritis and asthma; and bowel irregularities and digestive problems. High levels of stress have also been identified as a key risk factor for heart disease and stroke.

So, what's the best way to deal with all this unhealthy stress? Should you pack up all your belongings and move into the nearest cave, or become a monk and meditate all day? Far from it! By following the simple guidelines outlined in this chapter you'll be well on the way to substantially lowering your stress levels.

pain can often be worse than physical pain—but at the same time I also learned firsthand that emotional pain really is self-induced.

These days, when a situation arises in my life that could be stressful, I like to ask myself this simple question: *"Is getting worried about it going to help or hinder the situation?"* I soon realize that no matter what the problem is, worrying about it certainly won't help—but turning it into a challenge will. In other words, instead of crying over spilt milk I just clean it up and get on with my life.

Obviously, all situations aren't going to be so easy to deal with, but always remember that no matter what the situation is, worrying about it definitely won't help—*it will only make it worse.*

In the end you're the one in control and it's up to you how you deal with any situation that arises in your life. However, by having a more optimistic attitude and seeing challenges instead of problems, you'll find it much easier, not only to deal with stress, but not to let a situation turn stressful in the first place.

Looking for Positives in the Worst of Situations

Having a positive outlook on life and turning life's curveballs into challenges may seem like a relatively straightforward thing to accomplish with life's minor ups and downs. But what about really major, life-changing events like the death of a loved one, losing your job, going through a divorce, or a major accident?

How is it possible in these circumstances simply to look for positives and turn these events into challenges? Actually, in exceptional circumstances like these it's more important than ever to have an optimistic outlook.

I think someone who really epitomizes seeing the positives in the worst of situations is Alex Zanardi, a champion Italian race car driver who found fame when he won the prestigious and grueling CART motor racing series back-to-back in 1997 and 1998. But unfortunately Zanardi's outstanding career was cut abruptly short during the 2001 CART World Series. While leading the race at the American Memorial 500 in Lausitz, Germany, Zanardi pulled in to make a routine pit stop with thirteen laps to go. As he exited the pits his car skidded, lost control, and veered across the track into the path of a race car traveling at almost 200 miles an hour.

The horrific accident tore Zanardi's car in half and sprayed debris across the track. He was quickly rushed by helicopter to a Berlin hospital, but due to the severity of Zanardi's injuries doctors had to amputate both his legs above the knee.

Despite losing both his legs, the medical staff was amazed by Zanardi's quick recovery, as well as his mental resilience. In fact, less than a month after the accident Zanardi was conducting interviews with the media from his hospital bed. In one interview with the Associated Press he said in a strong and cheerful voice, "I can't complain. I'm in good condition . . . I lost my legs, but my upper body is strong, my energy is back and I move around with my arms and I'm pretty independent about everything."

Although he was highly optimistic, Zanardi was also realistic about his circum-stances. In an interview with the Italian magazine *Autosprint* he said, "I'm trying to get through this in the most positive way possible. I don't think about what I lost, but everything I've still got, which I've realized is a great deal. . . I've always looked forward and that's what I intend doing this time. There have been difficult moments and I know there will be more in the future, but with every day that goes by things are getting better. Even my legs, what's left of them, I'm learning to control my movements better. I want to, and I must, think positively. I've got a new life ahead of me and now I want to use all my energy to make the most of it."

Even though it looked like Zanardi's racing career was over, in 2003 Zanardi stunned everybody by reappearing at the same racetrack where he had nearly lost his life in 2001. Aided by a hand-operated brake and accelerator, he symbolically drove the thirteen laps he wasn't able to complete when he had last been on the track.

Later that year he drove a specially modified sports car at Monza in his first full race since the accident. Zanardi not only finished the race, but after starting near the back of the field he placed a competitive seventh. Then in 2007 Zanardi decided to take up handcycling. Amazingly, after only four weeks of training, he placed 4th place in the New York City Marathon in the handcycle division. Even more incredibly, in 2012, he won two golds and a silver at the Paralympic Games in London. Then in 2016 he again won two golds and a silver at the Paralympics in Rio de Janeiro.

Alex Zanardi's typically positive Mediterranean attitude toward adversity is a lesson for all of us when we go through rough patches in life. No matter how dire a situation may seem, having a positive, optimistic attitude and seeing a challenge instead of a problem will always be the best way of getting through it.

The Longevity Bonus

Having a more optimistic outlook toward life's ups and downs doesn't just benefit you now by reducing your stress levels; it can also benefit you in the future by increasing your life span. Scientists have long suspected that an optimistic outlook can help people live longer, and now two recent studies have confirmed just that.

One study of 160 centenarians (people who live to 100 and older) living in Boston found that most of them tended to have a similar mindset. According to Margery Silver, EdD, a neuropsychologist at Harvard Medical School and associate director of the study: "They are usually positive, optimistic people, who handle stress extremely well. They also tend to be resourceful and adaptable. There are people in our study who survived the Holocaust and others who went through other terrible hardships. They just were able to adapt to their situation, maintaining a positive attitude. When they have a problem or setback, they figure out a way to deal with it."

Another study, by researchers at the Mayo Clinic in Minnesota also found that people with a more optimistic view on life tended to have longer life spans. In the study, researchers compared results from a personality test taken by participants thirty years earlier with their subsequent mortality rates. It was found that those who scored high on optimism had almost 20 percent less risk of premature death than did those who scored high on pessimism.

"It confirmed our commonsense belief," reported Toshihiko Maruta, MD, a psychiatrist at the Mayo Clinic and lead author of the study, "it tells us that mind and body are linked and that attitude has an impact on the final outcome—death."

TRULY APPRECIATE THE PEOPLE AND THINGS AROUND YOU

Of course, it's always going to be a lot easier to be optimistic about life's up and downs when you have a positive frame of mind to begin with. But you can't simply force yourself into having a positive frame of mind; it's something that has to be developed naturally. But *how*?

From our own personal experience, we have found that a good way to start naturally developing a positive frame of mind is by not taking things for granted in life. It's a sad fact that many of us are so caught up in the routine of our day-to-day lives that we often neglect to truly appreciate life and those around us. We forget how important things are to us, and it's usually only after they're gone that we truly appreciate how much they're really worth to us.

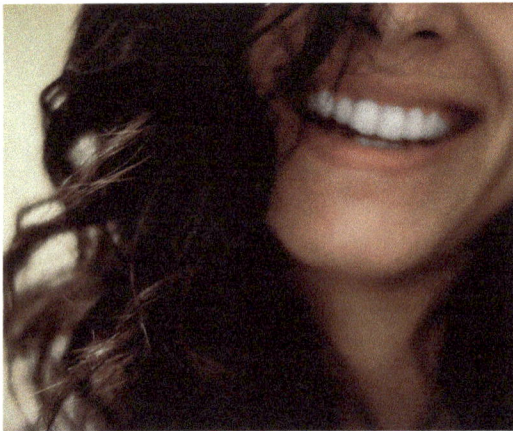

I've often read about people who've been diagnosed with terminal cancer and how suddenly they get a new appreciation of life and the things around them. Many of these people even say that, although they may be dying, they are actually "living" more than they ever have before.

By this, they mean they are seeing the world from a different perspective. Nothing can be taken for granted anymore, and even things that most of us would think of as trivial, such as the feeling of wind through your hair or the warmth of sun on your face, become much more important and special.

Stop and Smell the Roses

It doesn't have to take a terminal illness to heighten your appreciation of the people and the things around you. It's all about having the realization in your own life that time in this world, for all of us, really is quite fleeting—but rejoicing in this fact and seeing time as the precious commodity that it is. It's about realizing that once a day of your life is gone you can never have it back again, and thus making the most of it and appreciating all the wonderful things around you in life: the company of friends and loved ones, the taste and texture of good food, the smell of freshly baked bread, the storekeeper's smile, the sounds of children playing, the colorful marvels of nature, the fact that all your trillions of cells are working in remarkable harmony to keep you alive.

Having genuine gratitude for life and those around you truly enriches your spirit and makes life much more emotionally fulfilling. And, as a natural consequence, it's also a great way of creating a much more positive frame of mind.

PURSUE YOUR PASSIONS

Along with being grateful, another very important way you can develop a naturally positive frame of mind is by pursuing the things in life you feel truly passionate about. It's easy in life to sometimes feel like you're adrift on a huge ocean with no compass; but having a passion helps give you direction and brings more meaning to your life. To identify what your true passions are in life, simply follow your heart and really explore what fulfills and excites you.

You might have a passion for writing, cooking, decorating, animals, computers, helping others, sport, mathematics, teaching, crafts, music, or like me, your passion could be art. Whatever your passions are, be proactive and pursue them with vigor. And if you can find a way to turn your passion into your job, then you'll never have to "work" another day in your life.

That's exactly what my stepfather, Lindsay, did. When he was in his forties he felt "stressed out" and stuck in a rut working as a sales manager. However, one of the things he was really passionate about in life was home brewing. He would spend hours at a time out in the backyard shed brewing and bottling beer—and he *loved* every minute of it.

So he decided to quit his job, combine his sales experience with his passion for home brewing, and start his own home brew shop. He now owns and runs his own successful home brewing shop and, needless to say, he feels much more fulfilled and positive about life.

SET ASIDE "CALM TIME" EACH DAY

Enjoying good food and the rituals surrounding it, having a more optimistic attitude toward life, truly appreciating the people and things around you, and pursuing the things in life you are passionate about are all great ways of reducing stress and improving your emotional and spiritual well-being. But there is one other *very important* way you can substantially improve your emotional and spiritual well-being. We call it "calm time". Simply put, calm time is a special time just for you (or you can share it with someone close). It's a time to relax, rejuvenate, and reconnect with your spirit.

The Principle of Calm Time

Just as you need to sleep each day to be physically recharged, you also need time each day to de-stress, and recharge your emotional and spiritual energy.

For centuries Mediterraneans and Asians have made a point of setting aside special time to relax and rejuvenate their minds and bodies. The afternoon siesta in Italy, Spain, and Greece and meditation and tai chi in Asia are some good examples. But calm time can also be as simple as sitting in the garden admiring the beauty of nature, or relaxing in a hot bubble bath with candles and incense burning. As long as it's relaxing and enjoyable—it's *calm time.*

Trudy and I always make sure we set aside at least thirty minutes for calm time each day (not necessarily in one block of thirty minutes). We realize that this time of emotional and spiritual rejuvenation is just as important for our overall health and well-being as what we eat and how much we move.

Over the years we've discovered there are dozens of fun and enjoyable ways to relax, rejuvenate, and reconnect with our spirit—and we're sure you'll have no trouble regularly incorporating some of these ideas into your own life.

Soak in a hot bubble bath by candlelight. Shed your clothes and your daily concerns and relax in a good old-fashioned hot bath, full to the brim with creamy bubbles. Let all your tensions evaporate with the dissolving foam. Make sure your favorite music is playing in the background. And don't forget to accompany those burning candles with a stick of incense. If you don't have a bathtub, have a long relaxing soak under a hot shower instead.

See a funny film. Go to the cinema or rent a comedy movie and laugh until you cry. Laughter is one of the healthiest antidotes to stress. When you laugh, or even just smile, blood flow to the brain is increased, endorphins (painkilling hormones that give you a sense of well-being) are released, and levels of stress hormones drop. And besides, life's too serious, so laugh as long, loud, and often as you can.

Surf the Web. There are literally millions of words, pictures, sounds, videos, and animations out there in cyberspace. And for just a few dollars each month you can have unlimited access to it all (as long as you have a computer or similar device, of course). Everything from thousands of Mediterranean and Asian recipes to the latest Hollywood gossip is at your fingertips.

Keep a diary or journal. Writing down your feelings in a diary or journal can help you get in touch with your soul as well as relieve emotional stress. In a study conducted by psychologist James W. Pennebaker, PhD, from Southern Methodist University, participants wrote for twenty minutes a day over four consecutive days about issues or emotions that were causing them stress. When the study was completed, participants showed improved mental health and were better able to cope with stress.

Relax in the garden. Set up that old hammock, throw down a comfy rug, or just lounge on a patch of grass and soak up the sunshine (don't forget the sunscreen!). If you like to rejuvenate but also want to get more than a sunbath, why not get in touch with Mother Nature and get your hands dirty by tending to an herb garden or planting a tree? The garden is a wonderful sanctuary that is ideal for both mindless leisure activities and more practical pursuits. If your own garden is little more than a couple of pots on the window ledge, then head to a public park or garden nearby for some regular botanical therapy.

Visit parks, gardens, and nurseries. Stop and smell the flowers, play on the swings (you're never too old), or throw a Frisbee or ball around. Instead of heading straight to the office cafeteria at break time, relax by yourself or with a friend at the nearest park and take in the fresh air and scenery. Even the local plant nursery is a wonderful place to immerse yourself in the natural beauty of the plant kingdom—and you can even take a little piece home with you.

Have a massage. Enjoy a relaxing massage from the tips of your toes to the top of your scalp. Call your local salon for a rundown of their services and the types of massage offered. Or exchange favors with your partner and give each other a gentle massage with a little oil and lots of TLC. The soothing experience will give you a chance to revive sore muscles and leave your entire body feeling renewed.

Read or write poetry. Read works by your favorite poet. Make sure you find a relaxed room away from noise, and totally absorb yourself in the words as they unravel from the page. Or go a step further and write your own poetry.

Paint or draw a picture. Grab some crayons, pencils, oils, pastels, or ink and express yourself on paper, canvas, or paint digitally on a computer. If you think you're lacking in natural artistic ability, think about joining an art class. For inspiration, get art books from the library or bookstore, or visit your local art gallery.

Learn to play an instrument. Either take lessons or grab some sheet music and teach yourself at your own pace. If you used to play music in a school band, reacquaint yourself with your old instrument. Or maybe there's a closet rock star hidden somewhere...why not find out?

Learn another language. Learning to speak and write another language is a great way of increasing your life skills, and it's also a relaxing experience. Find a language that appeals to you on an emotional level and learn the language by yourself, or get your partner involved and learn together.

Plan your next vacation. Pick up a few vacation brochures at your local travel agent for some getaway ideas. Be adventurous and plan a trip to exotic, faraway places or maybe just a fun weekend away somewhere closer to home.

Watch a classic movie. Sink back in your sofa, dim the lights, and travel back to another time and place courtesy of the classic movie of your choice. Some of our favorites include *Wuthering Heights* (1939), *Rear Window* (1954), *It's a Wonderful Life* (1946), *Rebecca* (1940), *The Adventures of Robin Hood* (1938), *It Happened One Night* (1934), and *Some Like it Hot* (1959).

Visit the library. Take some time out and browse through the shelves for books and magazines that interest you. Read in the peace and quiet of the library or borrow some books to read at home.

Look through old photos and home movies. Dust off your old photos, or dig out your home movies. Get nostalgic and reminisce about old memories from your past (only good ones, of course!).

Go for a sightseeing drive. With a local map or street directory in hand, go exploring in your car. Most towns and cities have pleasant areas for a leisurely drive on a Sunday afternoon. Check out the local scenery, sights, and sounds and discover places that you've never been before.

Go to the zoo. Marvel at the animal kingdom firsthand. Watch the frenzy of animals at feeding time and take the opportunity to feed the animals. If there's no zoo in your area, find an animal sanctuary or reserve, feed some ducks or squirrels in the park, or just take a moment to watch any local native wildlife, including birds.

Play a fun leisure game. Darts, pool, table tennis, and bowling are always favorites.

Take up pottery. If you've ever seen the movie *Ghost* you'll appreciate that pottery can be a whole lot of fun. There's nothing quite like the feeling of slippery, wet clay oozing through your fingers. This stress relief alone makes pottery a worthwhile experience. The fact you can create your own pots, plates, vases, and cups is an added bonus!

Make love. Set aside a special time to relax and share intimacy with the one you love. Create the right mood with soft lighting, music, and perfume. Share your fantasies and experiment with different positions, locations, and times.

Take photos. It's a relaxing experience to enjoy pleasant surrounds and forever be able to capture the moment on film. Why not start up special albums and fill them full of different shots (for example, a nature album or a baby album)?

Get a pet. Whether it's a dog, cat, bird, or fish, a pet can play a vital role in stress relief. Pets can also be good for your heart. A Johns Hopkins Medical Center study found that fifty out of fifty-three people with pets were alive a year after their first heart attacks, while only seventeen of thirty-nine of those without pets lived a year.

Visit a museum or local art gallery. Walk among the exhibits and explore in detail the ones that interest you.

Play a board game. Monopoly®, chess, Trivial Pursuit®, checkers, and Scrabble® are some good examples.

Do a crossword puzzle. Completing a crossword not only enhances your knowledge of words, it's also a great way of relaxing and de-stressing.
Play a game of cards. Try your hand at solitaire or get together with friends for a game of poker or gin rummy.

Meditate. Meditation is a quick and relaxing way to take your mind away from troubling and stressful thoughts. Go deep within yourself or just catch a few quiet moments in the solitude of a private room. For information on different meditation techniques you can purchase a book on the subject or research under "meditation" and "breathing techniques" on the Internet.

Book into a day spa. Day spas provide a little bit of luxury for everyone. Try one of the beauty treatments and other self-indulging services that are offered.

Chill out at the beach. Listen to the sounds of the ocean, drench yourself in the refreshing surf, or just read your favorite novel on the warm sand.

Write a letter or e-mail. Whether you want to catch up with an old friend or find out the latest family gossip, take the time to share your news in a letter. For something more immediate than snail mail, why not e-mail your thoughts instead?

Phone friends or family. Have a good old gossip with a friend or family member. Or maybe a long and personal chat with someone more intimate.

Listen to your favorite music. Select music to suit your mood. Give yourself a chance to put your feet up, then sit back, close your eyes, and be taken away by the music, lyrics, and memories.

Read a book or magazine. What are you in the mood for—a thriller, a romance, or maybe a mystery? Or perhaps a nonfiction title or glossy magazine is more your style. Find somewhere relaxed and quiet (snuggled in bed is always a good option) and read it cover to cover.

Soak your feet. Give your feet a treat and fill a bowl with warm water and a few drops of aromatherapy oil of your choice. Let the warm water soothe away the day's tensions and leave your feet super-soft.

Relax in front of an open fireplace. Watch the burning logs, listen to the crackling, and allow the warmth to penetrate your inner being.

Practice tai chi. Tai chi is practiced by millions of Chinese and Japanese every day, and in recent years this ancient martial art has become increasingly popular in the West. The slow, controlled, dancelike movements of tai chi can be helpful in achieving a state of total relaxation of the whole body, which helps to quiet the mind and promote relaxation. A study in China observed a group of 120 people between 50 and 80 years of age who had practiced tai chi for many years. They found that after practice, 92 percent of the group became noticeably more cheerful and optimistic.

Practice yoga. Yoga originated in India over three thousand years ago. Although there are several distinct styles of yoga, the style familiar to most of us in the West is called *hatha yoga*. This style of yoga involves practicing a variety of static postures or *asanas*. These postures stretch, strengthen, and align the body, and increase flexibility. The practice of yoga also helps relieve physical and emotional stress and helps bring about a sense of inner peace, balance, and "oneness." To learn more about practicing yoga you can go to special classes in your neighborhood or learn positions from the Internet or a book (*Yoga for Dummies* is a good book for beginners).

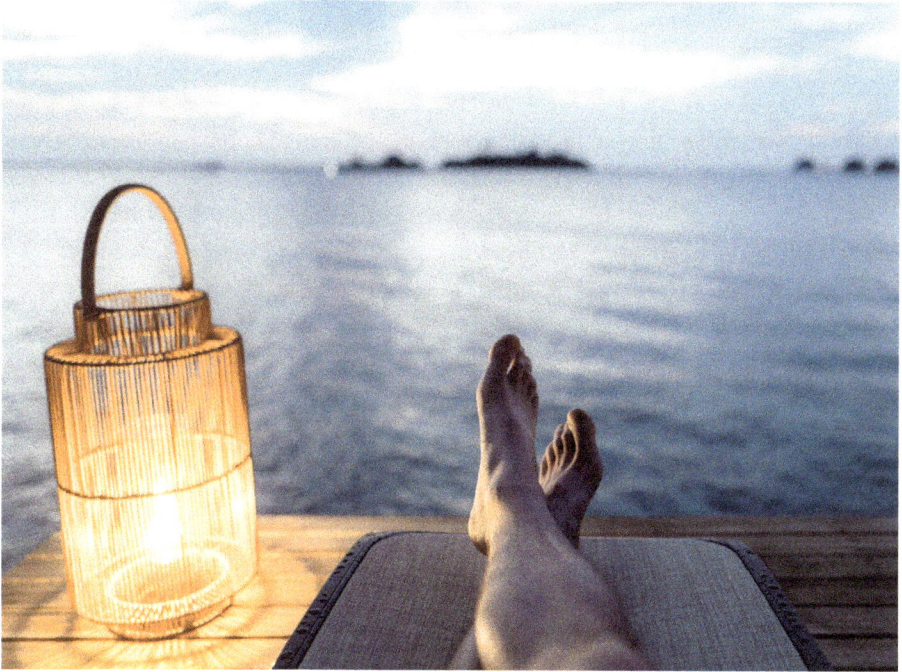

CHAPTER 9

The MediterrAsian Balanced Meal System

For thousands of years the peoples of the Mediterranean and Asia have never counted carbohydrate or fat grams, referred to a glycemic index, or separated their food into proteins and starches. And they certainly haven't counted calories. Instead, they've simply eaten a wide variety of delicious foods until they felt full and satisfied. Yet the great majority of them managed to stay lean and fit. What can explain this extraordinary paradox?

Well, one reason could be that Mediterraneans and Asians have traditionally burned off some of the calories they consume by being physically active as part of their day-to-day lives. But there's another very important reason—*how they balance their meals*.

Instead of eating lots of high-calorie processed foods, red meats, and junk foods like we do in the West, the majority of foods Mediterraneans and Asians have traditionally eaten consists of minimally processed foods as close to their natural state as possible. These foods—vegetables, grains, legumes, fruits, and lean protein sources such as fish, poultry, and seafood—are all bulky, high in volume, and filling, but are generally only low to moderate in calories. In simple terms, this means that if you eat a traditional Mediterranean or Asian-style meal instead of a typical Western-style meal, you'll be able to eat *more* food while consuming *fewer* calories.

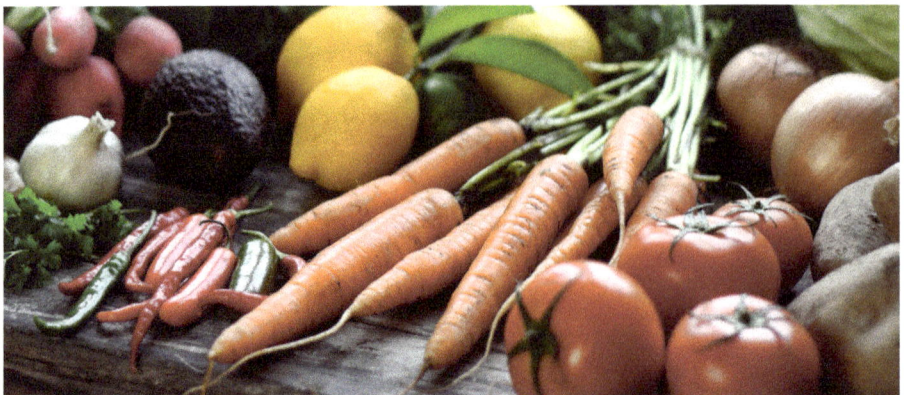

As an example, let's compare a Western-style meal, a Mediterranean-style meal, and an Asian-style meal:

WESTERN-STYLE MEAL	MEDITERRANAN-STYLE MEAL	ASIAN-STYLE MEAL
1 quarter-pound burger with cheese	Sicilian salmon and pasta with roasted red pepper, zucchini, basil and pine nuts	Bowl of fragrant broccoli and mushroom soup
1 large fries	1 slice crusty whole grain bread drizzled with 1/2 tablespoon extra virgin olive oil	Rice paper roll stuffed with chicken breast, snow pea sprouts and peppers, and served with a soy-sesame dipping sauce
	Large salad with tomatoes, olives, romaine lettuce and red onion, served with olive oil and balsamic vinaigrette	Cantonese shrimp, cashew nut and mixed vegetable stir-fry served over steamed long-grain rice
1 large soda	1 glass red wine	1 glass cold beer
1 ice cream sundae	Bowl of mixed berries served with a scoop of sorbet	Fresh fruit salad with mango, lychees and pineapple
Calories: 1,679	Calories: 860	Calories: 810

How's that for a comparison? If you eat a traditionally balanced Mediterranean or Asian-style meal instead of a typical burger and fries meal, you'll end up eating close to twice the volume of food, but around half the calories. And unlike the burger and fries meal, the Mediterranean and Asian-style meals aren't riddled with saturated and hydrogenated fat, sugar, and other nasties. Instead, they're overflowing with essential vitamins and minerals as well as many other health-giving nutrients and compounds such as phytochemicals, antioxidants, omega-3 fatty acids, and soluble and insoluble fiber.

The Mediterranean- and Asian-style meals also boost your fat-fighting metabolism, and ensure that your blood sugar levels stay balanced for sustained energy and concentration. And just as important, this food isn't only nutritious, it's also *delicious*, so your mind and senses will be satisfied too—which is incredibly important!

BALANCING ALL YOUR MEALS THIS WAY

How do you balance all your meals like the Mediterranean and Asian examples above so they're nutritious, filling, and delicious but only moderate in calories? Well, it's actually a lot easier than you may think. As a matter of fact, it's as easy as following these five simple steps when you prepare or purchase a meal:

Step 1: Go with the grains. Include a grain-based food such as rice, pasta, bread, noodles, bulgur, or couscous in each meal.

Step 2: Value your vegetables. Include a variety of colorful vegetables in each meal and/or have a salad or vegetable-based soup on the side.

Step 3: Pick your protein. Include a moderate amount of protein-based foods in each meal—preferably fish (any variety, but particularly fattier types of fish like salmon, tuna, mackerel, sardines, and anchovies, which are rich in omega-3s) and seafood (such as shrimp, scallops, crab, oysters, clams, mussels, and squid), legumes (beans, peas, and lentils), nuts, or chicken. Use eggs moderately and red meat (beef, pork, and lamb) only occasionally.

Step 4: Favor the good fats. Plant oils (particularly monounsaturated vegetable oils like olive and peanut oil) and fish oils (from the fish you eat) should make up the majority of fat in each meal. Dairy products such as cheese and yogurt can be used in moderate amounts and butter should be used only occasionally or in very small amounts.

Step 5: Savor the seasonings. Use a wide variety of herbs, spices, condiments, and seasonings to add flavor, color, and depth to each meal.

We call this simple five-step meal preparation system the *MediterrAsian Balanced Meal System*, or MBMS for short. By using this simple yet powerful system you'll never have to worry about not getting the right balance of food, because the MBMS is based directly on how Mediterraneans and Asians have instinctively been balancing their meals for thousands of years. So by designing your meals according to this system, you'll not only become leaner while eating lots of food, you'll also automatically be following the healthiest diet in the world!

You can use the guidelines of the MBMS when you prepare your own meals or when you eat out, and it can even be used to adapt typically less healthy foods like burgers and hot dogs into far healthier versions that taste just as good. (We'll show you how shortly).

USING THE MBMS IN REAL LIFE

It's easy to create a huge range of delicious and nutritious Mediterranean and Asian-style meals using the guidelines of the MBMS. For example, by mixing and matching grains, vegetables, proteins, fats, seasonings, and fruit for the Mediterranean and Asian dishes listed below, it's possible to come up with literally thousands of different meal combinations.

Pasta Dishes:

Go with the grains. Choose a type of pasta. It comes in over four hundred varieties, but some of the most useful include spaghetti, lasagna, fusilli (corkscrew shape), fettuccine (flat, ribbonlike), penne (tubular with ends cut on diagonal), farfalle (bow-tie shape), and conchiglie (shells).

Value your vegetables. Tomatoes, onions, garlic, bell peppers (red, green, yellow, and orange), mushrooms, broccoli, zucchini, artichokes, arugula, celery, carrots, chilies, spinach, asparagus, and eggplant are some good choices.

Pick your protein. Good choices include tuna or salmon (fresh or canned), anchovies, fresh sardines, dried and fresh beans (cannellini beans, chickpeas, fresh green beans, and fava beans are particularly good choices), chicken, nuts (walnuts, pine nuts, and pistachios), and seafood like shrimp, crab, scallops, clams, mussels, squid, and octopus. Use meats like ground beef, salami, prosciutto, and pancetta only occasionally, or in small amounts as a flavor and texture enhancer.

Favor the good fats. Use olive oil as your principal cooking fat. If you're having cheese with your pasta meal, opt for a strong-flavored variety like Parmesan so a little goes a long way.

Savor the seasonings. Sun-dried tomatoes, olives, vinegars (like balsamic and red wine), capers, red and white wine, basil, oregano, rosemary, flat-leaf parsley, sea salt, and freshly ground black pepper can all be used in various combinations.

(For examples of MediterrAsian-balanced pasta dishes, see page 141.)

Stir-Fries:

Go with the grains. A stir-fry is typically mixed or served with rice or noodles.

Value your vegetables. Broccoli, scallions, garlic, ginger, red and green bell peppers, zucchini, chili, celery, bean sprouts, cabbage (including Chinese cabbage), asparagus, cauliflower, carrots, mushrooms (fresh or dried), sweet corn, and Asian greens (such as bok choy, gai lan, and choy sum) are some good choices.

Pick your protein. Good choices include firm white fish (like snapper, cod, and haddock), fresh tuna or salmon, tofu, chicken, nuts (almonds, cashews, or peanuts) and seafood like shrimp, crab (or surimi), squid, and scallops.

Favor the good fats. Use peanut oil as your main cooking fat.

Savor the seasonings. Soy sauce, fresh cilantro, five-spice powder, oyster sauce, rice wine, black bean sauce, hoisin sauce, and toasted sesame oil can all be used in various combinations.

(For examples of MediterrAsian balanced stir-fries, see page 155.)

Indian Curries:

Go with the grains. An Indian curry is typically served over rice (basmati is a good traditional variety) or with Indian breads such as *naan* or *chapati*.

Value your vegetables. Broccoli, cauliflower, garlic, ginger, tomatoes, carrots, scallions, eggplant, cucumber, cabbage, spinach, red and green bell peppers, and chilies are some good choices.

Pick your protein. Good choices include firm white fish, salmon, tuna, chicken, lentils, chickpeas, almonds, green beans, fresh or dried peas, and seafood like shrimp and scallops.

Favor the good fats. Use peanut or canola oil as your cooking fat. Use only moderate amounts of coconut milk and yogurt.

Savor the seasonings. Fresh coriander and mint, tamarind, dried spices (including cumin, turmeric, coriander, cinnamon, and chili powder), and fruit and vegetable relishes and chutneys can all be used in various combinations.

(For examples of MediterrAsian-balanced Indian curries, see page 173.)

Sushi Rolls:

Go with the grains. Rice is an integral part of sushi because it makes up the largest part of the filling. A short-grain rice is the best variety to use.

Value your vegetables. Nori (thin sheets of seaweed used to wrap sushi rolls), cucumber, bean sprouts, carrots, mushrooms (like shiitake and enoki), avocado, snow peas, and snow pea sprouts are some good choices.

Pick your protein. Good choices include very fresh raw salmon or tuna, smoked salmon, fish roe, tofu, and seafood like shrimp, squid, and crab (or use surimi as a crab substitute).

Favor the good fats. No fat or oil is used in the preparation of sushi, so the good fats come mainly from the omega-3 rich fish.

Savor the seasonings. Wasabi (hot Japanese horseradish paste), soy sauce, pickled ginger (*gari*), pickled radish (*daikon*), rice vinegar are all possibilities.

(For examples of MediterrAsian-balanced sushi rolls, see page 216.)

Pizza:

Go with the grains. Choose a base for your pizza. Opt for either a premade pizza base (thin is traditional) or large whole grain pita bread as the base.

Value your vegetables. Tomato-based sauce and tomatoes, onion, garlic, bell peppers (red and green), mushrooms, eggplant, broccoli, zucchini, artichoke hearts, spinach, and asparagus are some good choices.

Pick your protein. Opt mainly for anchovies, tuna, smoked salmon, shrimp, scallops, smoked oysters, diced chicken, clams, and squid. We've also found that sliced soy hot dogs add a smoky sausage flavor to pizza without adding saturated fat. Use meaty toppings like ground beef, pepperoni, and salami only occasionally, or more as a garnish.

Favor the good fats. You can add flavor and texture to your pizza by drizzling the top with a little extra virgin olive oil. Don't drown your pizza in cheese either, just lightly cover it—and use a good pizza cheese like mozzarella so you get both flavor and texture.

Savor the seasonings. Sun-dried tomatoes, olives (many varieties), capers, basil, oregano, rosemary, flat-leaf parsley, sea salt, and freshly ground black pepper can all be used in various combinations.

(For examples of MediterrAsian-balanced pizzas, see page 168.)

MEDITERRASIAN MAKEOVERS

The examples above show you how the MBMS can be used to create lots of different traditional Mediterranean and Asian dishes. But it's not only Mediterranean and Asian meals that can be put together using the guidelines of the MBMS. Many Western-style meals can also be easily adapted to follow MBMS guidelines. Following are some examples.

Burgers:

Burgers have gotten a very bad reputation for being unhealthy and fattening. But when you think about it, if you remove the meat patty from a burger with cheese, what you're left with is basically a cheese and salad roll. So the key to making a burger far healthier is to find a healthy yet tasty alternative to the meat patty. You can also add more bulk, flavor, and nutrients to the burger by including more vegetables (which are naturally very low in calories).

Go with the grains. Choose a burger bun, regular or whole grain.

Value your vegetables. Fill your burger with lots of vegetables, including thinly sliced onions, tomatoes, lettuce, and pickles.

Pick your protein. Instead of using a beef patty to make your burger, opt for a soy, lentil, bean, fish, or chicken-based patty.

Favor the good fats. Cook the burger patties in a little canola, peanut, or light olive oil. If you add mayonnaise to your burger, use it more sparingly and preferably use an olive oil-based mayo. If you're having cheese with your burger, use a strong cheese such as sharp cheddar so a little goes a long way.

Savor the seasonings. Add flavor to your burger with condiments and sauces like ketchup, mustard (many varieties), BBQ sauce, relish, chutney, salsa, chili sauce, pepper, or horseradish.

Sandwiches and Subs:

By making a few sensible choices when you're constructing a sandwich, you can easily keep the calories down while increasing the bulk and the flavor—in other words, you can eat a bigger, tastier sandwich while consuming fewer calories!

Go with the grains. Choose a bread, preferably a whole grain variety. Vary the type of bread you use—some examples include sliced whole grain bread, pita bread, Middle Eastern lavash bread, rolls (many different types), French baguettes, Italian breads (like focaccia or ciabatta), or Turkish *pide* bread.

Value your vegetables. Pack your sandwich with a generous serving of any combination of salad vegetables you like—lettuce (iceberg, romaine, or other varieties), tomatoes, onions, bell peppers (red, green, orange, or yellow), carrots, sprouts (such as alfalfa, mung bean, or snow pea), cucumber, celery, sweet corn kernels, mushrooms, scallions, and char-grilled and marinated vegetables such as eggplant, peppers, or zucchini.

Pick your protein. Use red meat and meat products on your sandwich only occasionally. Opt instead for canned tuna, salmon (canned or smoked), mashed canned sardines, roast chicken or turkey, shrimp (fresh or canned), crab (or surimi). Canned beans are another versatile and healthy high-protein sandwich filling. Hard-boiled eggs can be used in moderation.

Favor the good fats. Spread your bread lightly with olive oil-based margarine (preferably trans fat free). You can also use avocado or hummus. If you add mayonnaise to your sub or sandwich, use it more sparingly (the same goes for other creamy dressings such as seafood cocktail sauce). And if you have cheese on your sandwich, use a strong variety like sharp cheddar so a little goes a long way.

Savor the seasonings. To add extra flavor to your sandwich there are plenty of condiments to choose from—mustard (lots of varieties), olives, chutney, relish, horseradish, salsa, pickles, sun-dried tomatoes, cranberry sauce, pesto, sweet chili sauce, freshly ground black pepper, lemon juice, and vinegar are some good examples.

Hot Dogs:

A normal hot dog is simply oozing with saturated fat. But you can enjoy all the wonderful flavors of a hot dog without any of the guilt by applying the guidelines of the MBMS.

Go with the grains. Choose a hot dog roll, regular or whole grain.

Value your vegetables. As well as onions, there are lots of other vegetables you can add to hot dogs, including sautéed red and green bell peppers, mushrooms, and garlic. Alternatively, have a serving of coleslaw with your hot dog.

Pick your protein. Instead of using a meat-based hot dog, opt for a soy-based hot dog.

Favor the good fats. The best way to cook a hot dog is in the microwave or in plenty of hot boiling water, so fat isn't required in the cooking process. By eating a soy-based hot dog instead of a meat-based one, you're already going with the good fats. If you have cheese on your hot dog, use a strong variety like sharp cheddar so a little goes a long way.

Savor the seasonings. Add flavor to your hot dog with condiments and sauces like ketchup, mustard (many varieties), BBQ sauce, chili sauce, relish, salsa, and chutney

Barbecues:

At a typical Western barbecue the focus is squarely on the meat. A MediterrAsian-balanced barbecue, on the other hand, divides the focus between the grilled food and the bread and side dishes.

Go with the grains. Serve bread (such as sliced whole grain bread, pita, lavash, ciabatta, and baguette) or bread rolls on the side.

Value your vegetables. Have a salad on the side, add vegetable pieces to kebabs, or cook up some vegetables on the grill (bell peppers, onion, eggplant, mushrooms, and zucchini grill up particularly well).

Pick your protein. Instead of the usual steak and sausages, opt mainly for salmon, tuna or swordfish steaks and soy-based sausages. Other alternatives include soy-, fish- or chicken-based burger patties; any kind of firm fresh fish; and seafood like shrimp, squid, scallops, and mussels.

Favor the good fats. Use peanut or canola oil as your cooking fat. Instead of serving bread with butter or margarine, have a small dish of extra virgin olive oil for dipping or drizzling. Alternatively, use a trans fat-free margarine made from olive or canola oil.

Savor the seasonings. Add flavor to the grilled food either with a marinade (which can used for basting and marinating) or with condiments and sauces like ketchup, mustard (many varieties), barbecue sauce, relish, salsa, and chutney.

EATING OUT: A WORLD OF CHOICE

One of the joys of eating MediterrAsian-balanced meals is that you don't have to prepare them all at home. We enjoy going out to restaurants and getting takeouts weekly while still applying the principles of the MBMS—here's how.

Restaurants

Without a doubt, dining out should be a highly pleasurable experience. Why spend good money at a restaurant and leave feeling unsatisfied? Why spend an evening out with friends if you can't enjoy the pleasure of eating with everyone else?

Eating a MediterrAsian-balanced meal when you dine out at a restaurant is incredibly simple. Actually, we're willing to bet that a lot of your favorite restaurant food is already based on Mediterranean and Asian cuisine. Think of the countries of the Mediterranean and Asia and you can probably match it up with a favorite restaurant. Some examples include Italian, Indian, Greek, Thai, Chinese, Lebanese, Provençal, Vietnamese, Turkish, and Japanese. And these restaurants often have a takeout section, and many even deliver, so you can also enjoy these foods in the comfort of your own home.

But just because a meal is from a Mediterranean- or Asian-style restaurant doesn't necessarily mean it will be MediterrAsian-balanced. Many of the meals in these restaurants are actually based on the banquet foods that are eaten in these countries, and not necessarily the staple meals that are eaten by people every day. That's why many people who dine out regularly at these restaurants wonder why they gain weight—Mediterraneans and Asians would most certainly gain weight too if they ate banquet foods every day!

At the same time, many Mediterranean and Asian restaurants have adapted their meals for a Western palate. In other words, there's now usually lots of red meat, fried food, and creamy-style sauces on the menu.

With all that said, you should still have no problem finding lots of dishes in Mediterranean and Asian-style restaurants that will be traditionally balanced—it's just a matter of looking. If you keep in mind the guidelines of the MBMS when you're reviewing the menu it will make things a lot easier.

Here are some good examples of what types of meals to keep an eye out for at various Mediterranean- and Asian-style restaurants:

Italian

- Pasta dishes with fish, shellfish, chicken, legumes, and vegetables served with a tomato-based sauce like marinara or pomodoro, or an olive oil and herb-based sauce like pesto or salsa verde
- Thin-base pizza (which is traditional) topped with vegetables and different kinds of fish and shellfish like anchovies, salmon, shrimp and clams
- Vegetable-, seafood-, chicken-, or bean-based risotto
- Grilled fish, poultry, and vegetables served with rice, pasta, polenta (cornmeal), or bread and salad
- Fish, shellfish, chicken, vegetable, and bean dishes cooked in tomato-, wine-, or stock-based sauces served with ciabatta or focaccia bread on the side
- Vegetable- and legume-based salads served with olive oil vinaigrette
- Vegetable-, fish-, shellfish-, poultry-, and bean-based soups
- Bruschetta (garlic and olive oil toasts) topped with grilled or roasted vegetables (like tomatoes and peppers) and drizzled with a little olive oil
- Antipasti (appetizers) such as marinated vegetables, olives, sun-dried tomatoes, and small amounts of cheese and cold meat (like shaved ham or salami)
- A fruit platter, or gelato served with fresh fruit

Greek and Middle Eastern

- Fish, shellfish, poultry, vegetables, and legumes cooked in sauces based on wine, stock, tomato, and yogurt
- Traditional Greek salad (*horiatiki salata*) with tomatoes, cucumbers, feta cheese, kalamata olives, and red onion
- Fish, shellfish, or poultry grilled, baked, or poached with onions, tomatoes, peppers, garlic, and other vegetables and served over rice or bulgur
- Grape leaves stuffed with rice, vegetables, and pine nuts or pistachios
- Legume, fish, shellfish, or poultry-based pilaf
- Meze (traditional Greek/Middle Eastern appetizer dishes similar to Italian antipasto)
- Chicken-, falafel-, and seafood-based gyros served with salad
- Pita bread stuffed with grilled chicken, falafel, or shrimp and vegetables
- Tabbouleh (tomato, bulgur, parsley, and mint salad)
- Fish-, shellfish-, poultry-, or legume-based pasta dishes
- Vegetable-, bean-, and lentil-based soups
- Crusty bread sticks or pita bread dipped into baba ghanoush (smoky eggplant dip), hummus (chickpea and sesame dip), or tzatziki (yogurt-cucumber dip)
- Rice pudding served with fruit and crushed nuts

French Provençal

- Niçoise salad (with tuna, tomatoes, potatoes, olives, sliced boiled eggs, and lettuce)
- Bouillabaisse (fish and shellfish stew)
- Pan bagnat (bread stuffed with Niçoise salad)
- Crêpes stuffed with fish, shellfish, poultry, or beans
- Toasted baguette spread with tapenade (olive, garlic, and caper spread)
- Roasted, grilled, or stuffed eggplant, artichokes, zucchini, and tomatoes
- Vegetable, bean, and lentil soups (such as soupe au pistou)
- Ratatouille (a vegetable stew traditionally made with tomatoes, bell pepper, eggplant, and zucchini that goes wonderfully served on the side of grilled or baked fish, chicken, or shellfish)

- Salade verte (green salad served with any combination of fresh leaves, including endive, arugula, spinach, and watercress) dressed with vinaigrette
- Grilled, broiled, steamed, roasted fish, shellfish, or chicken dishes
- Crudités (fresh raw vegetable pieces) with white bean dip
- Fresh fruits in liqueur like Cointreau or Grand Marnier.
- Fruit filled Crêpes

Spanish

- Paella (saffron-infused rice dish with any combination of seafood, chicken, beans, and vegetables)
- Tortilla de patatas (an egg dish with potatoes, similar to an omelet)
- Tapas—small appetizer dishes (which could include garlic shrimp, steamed mussels, fried squid, marinated mushrooms and artichokes, olives, and roasted marinated red peppers)
- Vegetable soups like gazpacho (chilled tomato and cucumber soup) and seafood soups (which include mussels, shrimp, and fish)
- Tomato-based stews made with fish, shellfish, or beans and vegetables like potatoes, bell peppers, and zucchini
- Grilled tuna or salmon skewers with vegetables (such as mixed peppers, tomatoes, red onions, potatoes) and Spanish-style tomato sauce
- Chickpea salad with roasted peppers and capers
- Hogazas (thick slices of bread with toppings like tomato, ham, red peppers, and anchovies)
- Bean stews made with any combination of white beans, fava beans, or chickpeas
- Vegetable, bean, or seafood soup served with crusty bread
- Fruit compotes using fruit such as plums, cherries, apricots, and peaches

North African (including Moroccan and Tunisian)

- Tagine (stew) made with combinations of fish, beans (like chickpeas), chicken, vegetables, nuts, fruits, herbs, and spices served over couscous
- Soups made with vegetables, chickpeas, and lentils
- North African baked fish flavored with chermoula (Moroccan spice mixture) and served with vegetables and rice or couscous

- Salads like couscous and vegetable salad, orange and black olive salad, carrot salad, or bean salad
- Bean dips like ful nabed (lima bean puree) and bessara (white bean dip) served with pita bread
- Vegetables (like peppers and eggplants) stuffed with couscous (or rice) nuts and vegetables
- Chakchouka (a North African cousin of Provençal ratatouille—a mixture of peppers, onions, and tomatoes fried in olive oil with herbs, spices, and eggs)
- Seafood or chicken bastilla—a spiced phyllo pastry pie
- Sweet couscous with almonds, honey, cinnamon, and dried or fresh fruits
- Oranges with dates, pistachio nuts, rosewater, and cinnamon

Southeast Asian (including Thai, Vietnamese, Malaysian, and Indonesian cuisine)

- Steamed, grilled, poached, or baked fish, shellfish, poultry, tempeh, and tofu dishes served over rice or noodles
- Vegetable, fish, or shellfish soups like Tom yum goong (Thai hot and sour shrimp soup) or Soto Ayam (spicy Malaysian chicken soup)
- Red, green, or yellow Thai curry with vegetables and fish, shellfish, poultry, or tofu served over rice
- Steamed spring rolls filled with shrimp, chicken, or crab and vegetables
- Vietnamese-style fresh rice paper rolls filled with vegetables and chicken or seafood
- Indonesian satay (marinated skewers) with chicken, fish, or shellfish
- Gado gado (cooked vegetable salad with peanut sauce)
- Kha Phat (Thai fried rice) with shrimp, crab, tofu, chicken, or squid
- Pad Thai (stir-fried noodle, shrimp, and vegetable dish)
- Nasi goreng (Indonesian fried rice) with chicken or seafood and vegetables
- Mie goreng (Indonesian fried noodles) with chicken or seafood and vegetables
- Laksa (Malaysian spicy noodle soup) with fish, shellfish, tofu, or chicken and vegetables

Indian

- Fish-, shellfish-, chicken-, lentil-, or chickpea-based curries served over rice and accompanied with relish, chutney, and raita (yogurt and cucumber)
- Dahl (lentil curry) served over rice or accompanied with breads like naan or chapati
- Fish, chicken, or shrimp cooked Tandoori-style (marinated and baked) or vindoori-style (marinated and braised) and served over rice or with bread
- Lentil-, bean-, fish-, shellfish-, and vegetable-based soups
- Vegetable-based curries like pea and potato curry served over rice with naan or chapati bread
- Vegetable-based salads like tamatar salat (tomato salad with mint and scallions)
- Pilau (a rice dish similar to a Middle Eastern pilaf) made with vegetables and fish, shellfish, or beans like chickpeas
- Grilled, baked, or poached fish, shellfish, or chicken served in tomato-, yogurt-, or stock-based sauces
- Murgh Tikka (skewered barbecued chicken) served with rice and a vegetable side dish

Chinese

- Stir-fried seafood, fish, chicken, or tofu (called bean curd in China) and vegetables served over rice or noodles
- Soups such as crab and sweet corn soup, chicken noodle soup, or hot and sour soup
- Chow mein made with vegetables and either fish, shellfish, tofu, or chicken (or a combination)
- Roasted lemon chicken served with vegetables over rice
- Fried rice made with shrimp (or other shellfish), fish, or chicken and vegetables
- Braised fish, shellfish, tofu, or chicken with vegetables served over rice or noodles
- Fish, vegetables, shellfish, or tofu with sweet and sour sauce served over rice or noodles
- Steamed spring rolls and dumplings filled with vegetables and seafood or chicken

- Noodle salad in sesame sauce
- Fresh fruit and fortune cookies

Japanese

- "Yaki" (broiled or grilled) or "nimono" (simmered) dishes with fish, shellfish, or chicken and vegetables served with rice or noodles (udon or soba)
- Sashimi (slices of raw fish such as tuna, salmon, whitefish, and mackerel) served with rice and vegetables on the side
- Sushi made with vegetables and your choice of fish and shellfish
- Soups like miso or sakana ushiojiru (fish broth)
- Hot pots like yosenabe (simmered seafood/chicken with vegetables)
- Steamed rice and noodles topped with vegetables and fish, tofu, or chicken
- Teriyaki salmon, tuna, shellfish, or chicken served with vegetables and rice or noodles
- Tempura (lightly battered and deep-fried seafood and vegetables) is good in moderation
- Hot or cold soba (buckwheat) noodles with vegetables and seafood
- Fresh fruit platter

FAST-FOOD OUTLETS

Restaurant cuisine isn't the only type of food you can enjoy when you eat out. Armed with your knowledge of the MBMS, it's also possible to eat at popular Western fast-food outlets.

Pizzas

The great thing about ordering a pizza is that you can add or take away ingredients. This means it's quite possible to turn a Western-style pizza into more of a MediterrAsian-balanced meal. The key is to load up on the vegetables and choose healthy protein sources with your pizza. So instead of going for the meat-lovers pizza, opt instead for the seafood-lovers pizza. Beans and chicken are also good high-protein toppings. Also opt for the traditional Italian thin-based pizza instead of the Western pan-pizza, which contains far more calories in the crust.

Fast-food pizza outlets also tend to go overboard with the cheese, so when you order your pizza tell them to halve the cheese and double the vegetables. This will make the pizza more flavorful and filling while keeping the calories and saturated fat down. A fresh salad with an olive oil-based dressing is also a good accompaniment to pizza.

Burgers

When you eat a burger at a fast food outlet, no matter how much you try to balance it, it's still going to be a high-calorie treat. But there are ways of minimizing the damage and making the burger more MediterrAsian-balanced.

For a start you could opt for a chicken- or fish-based burger instead of a beef-based one because this will reduce your intake of saturated fat and calories. A Filet-O-Fish, for example, contains less than half the saturated fat of a Big Mac, and a Premium Grilled Chicken Classic Sandwich contains less than a quarter of the saturated fat. Fish- and chicken-based burgers also generally contain between 150 and 250 calories fewer than a typical beef-based burger. And make sure to order a burger that comes with lots of salad veggies, including lettuce, tomatoes, onions, and pickles. These not only make the burger more filling and tasty but they add essential vitamins and minerals.

French fries also contain lots of calories as well as bad fat, so consume these foods in moderation. (In other words, order the small fries instead of the large fries.)

Sandwiches and Subs

Sandwich shops and delis are some of the easiest places to get a quick MediterrAsian-balanced meal because the sandwich is constructed according to your own wishes. This means that all you have to do is follow the guidelines for making your own MediterrAsian-balanced subs and sandwiches at home (see page 102) except the difference is that someone else is conveniently making it for you, and you don't have to shop for the ingredients!

So far we've talked about how to balance your meals according to the MBMS. But it's very important to remember that all your meals don't have to be MediterrAsian-balanced. As long as it's in moderation, sometimes an unbalanced meal like a beef burger or fried chicken is fine. However, if you try to make the majority of your meals MediterrAsian-balanced—or at least try to follow as many of the five steps as possible—the health-giving benefits will be far more substantial.

And you'll find that because MediterrAsian-style food is so delicious and filling, it really doesn't make sense to cheat much, because it feels like you're cheating the whole time anyway!

CHAPTER 10

A 14-day example of MediterrAsian living

In our opinion, most diets are destined to fail in the long run for two main reasons: *deprivation and complication*. No matter how much a diet will try to cover up the fact that it's depriving you, deep down they all are—whether it's depriving you of fat, or carbohydrates, or simply food.

What's your first reaction when you're deprived of something? You end up wanting it twice as much, don't you? At the same time, it takes steely discipline to stay on a diet because, invariably, they're complicated and time-consuming.

But compare this to how the peoples of the Mediterranean and Asia having been living for the past few thousand years. Instead of strict diets, they've simply eaten lots of good food until they felt full and satisfied; instead of grueling exercise routines they've simply moved as a consequence of their everyday lives; and they've also made sure to set aside time each day to relax and rejuvenate—by themselves and with the company of friends and loved ones. Talk about the total opposite of deprivation and complication!

And we truly believe it's this *healthy balanced lifestyle*—incorporating wholesome food, natural movement, and emotional calm time—that equates to a healthy body, mind, and spirit and lays down solid foundations for achieving a long, disease-free life.

THE FOURTEEN-DAY PLAN

To give you an example of how to incorporate this healthy balanced lifestyle into your own life, we've designed a fourteen-day plan based on how we live day to day. The plan includes all the meals, snacks, and drinks for a full fourteen days, and it also includes lots of tips and ideas on how you can easily incorporate natural movement and calm time into your daily life.

It's important to remember that this is just an example of how to live. If you want to follow it to the letter that's up to you—but we think a far better approach is to mix and match the meals, and adapt the plan to fit into your own life and your own circumstances.

Breakfast
- A bowl of whole grain breakfast cereal (for example, oatmeal, Bran Flakes®, Wheaties®, All-Bran®, Shredded Wheat®, untoasted muesli, and wheatbiscuit cereals such as Weet-bix® and Weetabix®) with soy or regular milk

Lunch
- Sandwich or 6-inch sub on whole grain bread (homemade or store-bought): Tuna, chicken, crab, or turkey with lettuce, tomatoes, sliced onions, cucumber, grated carrot, peppers or other vegetables and mustard, mayo, olives, pickles, or preserved chili as flavor enhancers

- 1 fresh peach

Dinner
- Pesto Chicken Pizza (page 172)

Dessert
- 2 sliced kiwi fruit topped with a scoop of your favorite ice cream

Snacks
- Choose 2-3 separate snacks from the MediterrAsian-Friendly Snacks list on page 127 and enjoy them throughout the day between meals.

Beverages
- 1 to 2 cups of tea or coffee
- 1 to 2 glasses of wine or beer
- Plenty of water

Natural Movement
- Be physically active for at least 20 minutes. Choose from the Natural Movement Ideas on page 71, or come up with your own.

Calm Time
- Physically and emotionally relax for at least 30 minutes. Choose from the Calm Time Ideas on page 89, or come up with your own.

▶ Day 2

Breakfast
- Half a medium can of baked beans, heated and served on two slices of lightly buttered whole grain toast

- 1 fresh orange

Lunch
- Savory Salmon Spread Sandwich: Spread 2 tablespoons of Savory Salmon Spread (page 292) on a slice of whole grain bread. Top with 4 sliced cucumber rounds and half a cup of shredded lettuce. Sandwich together with another slice of whole grain bread and cut in half to serve.

- A small bunch of grapes

Dinner
- Lemony Tuna, Olive, and Vegetable Pasta (page 145)

Dessert
- Pears with Peach Ricotta Whip and Almonds (page 308)

Snacks
- Choose 2-3 separate snacks from the MediterrAsian-Friendly Snacks list on page 127 and enjoy them throughout the day between meals.

Beverages
- 1 to 2 cups of tea or coffee
- 1 to 2 glasses of wine or beer
- Plenty of water

Natural Movement
- Be physically active for at least 20 minutes. Choose from the Natural Movement Ideas on page 71, or come up with your own.

Calm Time
- Physically and emotionally relax for at least 30 minutes. Choose from the Calm Time Ideas on page 89, or come up with your own.

▶ Day 3

Breakfast
- Tomato and cheese toasts: Toast two slices of whole grain bread and melt a little sliced cheese on top, then arrange some sliced tomato on top and garnish with salt and freshly ground black pepper.

- 1 apple

Lunch
- Turkish Chickpea Salad Wrap (page 244)

- 6 dried apricots

Dinner
- Mushroom, Bacon, and Walnut Risotto (page 194)

Dessert
- A cup of strawberries topped with ½ cup of Greek yogurt and 1 teaspoon honey

Snacks
- Choose 2-3 separate snacks from the MediterrAsian-Friendly Snacks list on page 127 and enjoy them throughout the day between meals.

Beverages
- 1 to 2 cups of tea or coffee
- 1 to 2 glasses of wine or beer
- A glass of freshly-squeezed juice
- Plenty of water

Natural Movement
- Be physically active for at least 20 minutes. Choose from the Natural Movement Ideas on page 71, or come up with your own.

Calm Time
- Physically and emotionally relax for at least 30 minutes. Choose from the Calm Time Ideas on page 89, or come up with your own.

▶ Day 4

Breakfast	• Creamy Fruit and Nut Oatmeal (page 277) • 1 fresh orange
Lunch	• Chicken salad sandwich: Combine 5 ounces (140g) shredded cooked chicken breast with sliced tomato, shredded lettuce, sliced cucumber, and a tablespoon of mayo on multigrain bread (2 slices). • ¼ small cantaloupe (rockmelon)
Dinner	• Shrimp, Bok Choy, and Snow Pea Stir-Fry (page 156)
Dessert	• 1 sliced banana topped with a scoop of your favorite ice cream
Snacks	• Choose 2-3 separate snacks from the MediterrAsian-Friendly Snacks list on page 127 and enjoy them throughout the day between meals.
Beverages	• 1 to 2 cups of tea or coffee • 1 to 2 glasses of wine or beer • Plenty of water
Natural Movement	• Be physically active for at least 20 minutes. Choose from the Natural Movement Ideas on page 71, or come up with your own.
Calm Time	• Physically and emotionally relax for at least 30 minutes. Choose from the Calm Time Ideas on page 89, or come up with your own.

▶ Day 5

Breakfast	• Sardine Toast Topper (page 275) • 1 tangerine
Lunch	• Go to a sushi bar and order 8 pieces of sushi and a bowl of miso soup; finish with a simple fresh fruit salad.
Dinner	• Moroccan Stew with Couscous (page 187)
Dessert	• Tunisian Orange, Date, and Pistachio Salad (page 309)
Snacks	• Choose 2-3 separate snacks from the MediterrAsian-Friendly Snacks list on page 127 and enjoy them throughout the day between meals.
Beverages	• 1 to 2 cups of tea or coffee • 1 to 2 glasses of wine or beer • Plenty of water
Natural Movement	• Be physically active for at least 20 minutes. Choose from the Natural Movement Ideas on page 71, or come up with your own.
Calm Time	• Physically and emotionally relax for at least 30 minutes. Choose from the Calm Time Ideas on page 89, or come up with your own.

▶ Day 6

Breakfast	• Italian-Style Scrambled Eggs (page 273)
	• A small handful of cherries
Lunch	• Savory Tuna Melt: Toast 2 slices of whole grain bread, then top each slice with 2 tablespoons of Savory Tuna Spread (page 293) and a little sliced cheddar cheese. Place under a hot broiler for a minute, or until the cheese is bubbling and golden brown.
	• 6 dried apricots
Dinner	• Night out at a Mediterranean or Asian restaurant (such as Greek, Italian, Chinese, Spanish, Japanese, Indian, Thai, and Moroccan): Order traditional dishes based around fish, seafood, chicken, legumes, grains, and vegetables.
Dessert	• Choose a fruit-based dessert.
Snacks	• Choose 2-3 separate snacks from the MediterrAsian-Friendly Snacks list on page 127 and enjoy them throughout the day between meals.
Beverages	• 1 to 2 cups of tea or coffee
	• 1 to 2 glasses of wine or beer
	• Plenty of water
Natural Movement	• Be physically active for at least 20 minutes. Choose from the Natural Movement Ideas on page 71, or come up with your own.
Calm Time	• Physically and emotionally relax for at least 30 minutes. Choose from the Calm Time Ideas on page 89, or come up with your own.

Breakfast	• Toast two slices of whole grain bread, each slice topped with a tablespoon of natural peanut butter. • 1 nectarine
Lunch	• Chicken and Avocado Salad Wraps: Spread 1 tablespoon of mayonnaise in a horizontal line down the middle of a whole grain flat bread (such as pocketless pita bread or a flour tortilla). Arrange ½ cup of shredded pre-cooked chicken breast, ½ cup of torn lettuce, ¼ sliced avocado, 1 tablespoon of finely chopped green bell pepper and ½ of a sliced tomato evenly on top. Season with salt and pepper and roll up. • 2 kiwi fruit
Dinner	• Salmon Kedgeree (page 199)
Dessert	• 1 sliced banana topped with ½ cup of Greek yogurt and a teaspoon of honey
Snacks	• Choose 2-3 separate snacks from the MediterrAsian-Friendly Snacks list on page 127 and enjoy them throughout the day between meals.
Beverages	• 1 to 2 cups of tea or coffee • 1 to 2 glasses of wine or beer • Plenty of water
Natural Movement	• Be physically active for at least 20 minutes. Choose from the Natural Movement Ideas on page 71, or come up with your own.
Calm Time	• Physically and emotionally relax for at least 30 minutes. Choose from the Calm Time Ideas on page 89, or come up with your own.

▶ Day 8

Breakfast
- Bruschetta with Tomato, Mozzarella, and Anchovy (page 245)

- 1 sliced apple

Lunch
- Savory Tuna Spread Sandwich: Spread 2 tablespoons of Savory Tuna Spread (293) on a slice of whole grain bread. Top with 4 sliced cucumber rounds and half a cup of shredded lettuce. Sandwich together with another slice of multigrain bread and cut in half to serve.

- 3 plums

Dinner
- Tofu and cashew chow mein (page 209)

Dessert
- Asian-style fruit Salad (page 311)

Snacks
- Choose 2-3 separate snacks from the MediterrAsian-Friendly Snacks list on page 127 and enjoy them throughout the day between meals.

Beverages
- 1 to 2 cups of tea or coffee
- 1 to 2 glasses of wine or beer
- Plenty of water
- A glass of freshly-squeezed juice

Natural Movement
- Be physically active for at least 20 minutes. Choose from the Natural Movement Ideas on page 71, or come up with your own.

Calm Time
- Physically and emotionally relax for at least 30 minutes. Choose from the Calm Time Ideas on page 89, or come up with your own.

Breakfast
- A bowl of whole grain breakfast cereal (for example, oatmeal, Bran Flakes®, Wheaties®, All-Bran®, Shredded Wheat®, untoasted muesli, and wheatbiscuit cereals such as Weet-bix® and Weetabix®) with soy or regular milk

Lunch
- Curried Egg and Salad Sandwich: In a small bowl mash 1 hard-boiled egg with a fork and stir in ½ tablespoon of mayonnaise, ¼ teaspoon of curry powder, and a pinch each of salt and pepper until well combined. Spread the curried egg mixture evenly over 1 slice of whole grain bread and top with ½ cup shredded lettuce and half a grated carrot. Sandwich together with another whole grain bread slice and cut in half to serve.

- 1 mandarin

Dinner
- Sicilian Tuna and Basil Pizza (page 171)

Dessert
- Mango with Lime Syrup and Toasted Coconut (page 305)

Snacks
- Choose 2-3 separate snacks from the MediterrAsian-Friendly Snacks list on page 127 and enjoy them throughout the day between meals.

Beverages
- 1 to 2 cups of tea or coffee
- 1 to 2 glasses of wine or beer
- Plenty of water

Natural Movement
- Be physically active for at least 20 minutes. Choose from the Natural Movement Ideas on page 71, or come up with your own.

Calm Time
- Physically and emotionally relax for at least 30 minutes. Choose from the Calm Time Ideas on page 89, or come up with your own.

▶ Day 10

Breakfast
- Half a medium can of baked beans served on two slices of lightly buttered whole grain toast

- 1 orange

Lunch
- Sandwich or 6-inch sub sandwich on whole grain bread (homemade or store-bought): Tuna, chicken, crab, or turkey with lettuce, tomatoes, sliced onions, cucumber, grated carrot, peppers or other vegetables and mustard, mayo, olives, pickles, or preserved chili as flavor enhancers

- 1 banana

Dinner
- Thai Red Chicken Curry (page 174)

Dessert
- Strawberry and blueberry fruit salad: Combine 6 hulled sliced strawberries, ¼ cup of blueberries, 1 teaspoon of sugar, and a tablespoon of water in a bowl. Toss together and serve with a scoop of your favorite ice cream.

Snacks
- Choose 2-3 separate snacks from the MediterrAsian-Friendly Snacks list on page 127 and enjoy them throughout the day between meals.

Beverages
- 1 to 2 cups of tea or coffee
- 1 to 2 glasses of wine or beer
- Plenty of water

Natural Movement
- Be physically active for at least 20 minutes. Choose from the Natural Movement Ideas on page 71, or come up with your own.

Calm Time
- Physically and emotionally relax for at least 30 minutes. Choose from the Calm Time Ideas on page 89, or come up with your own.

▶ Day 11

Breakfast	• A bowl of oatmeal topped with ½ chopped apple and a sprinkle of cinnamon
	• 1 tangerine
Lunch	• Tuna and Sweet Chili Wraps (page 242)
	• 2 fresh apricots
Dinner	• Pasta Puttanesca (page 143)
Dessert	• Fruit and Nut Platter: Combine ½ sliced apple, 2 dried figs, a handful of grapes, 6 walnut halves, and 10 almonds on a platter
Snacks	• Choose 2-3 separate snacks from the MediterrAsian-Friendly Snacks list on page 127 and enjoy them throughout the day between meals.
Beverages	• 1 to 2 cups of tea or coffee • 1 to 2 glasses of wine or beer • Plenty of water
Natural Movement	• Be physically active for at least 20 minutes. Choose from the Natural Movement Ideas on page 71, or come up with your own.
Calm Time	• Physically and emotionally relax for at least 30 minutes. Choose from the Calm Time Ideas on page 89, or come up with your own.

▶ Day 12

Breakfast
- A bowl of whole grain breakfast cereal (for example, oatmeal, Bran Flakes®, Wheaties®, All-Bran®, Shredded Wheat®, untoasted muesli, and wheatbiscuit cereals such as Weet-bix® and Weetabix®) with soy or regular milk, topped with strawberries or blueberries

Lunch
- Italian-Style Chicken Sandwich with Pesto Mayonnaise (page 239)

- 1 banana

Dinner
- Salad plate with canned salmon: Arrange 5 ounces (140g) of canned Alaskan salmon on a plate with 1 tomato (cut into wedges), 10 cucumber slices, a handful of your favorite lettuce, ½ grated carrot, 6 kalamata olives, and 4 red onion slices. Drizzle the vegetables with a tablespoon each of balsamic vinegar and extra virgin olive oil, and season with sea salt and freshly ground black pepper. Serve with a thick slice of crusty whole grain bread on the side.

Dessert
- Strawberries and Mascarpone Cheese (page 309)

Snacks
- Choose 2-3 separate snacks from the MediterrAsian-Friendly Snacks list on page 127 and enjoy them throughout the day between meals.

Beverages
- 1 to 2 cups of tea or coffee
- 1 to 2 glasses of wine or beer
- Plenty of water

Natural Movement
- Be physically active for at least 20 minutes. Choose from the Natural Movement Ideas on page 71, or come up with your own.

Calm Time
- Physically and emotionally relax for at least 30 minutes. Choose from the Calm Time Ideas on page 89, or come up with your own.

Breakfast	• Tuna, Pea and Corn Frittata (page 275)
	• 1 orange
Lunch	• Vegetable and Almond Soup: Heat up ½ can of good-quality store-bought vegetable soup; when warm, transfer to a blender and add 2 tablespoons of almond meal, blend, then reheat and serve in a bowl with a thick slice of whole grain country bread.
	• 1 peach
Dinner	• Night out at a Mediterranean or Asian restaurant (such as Greek, Italian, Chinese, Spanish, Japanese, Indian, Thai, and Moroccan). Order traditional dishes based around fish, seafood, chicken, legumes, grains, and vegetables.
Dessert	• Choose a fruit-based dessert.
Snacks	• Choose 2-3 separate snacks from the MediterrAsian-Friendly Snacks list on page 127 and enjoy them throughout the day between meals.
Beverages	• 1 to 2 cups of tea or coffee
	• 1 to 2 glasses of wine or beer
	• Plenty of water
Natural Movement	• Be physically active for at least 20 minutes. Choose from the Natural Movement Ideas on page 71, or come up with your own.
Calm Time	• Physically and emotionally relax for at least 30 minutes. Choose from the Calm Time Ideas on page 89, or come up with your own.

▶ Day 14

Breakfast
- Smoked Salmon Bruschetta (page 272)

- A handful of cherries

Lunch
- Ham salad sandwich: Combine a thin slice of ham with sliced tomato, shredded lettuce, a little diced red onion, and a teaspoon of your favorite mustard on lightly buttered whole grain bread (2 slices).

- 1 nectarine

Dinner
- Japanese-Style Grilled Marinated Tuna (page 236) with Japanese Soba Noodle Salad (page 261)

Dessert
- Mango, Grape, and Honeydew Melon Salad (page 308) served with ½ cup Greek yogurt and a teaspoon of honey

Snacks
- Choose 2-3 separate snacks from the MediterrAsian-Friendly Snacks list on page 127 and enjoy them throughout the day between meals.

Beverages
- 1 to 2 cups of tea or coffee
- 1 to 2 glasses of wine or beer
- Plenty of water
- A glass of freshly-squeezed juice

Natural Movement
- Be physically active for at least 20 minutes. Choose from the Natural Movement Ideas on page 71, or come up with your own.

Calm Time
- Physically and emotionally relax for at least 30 minutes. Choose from the Calm Time Ideas on page 89, or come up with your own.

▶ MediterrAsian-Friendly Snack Ideas

- Piece of fruit (such as an orange, apple, pear or peach)
- Small bowl of fresh fruit salad topped with a little fruit yogurt
- Handful of berries like strawberries or raspberries
- Wedge of melon
- Small bunch of grapes
- Handful of cherries
- Small fruit platter
- Sliced apple or pear with a little thinly sliced Parmesan cheese
- Mashed banana spread on a slice of whole grain bread or a whole grain cracker and dusted lightly with cinnamon
- ½ cup Greek yogurt with 1 teaspoon honey
- Handful of dried figs and pistachios
- Handful of dried dates and walnuts
- Handful of dried apricots and cashew nuts
- Handful of nuts (such as walnuts, almonds, cashews, peanuts, pistachios, and macadamias)
- Handful of slivered or flaked almonds and raisins
- Handful of toasted sunflower seeds
- Handful of pecans served with a little blue cheese (like gorgonzola)
- Handful of trail mix
- Whole grain cracker topped with a little thinly sliced sharp cheese, sliced tomato, sea salt, and freshly ground black pepper
- Whole grain cracker topped with smoked salmon, capers, dill, sea salt, freshly ground black pepper, and drizzled with lemon juice
- Whole grain cracker topped with 1 tablespoon of Savory Salmon Spread (page 292) or Savory Tuna Spread (page 293)
- Whole grain cracker topped with ricotta cheese and sun-dried tomatoes
- Whole grain cracker topped with a little goat cheese and sliced stuffed green olives
- Slice of whole grain bread or toast topped with 2 teaspoons of natural peanut butter
- Piece of bruschetta spread lightly with pesto
- Half dozen cherry tomatoes with 1 ounce (30 grams) of cubed cheddar cheese
- 6 olives and a little thinly sliced sharp cheese
- 3 jarred marinated bell pepper strips with a little finely sliced Parmesan cheese
- 8 canned smoked oysters
- 1 carrot, halved and spread with 1 tablespoon hummus
- Half a small can of baby shrimp wrapped in a lettuce leaf with half a sliced tomato and a teaspoon of mayonnaise
- Half a small can of tuna with sliced tomato and 4 olives
- Handful of pita wedges dipped in a little hummus
- Vegetable crudités served with a little hummus
- 2 dolmades (stuffed grape leaves)
- Handful of pretzels
- Cup of air-popped popcorn (popcorn is a whole grain!)
- Boiled egg lightly sprinkled with sea salt
- ⅓ cup cold baked beans
- Small bowl of your favorite whole grain breakfast cereal
- ½ ounce (15g) high-quality dark chocolate

CHAPTER 11

Living the MediterrAsian way: 11 lifestyle scenarios

Here are eleven lifestyle scenarios that show you how a MediterrAsian way of living can easily be adapted and customized to fit into any lifestyle, and any situation. These scenarios also highlight how fun, easy, and flexible it is to follow a MediterrAsian way of living on a day-to-day basis.

Relaxing Weekend at Home

Morning

BREAKFAST: For a breakfast with an Italian twist this morning, make Italian-Style Scrambled Eggs (page 273). Enjoy a good strong cup of coffee and finish off with a bowl of grapes topped with a dollop of fruit yogurt.

CALM TIME: Visit the library and browse for books. The quiet serenity of the library is a real break from noise pollution. Look for some interesting cookbooks based on Mediterranean and Asian cuisine for recipe ideas.

SNACK: 3 dried figs make the perfect chewy sweet treat.

Afternoon

LUNCH: Enjoy the beautiful weather by having an outdoor barbecue for lunch. Instead of the usual grilled beef steak and sausages, opt for grilled salmon steak and tender grilled shrimp. Serve this with a crusty whole grain roll and mixed salad leaves drizzled with a little extra virgin olive oil and balsamic vinegar. And what better way to wash down a hot barbecue than with a glass of icy cold beer. Finish the barbecue with some fresh sliced melon.

NATURAL MOVEMENT: After lunch has had a little time to go down, head to the local park with a friend and play Frisbee.

SNACK: A handful of creamy macadamia nuts will keep hunger at bay until dinner.

Evening

DINNER AND DESSERT: For something quick and tasty, cook up a Fragrant Shrimp and Vegetable Stir-Fry (page 163) Follow this with some sliced kiwi fruit and banana topped with a scoop of favorite ice cream.

NATURAL MOVEMENT: Before it gets dark, walk the dog and check out the beautiful sunset on the way home.

SNACK: A handful of pretzels.

CALM TIME: Dust off your old photo albums and have a nostalgic look through your past.

Hectic Weekend at Home

Morning

BREAKFAST: A Sardine Toast Topper (page 275) served with fresh juice and followed by some crispy sliced apple will make the perfect energy-filled start to the day.

NATURAL MOVEMENT: The first jobs of the day are to mow the lawn and get rid of some of those weeds that have accumulated in the backyard.

SNACK: Gardening is hungry work, so grab a handful of almonds and enjoy a refreshing mango.

Afternoon

NATURAL MOVEMENT: As part of your hectic day you have to do some shopping at the mall. As you drive into the parking lot you see dozens of people circling around trying to find the closest spot. Simply park at the far end of the lot and walk the extra distance. The people who are circling the mall look on jealously as you enter the mall before them.

LUNCH: At the mall pop into a sandwich shop and have them assemble a big MediterrAsian-balanced sandwich with roast chicken, peppers, tomatoes, pickles, lettuce, olives, mustard, and a little mayo on whole grain bread.

CALM TIME AND NATURAL MOVEMENT: After lunch, take ten minutes for yourself and window-shop your favorite stores.

SNACK: A juicy mandarin not only makes a sweet snack, it also quenches your thirst after all that exhausting window shopping.

Evening

DINNER AND DESSERT: Take a break from cooking tonight, and order in a MediterrAsian-balanced meal from the local Chinese restaurant instead, and wash it down with a cold beer. For dessert, carry on the Asian theme and have a fortune cookie, then some canned lychees and pineapple in natural juice with a scoop of your favorite ice cream.

SNACK: A couple of thin slices of sharp cheddar cheese and half a dozen olives.

CALM TIME: About 20 minutes before bedtime, find a quite place in the house by yourself, light a candle and incense, put on some soft music, and meditate. This not only calms your mind and helps you reconnect with your spirit, it also sets you up for an extra sound sleep.

Busy Work Day

Morning

BREAKFAST: Today is a busy day—deadlines are backing up and time is scarce, but it is important to be mentally focused for the busy day ahead, so quickly have a bowl of muesli topped with sliced kiwi fruit.

NATURAL MOVEMENT: You can't afford to get stuck in traffic and be late for work, so catch the bus instead. The five-minute walk to the bus stop isn't only a good opportunity for some natural movement, it also provides a chance to gather your thoughts for the day ahead. At work, instead of taking the elevator, simply walk up the four flights of stairs.

SNACK: Mid-morning, enjoy a biscotti and a cup of coffee.

Afternoon

LUNCH: Lunchtime and there's no time to lose. You need to keep your energy up and your hunger at bay—but there's only a short time for lunch, so pop into a Lebanese takeout and grab a pita bread stuffed with falafel, salad, and hummus, and drizzled with a little chili sauce. While still out and about, pop into the deli and grab a handful of succulent cherries for a sweet finish.

CALM TIME: On the way back to work, stop at the park for five minutes and take in the fresh air, the sounds of the birds singing, and the wonderful colors of nature.

SNACK: It's mid-afternoon and time to satisfy an attack of the munchies. A handful of cashew nuts and a dozen grapes soon fix that problem.

NATURAL MOVEMENT: Walk from work to the bus stop, then at the other end walk from the local bus stop to home.

Evening

DINNER AND DESSERT: Arriving home exhausted, you simply order in a MediterrAsian-friendly pizza. To accompany the meal have a glass of red wine, and for dessert enjoy some sliced strawberries with topped with ½ cup of fruit yogurt.

CALM TIME: It's been a taxing day. After dinner fill a large bowl with hot water, add a few drops of aromatherapy oil, and soak your feet for 20 minutes.

SNACK: A whole grain cracker topped with some thinly sliced cheese, sliced tomato, and a little freshly ground pepper and sea salt.

Relaxed Work Day

Morning

BREAKFAST: For something hot and sweet this morning, make a bowl of Creamy Oatmeal Fruit and Nut Oatmeal (page 277) and accompany it with a cup of coffee.

SNACK: A handful of mixed nuts and a glass of fresh juice satisfy the mid-morning munchies.

LUNCH: Take a little extra time in the morning to make a Curried Egg and Salad Sandwich (page 121) and keep it in the staff refrigerator to enjoy at lunch. Follow this with 6 fresh strawberries.

Afternoon

NATURAL MOVEMENT: Instead of talking to colleagues on the phone or via e-mail, walk up and down the stairs to talk to them. Not only does this slip in some natural movement, but it's nice to have the extra bit of human contact.

CALM TIME: At lunchtime, pop into a day spa close to work and have a rejuvenating 20-minute neck and shoulder massage.

SNACK: Treat yourself to 2 squares of good-quality dark chocolate.

NATURAL MOVEMENT: Straight after work, meet up with a friend and play a bit of tennis at your local sports club.

Evening

DINNER AND DESSERT: Quickly whip up some Pasta with Arugula, Fava Beans & Prosciutto (page 152) and serve it with a simple green salad and a glass of red wine. For dessert have a slice of fruit cake.

SNACK: A cup of air-popped popcorn.

CALM TIME: Snuggle up in bed with your favorite book and slowly drift off to sleep.

Weekday with the Kids

Morning

BREAKFAST: It's got to be something quick and nourishing this morning, so enjoy a bowl of Raisin, Apricot, and Almond Muesli (page 279).

NATURAL MOVEMENT: Walk to the bus stop to see your older kids off to school. Take along the youngest in a stroller, which adds intensity to the walk.

SNACK: While out and about, pop into the store and pick up a small bag of jellybeans.

NATURAL MOVEMENT: There's lots of energetic cleaning and tidying around the house to be done, including making beds, picking up toys, hanging out the washing, and vacuuming the floors.

Afternoon

LUNCH: For lunch thaw some frozen precooked shrimp in hot water for five minutes and make up a shrimp and salad sandwich on whole grain bread. For a sweet finish have three fresh, juicy plums.

CALM TIME AND NATURAL MOVEMENT: With the chores out of the way it gives you a good opportunity to have a relaxing play with the little one.

SNACK: A slice of whole grain bread spread with natural peanut butter.

Evening

DINNER AND DESSERT: Use that premade fresh pesto purchased from the deli this morning when you walked the kids to the bus stop to quickly make up Pesto Pasta with Salmon, Broccoli, and Roasted Red Pepper (page 148). Accompany this with a glass of red wine. For dessert enjoy some Mango, Grape, and Honeydew Melon Salad (page 308) served with a scoop of gelato.

CALM TIME: While your other half looks after the kids, pop away into the bedroom, open up your soul, and write down your thoughts, feelings, and observations in a private journal.

SNACK: Over a favorite TV show, enjoy a handful of pistachio nuts and 4 dried dates.

Weekend with the Kids

Morning

BREAKFAST: For a quick, hearty, and healthy breakfast that everyone will enjoy, make up some baked beans on whole grain toast. Wash this down with a cold glass of orange juice and finish off with a fresh peach.

NATURAL MOVEMENT: The car is looking pretty grubby and the kids are looking bored—what a great opportunity to fix both problems at once and clean the car together! Not only will the car end up clean and shiny, you'll also have lots of fun getting wet and having water fights in the process.

SNACK: A small piece of lightly buttered fruit cake with a cup of tea is just what's needed to see you through to lunchtime.

Afternoon

LUNCH: For lunch, keep the kids happy by making Whole Wheat Pita Pockets with Chicken, Hummus and Mediterranean Salsa (page 244), but get the kids involved in the preparation and cooking. This isn't only a good bonding experience—it also cuts cooking time in half! After lunch enjoy ½ cup of strawberry yogurt.

NATURAL MOVEMENT: After lunch take the kids to the local zoo and have a good walk around checking out all the different animals.

SNACK: A handful of cashews will satisfy your hunger and help keep energy levels up.

CALM TIME: Late afternoon call up a close friend and have a relaxing chat.

Evening

DINNER AND DESSERT: Make a Sicilian Tuna and Basil Pizza (page 171), and wash it down with a glass of red wine. For dessert have something fun and colorful—chunks of papaya and pineapple topped with Greek yogurt and passionfruit.

CALM TIME: After dinner surf the net with the kids.

SNACK: A handful of Brazil nuts.

Dinner Party

Morning

BREAKFAST: Dinner guests will be arriving at 7:30 P.M., and the predinner party jitters make the thought of eating a big breakfast unappealing. But you need plenty of energy for the day ahead, so have a small bowl of your favorite whole grain cereal topped with sliced strawberries.

NATURAL MOVEMENT: The place needs a good dust and tidy up before the guests arrive so pop on your cleaning clothes and set to work transforming your house through a "cardio-cleaning blitz."

SNACK: Relax for 10 minutes and have a biscotti with a cup of coffee.

Afternoon

LUNCH: Whip up a tuna sandwich with lettuce and tomato on whole grain bread, then finish with a juicy nectarine.

NATURAL MOVEMENT: Time to grab some last-minute fresh ingredients from the local store. Instead of spending time warming up the car, opening and closing the garage door, and having to find a parking spot at the other end, walk instead (it's only a 15-minute round trip on foot anyway and it's nice to get some fresh air after being stuck in the house all morning). At the store, pick up a copy of your favorite magazine.

CALM TIME: After finishing the cleaning and other chores, there's still plenty of time before you need to start preparing for the night ahead. So slip away into the peace and calm of the bedroom and have a 20-minute browse through the magazine you picked up at the store.

SNACK: A handful of almonds and a small bunch of grapes boost energy for the dinner preparation and help to keep you mentally focused for the night ahead.

DINNER AND DESSERT: All week you've been thinking about what food to serve at the dinner party. Opt for a Mediterranean theme—Greek—and serve Greek Shrimp with Feta (page 183) and Greek Salad (page 261) with fresh crusty bread. For dessert it has to be something sweet and yummy, so try Mixed Berry Coulis with Greek Vanilla Yogurt (page 310).

Everyone at the dinner party thinks you've been slaving away in the kitchen all day, but little do they know it's taken only a little over an hour to prepare and cook the lot. And no one can believe that the decadent and delicious food they're eating is also incredibly good for them.

SNACK: Too full from dinner to even contemplate having something to eat? Instead have a soothing cup of antioxidant-rich tea.

CALM TIME: It's been a tiring but ultimately very exhilarating day. Reflect on the successful night while having a long, hot, calming soak in the shower.

Romantic Weekend

Morning

BREAKFAST: For a special breakfast for you and your loved one, prepare scrambled eggs with smoked salmon on whole grain English muffins. Accompany this with coffee and juice.

CALM TIME: Relax into the morning by reading the local weekend paper, paying particular interest to the food, social, travel, and living sections.

SNACK: A crunchy sliced apple and a little thinly sliced Parmesan cheese.

Afternoon

LUNCH: Go for a long drive to somewhere scenic and relaxing and find a pretty, grassy area and set up a picnic blanket. For your romantic picnic have an Italian-Style Chicken Sandwich with Pesto-Mayonnaise (page 239) and a selection of sliced cheeses, crackers, and fresh and dried fruit, all washed down with a bubbly glass of champagne.

NATURAL MOVEMENT: After lunch make the most of the wonderful outdoors and go for a scenic walk.

SNACK: A handful of walnuts will help get you through to dinner.

Evening

DINNER AND DESSERT: To carry on the romance of the day, go to a restaurant for dinner. The Italian place up the road serves salmon risotto to die for. On the side have some crusty bread drizzled with a little extra virgin olive oil and wash it all down with a glass of red wine. For dessert have something special and order tiramisu (a luxurious dessert made with coffee- and chocolate-infused sponge cakes and mascarpone cheese) accompanied with fresh sliced melon.

CALM TIME AND SNACK: After returning home from dinner, light a couple of candles and a stick of incense and have a nice long soak in the bath with your partner, and feed each other grapes.

NATURAL MOVEMENT: After the bath retire to the bedroom to do what comes naturally!

Party Night

Morning

BREAKFAST: There's a big party tonight but all you can think about right now is how hungry you are for a substantial and savory breakfast. So make an Italian-Style Pan-Fried Sandwich (page 279) and wash it down with a cup of coffee. Afterward have 3 juicy plums.

CALM TIME: Sink back in a comfy chair and have a relaxing read for 20 minutes.

SNACK: A handful of almonds.

NATURAL MOVEMENT: Because there might be some dancing at the party tonight, get in a little practice—pop on your favorite music and dance around the house.

Afternoon

LUNCH: For lunch heat up a bowl of Minestrone Soup (page 252), frozen from when you made it a fortnight ago. Finish with a sliced banana topped with a dollop of fruit yogurt.

CALM TIME: To relax your body and calm your mind before the party tonight, put on some loose and comfortable clothes, lay a towel down on the floor, and practice yoga for 20 minutes.

SNACK: A handful or two of pretzels.

Evening

DINNER AND DESSERT: There are going to be lots of snacks at the party so have a relatively light dinner and put together a Salade Niçoise (page 269) with a little crusty whole grain bread on the side. For dessert opt for something easy and simply have an orange.

SNACK: For the party bring along a selection of vegetable crudités accompanied with homemade hummus (page 288) for dipping. You end up going a little overboard on your alcohol intake, but that's fine because parties only happen occasionally, and besides you'll be back to your healthy moderate drinking habits tomorrow.

NATURAL MOVEMENT: Good thing you practiced your dance moves earlier today because as the night wears on and everyone gets more and more relaxed, the evening turns into a dance party!

At 30,000 Feet

Morning

BREAKFAST: You're going on a long flight later today and you realize you'll need lots of energy for packing your bags and lugging them around, so start the day with a generous bowl of Raisin, Apricot, and Almond Muesli (page 279).

CALM TIME: It's a lovely sunny morning so go out into the backyard, stand under the dappled shade of a tree, and relax your mind and body by practicing tai chi.

SNACK: 2 succulent fresh apricots.

NATURAL MOVEMENT: Pack your bags and carry them out to the car.

Afternoon

LUNCH: Don't eat anything too rich before the flight. Luckily there's a Japanese restaurant close to the airport that serves great lunches; so stop in and have a warming bowl of miso soup, a selection of fresh tuna, salmon, and shrimp sushi, and finish with a bowl of fresh fruit salad.

NATURAL MOVEMENT: When you arrive at the airport, carry your bags up to the counter. After you've checked your luggage, have a good walk around the airport checking out the duty-free stores.

SNACK: It's more than an hour until your flight, so grab a small chocolate bar from a newsstand.

Evening

DINNER AND DESSERT: You made sure to request a seafood meal for the flight. Luckily, this means you get your meal before everyone else, and your meal also is healthier and just as tasty. Accompany your meal with a glass of wine.

CALM TIME: Completely relax and make the most of the entertainment on the plane including movies, magazines, and audio broadcasts.

SNACK: Buzz a flight attendant and ask for a package of pretzels.

On Vacation

Morning

BREAKFAST: After a sleep-in, enjoy breakfast at a local café. Order a smoked salmon bagel (spread thinly with cream cheese and topped with dill and capers), some grilled tomatoes, and a cappuccino. Finish with a refreshing fruit salad with a dollop of Greek yogurt.

NATURAL MOVEMENT AND CALM TIME: What better way to familiarize yourself with a new place than a bit of sightseeing. You've thought ahead and already booked a guided walking tour. While on the tour, take lots of photos to capture the memories forever.

SNACK: A handful of sweet and chewy dates.

Afternoon

LUNCH: For something quick and familiar, grab lunch from a burger bar. Instead of going straight for the beef burger with cheese, order something equally tasty but more MediterrAsian-balanced: a grilled chicken burger with lots of salad veggies, including lettuce, tomatoes, onions, and pickles. Finish with a juicy pear.

CALM TIME AND NATURAL MOVEMENT: There are so many new stores to discover and souvenirs to be collected, so go on a relaxing shopping spree.

SNACK: A handful of macadamia nuts and a dozen grapes will provide even more energy for sightseeing and shopping.

Evening

DINNER AND DESSERT: There is no shortage of Chinese, Italian and Indian restaurants nearby. Opt for Indian food and enjoy a spicy shrimp and almond curry served over basmati rice with a vegetable side dish and naan bread. Wash it all down with a glass of cold beer.

CALM TIME: Back at the hotel, relax into the night by watching a funny movie.

SNACK: A small bag of baked corn chips make a great accompaniment to the movie.

CHAPTER 12

PASTA DISHES

Pasta Primavera

SERVES 4-6

A vegetable-packed pasta dish with asparagus, cherry tomatoes, mushrooms, peas, and green beans, combined with toasted pine nuts and topped with Parmesan cheese.

4 tablespoons pine nuts

14 oz (400g) dried pasta of your choice (penne works well)

6 tablespoons extra virgin olive oil

2 red onions, finely chopped

4 cloves garlic, finely chopped

20 cherry tomatoes, halved

16 fresh asparagus spears, bottoms trimmed, cut into 2-inch pieces

24 green beans, ends trimmed, halved

1 cup frozen green peas, thawed

8 button mushrooms, sliced

4 tablespoons finely chopped fresh basil

½ cup white wine

2 teaspoons salt

1 teaspoon freshly ground black pepper

Grated Parmesan cheese

HEAT a skillet over medium heat; add the pine nuts and toast, stirring continuously, then set aside. BRING a large pot of water to a boil. ADD the pasta and cook according to package directions. WHILE the pasta is cooking, heat 4 tablespoons of the olive oil in a large skillet over medium heat and cook the onions, stirring occasionally, for 8 minutes. ADD the garlic and cook for another minute. ADD the tomatoes, asparagus, and green beans and cook, stirring regularly, for 2 minutes. ADD the peas, mushrooms, basil, wine, salt, and pepper; cover the skillet and cook for 5 minutes. ADD the remaining 2 tablespoons of olive oil and the toasted pine nuts and stir to combine all the ingredients. DRAIN the cooked pasta in a colander and put the vegetable mixture in the bottom of the empty pot. TOP with the hot pasta and toss together gently to combine well and heat through. SERVE the pasta topped with a little Parmesan cheese.

Variations: Substitute some or all of the vegetables with broccoli, carrots, zucchini, or fresh corn kernels.

Pasta Puttanesca

SERVES 4-6

Also known as "whore's pasta," this robust pasta dish originated in Naples, named after the local women of easy virtue. All the ingredients are just as easy to get your hands on, making this a quick and satisfying meal!

6 tablespoons extra virgin olive oil

2 onions, finely chopped

4 cloves garlic, finely chopped

8 anchovy fillets, chopped

1 teaspoon dried chili flakes

4 teaspoons capers, rinsed and drained

16 pitted black olives, quartered

28 ounces (800g) canned tomatoes, chopped

1 teaspoon salt

½ teaspoon freshly ground black pepper

14 oz (400g) spaghetti

2 tablespoons finely chopped fresh flat-leaf parsley

BRING a large pot of water to a boil. HEAT 4 tablespoons of the oil in a skillet over medium heat and cook the onions for 8 minutes, stirring occasionally. ADD the garlic and anchovies and cook for 1 minute, stirring to break up the anchovies. ADD the dried chili flakes, capers, olives, tomatoes, salt, and pepper, and bring to a boil. REDUCE the heat to medium-low and simmer, uncovered, for 10 minutes, stirring occasionally. WHILE the sauce is simmering, add the pasta to the boiling water and cook according to package directions. DRAIN the cooked pasta in a colander and put the sauce in the bottom of the empty pot. TOP with the hot pasta, parsley, and reserved 2 tablespoons of olive oil, and toss together gently to combine.

Variation: For a more protein-packed meal, add a 12 ounce (340g) can of tuna (drained and flaked) to the sauce at the end of cooking to heat through.

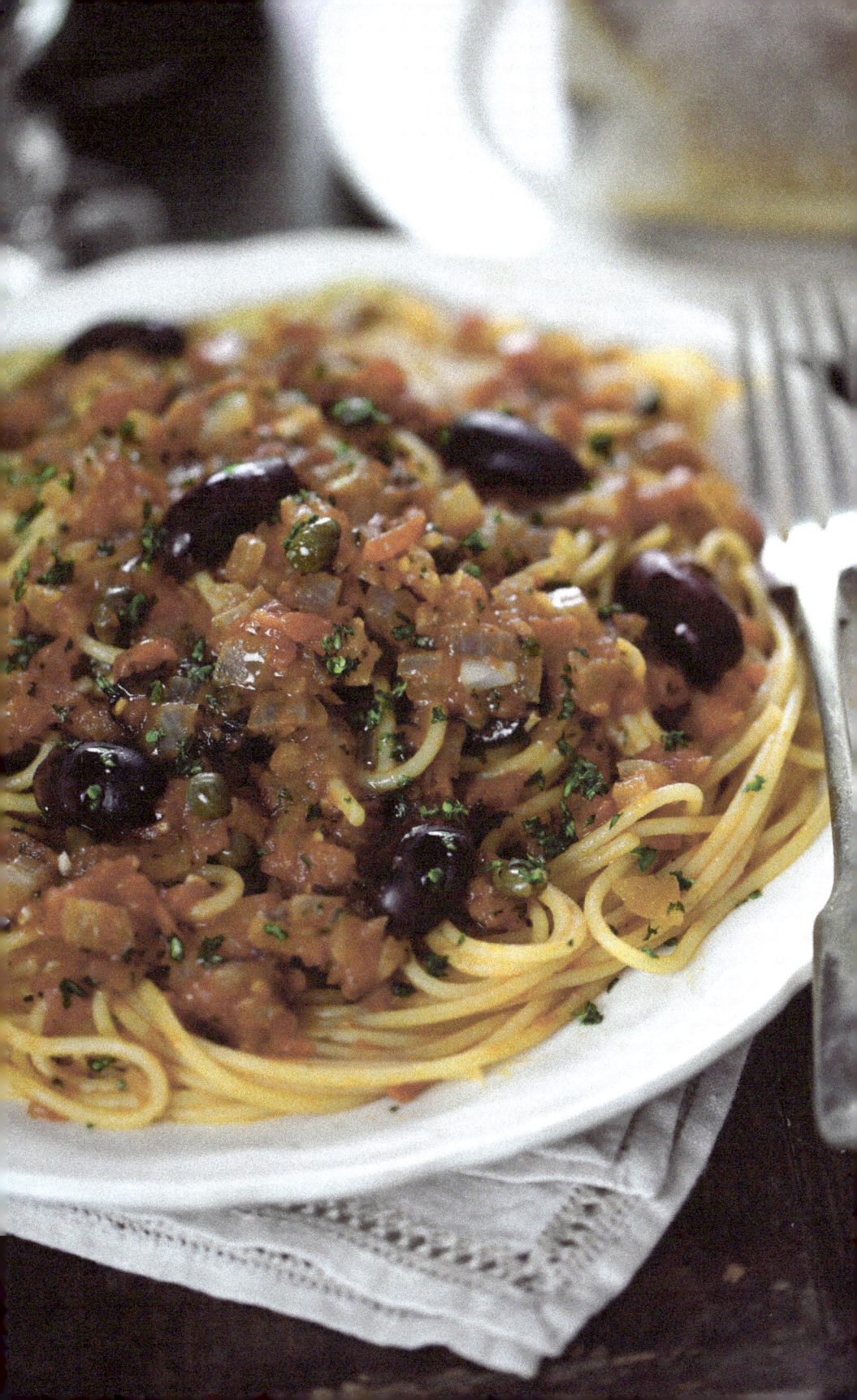

Lemony Tuna, Olive & Vegetable Pasta

SERVES 4-6

This pasta dish is extraordinarily easy to prepare and absolutely delicious to eat. Simply mix the ingredients together in a bowl while the pasta, beans, and red bell peppers cook in the same pot of boiling water. Put the uncooked sauce in the pasta pot and toss with the hot, drained pasta and vegetables to heat through.

14 oz (400g) pasta of your choice (fusilli works well)

24 green beans, ends trimmed and halved

2 red bell peppers, cut into thin strips

12 oz (340g) canned light tuna in olive oil, drained and broken into chunks

6 tablespoons extra virgin olive oil

4 tablespoons freshly squeezed lemon juice

16 pitted black olives, sliced

2 tablespoons chopped fresh flat-leaf parsley

2 tablespoons capers, rinsed, drained, and chopped

2 cloves garlic, minced

1 teaspoon freshly grated lemon zest

1 teaspoon salt

½ teaspoon freshly ground black pepper

BRING a large pot of water to a boil. ADD the pasta and cook according to package directions, adding the green beans and bell peppers to the pot for the final 8 minutes of cooking. WHILE the pasta is cooking, in a small bowl, mix together the tuna, olive oil, lemon juice, olives, parsley, capers, garlic, lemon zest, salt, and pepper. DRAIN the cooked pasta and vegetables in a colander, then put the tuna mixture in the bottom of the empty pot and top with the hot pasta and vegetables. TOSS together gently to combine well and heat through.

Simple Shrimp & Asparagus Pasta

SERVES 4-6

This garlicky shrimp and asparagus pasta can be whipped up in around 20 minutes. Perfect served with with a crisp salad on the side.

14 oz (400g) spaghetti

24 asparagus spears—woody ends removed and spears halved

5 tablespoons extra virgin olive oil

4 garlic cloves—finely chopped

32 large uncooked shrimp—peeled and deveined

2 tablespoons finely chopped fresh flat-leaf parsley

2 teaspoons salt

Lemon wedges for squeezing

BRING a large pot of lightly salted water to a boil. ADD the pasta and cook according to package directions, adding the asparagus to the pot for the final 5 minutes of cooking. WHILE the pasta is cooking, heat the oil in a large frying pan over a medium heat and add the shrimp and garlic. COOK for 3 minutes, tossing regularly. REMOVE from the heat and stir through the parsley and salt. ADD the drained pasta and asparagus and toss together gently to combine well. SERVE with lemon wedges for squeezing.

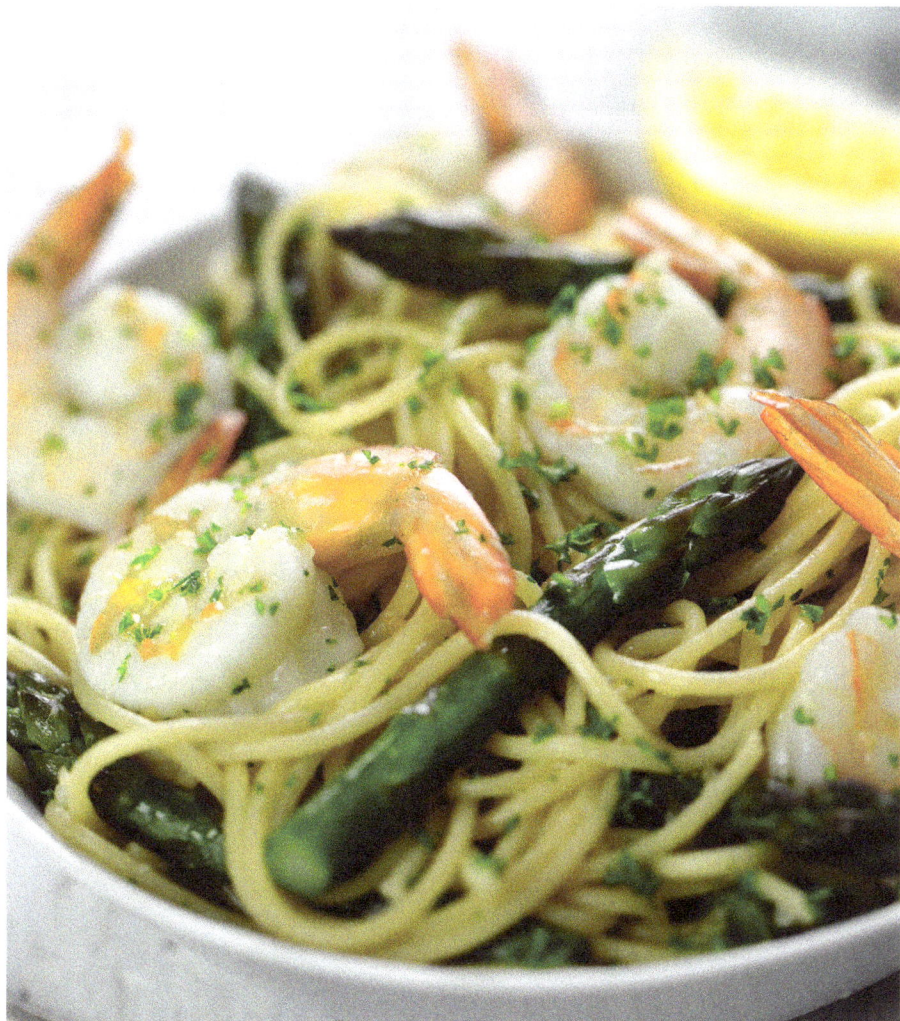

Sicilian Pasta with Broccoli, Raisins, & Pine Nuts

SERVES 4-6

This traditional Sicilian pasta dish combines the saltiness of anchovies with the sweetness of raisins.

4 tablespoons pine nuts

4 tablespoons extra virgin olive oil

2 onions, finely chopped

2 cloves garlic, finely chopped

8 anchovy fillets, chopped

2 cups canned tomatoes, chopped

2 tablespoons tomato paste

4 tablespoons raisins, soaked in ½ cup of hot water while you prepare the other ingredients

1 teaspoon salt

½ teaspoon freshly ground black pepper

14 oz (400g) pasta of your choice (farfalle or penne works well)

4 cups broccoli florets

½ cup grated Parmesan cheese

TOAST the pine nuts in a skillet over medium heat, stirring continuously, than set aside. BRING a large pot of water to a boil. HEAT the olive oil in a skillet over medium heat and cook the onions, stirring occasionally, for 8 minutes. ADD the garlic and anchovies and cook, stirring to break up the anchovies, for 1 minute. ADD the tomatoes, tomato paste, raisins and their soaking water, salt, and pepper. BRING to a boil, cover with a lid, reduce the heat to low, and simmer gently for 10 minutes. WHILE the sauce simmers, add the pasta to the boiling water and cook according to package directions, adding the broccoli to the pot for the final 6 minutes of cooking. DRAIN the cooked pasta and broccoli in a colander and put the sauce in the bottom of the empty pot. TOP with the hot pasta, broccoli, and toasted pine nuts and toss together gently to combine well. SERVE the pasta sprinkled with the Parmesan cheese.

Pesto Pasta with Salmon, Broccoli, & Roasted Red Pepper

SERVES 4-6

This dish takes very little time to prepare and cook, yet it's packed with flavor and nutrients.

14 oz (400g) pasta of your choice (penne or fusilli works well)

24 ounces (700g) uncooked salmon fillet, cut into bite-size pieces

4 cups broccoli florets

½ cup jarred roasted red bell peppers, roughly chopped

1½ cups pesto sauce, homemade (page 285) or store-bought

BRING a large pot of water to a boil. ADD the pasta and cook according to package directions, adding the salmon and broccoli to the pot for the final 5 minutes of cooking. DRAIN the cooked pasta, salmon, and broccoli in a colander, reserving 4 tablespoons of the cooking water in the pot. PUT the bell peppers and pesto in the bottom of the pot and top with the hot pasta, salmon, and broccoli. TOSS together gently to combine well and heat through.

Variation: Replace the salmon with bite-size pieces of chicken breast.

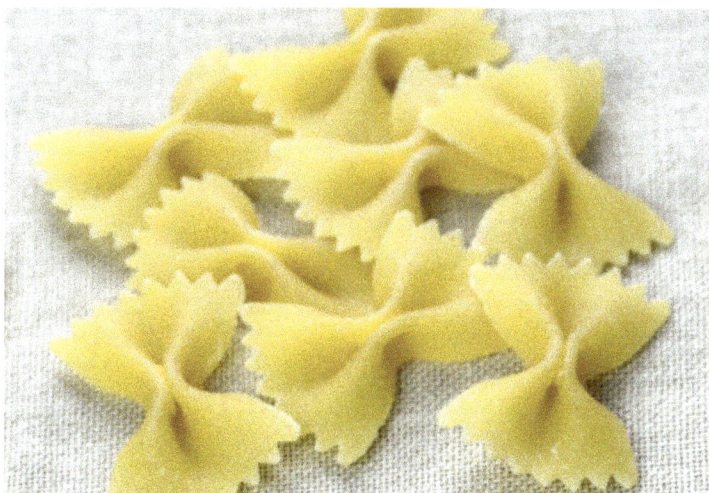

Greek-Style Pasta with White Beans, Walnuts, Spinach & Olives

SERVES 4-6

Pasta isn't something most people associate with Greece, but pasta was actually introduced to the Greeks by the Italians centuries ago and they've been enjoying it ever since. In this Greek-inspired pasta dish the robust flavors of the Kalamata olives and feta are really nicely counterbalanced by the sweet cherry tomatoes and delicately flavored cannellini beans. And the walnuts add a perfect contrasting crunch.

12 oz (340g) penne pasta

14 oz (400g) canned cannellini beans, rinsed and drained

4 cups fresh spinach, roughly chopped

3 cups cherry tomatoes, halved

⅓ cup extra virgin olive oil

3 tablespoons lemon juice

2 garlic cloves, minced

1 teaspoon salt

½ teaspoon freshly ground black pepper

2 tablespoons finely chopped fresh flat-leaf parsley

⅔ cup walnuts (raw or toasted), roughly chopped

16 Kalamata olives, pitted and halved

5 oz (150g) feta cheese, crumbled

COOK the pasta in a large pot of boiling water according to package directions, adding the cannellini beans, spinach and tomatoes in the final 2 minutes of cooking (making sure to bring the water back to a boil before timing the last 2 minutes). WHILE the pasta cooks, mix together the olive oil, lemon juice, garlic, salt, pepper and parsley in a small bowl. DRAIN the pasta, beans and vegetables, reserving 4 tablespoons of the pasta cooking water in bottom of the pot. RETURN the pasta, beans and vegetables to the pot with the dressing and toss gently to mix well. ADD the walnuts and olives and toss together until combined. SERVE with the crumbled feta on top.

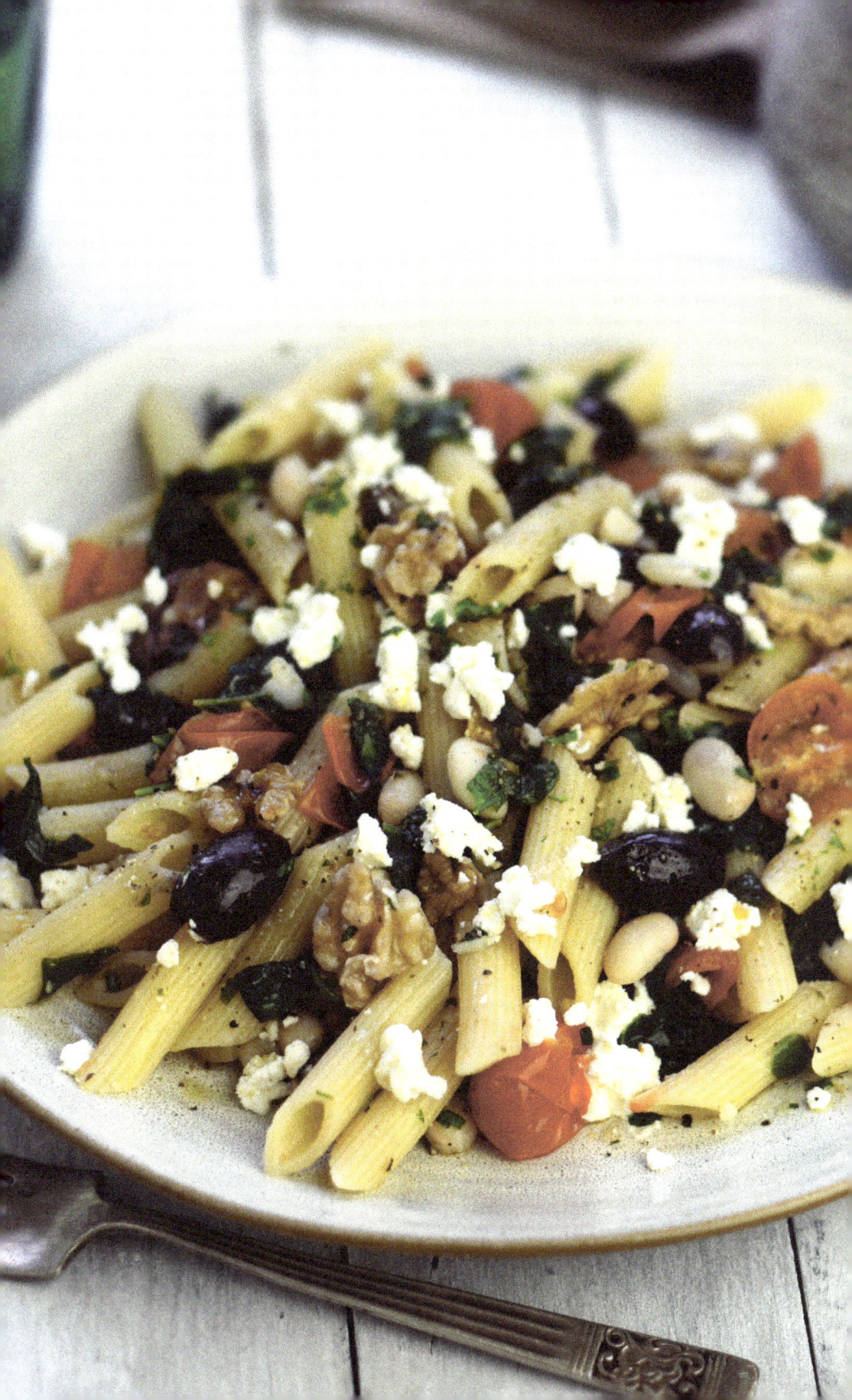

Pasta with Shrimp & Chili

SERVES 4-6

This simple recipe combines shrimp, chilies, and tomatoes with white wine to make a spicy sauce to toss with your favorite pasta.

4 tablespoons extra-virgin olive oil

2 green bell peppers, cut into thin strips

4 cloves garlic, finely chopped

4 small red chilies, deseeded and finely chopped

28 ounces (800g) canned tomatoes, chopped

1 cup white wine

14 oz (400g) pasta of your choice (fettuccine works well)

32 large uncooked shrimp (prawns), peeled

2 teaspoons salt

1 teaspoon freshly ground black pepper

2 tablespoons freshly squeezed lemon juice

2 tablespoons finely chopped fresh flat-leaf parsley

HEAT the olive oil in a skillet over medium heat and cook the bell pepper, stirring occasionally, for 6 minutes. ADD the garlic and chilies and cook for another minute. Add the tomatoes and white wine and simmer for 10 minutes. WHILE the sauce simmers, bring a large pot of water to a boil, add the pasta, and cook according to package directions. ADD the shrimp, salt, and pepper to the sauce and simmer, covered, for 5 minutes more, then stir in the lemon juice and parsley. DRAIN the cooked pasta into a colander and put the tomato-shrimp sauce in the bottom of the empty pot. TOP with the hot pasta and toss together gently to combine well.

Variations: Use scallops instead of shrimp, or replace the wine with good-quality fish stock.

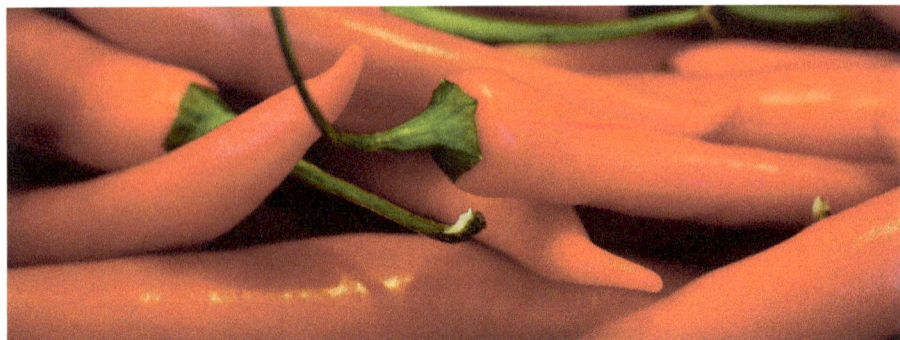

Pasta with Salsa Verde & Smoked Salmon

SERVES 4-6

Salsa verde, a classic Italian green sauce, is simply wonderful tossed with smoked salmon and pasta. The anchovies and smoked salmon in this recipe are good sources of healthy omega-3 fatty acids, and are handy alternatives to fresh fish.

14 oz (400g) pasta of your choice (spaghetti or fettuccine works well)

2 zucchini, cut into ¼-inch rounds

⅔ cup Salsa Verde (page 288)

7 oz (200g) sliced smoked salmon, cut thin into strips

BRING a large pot of water to a boil. ADD the pasta to the boiling water and cook according to package directions, adding the zucchini to the pot for the final 5 minutes of cooking. DRAIN the cooked pasta and zucchini in a colander, reserving 4 tablespoons of cooking water in the pot. PUT the salsa verde and salmon in the bottom of the pot and top with the hot pasta and zucchini. TOSS together gently to combine well and heat through.

Pasta with Arugula, Fava Beans & Prosciutto

SERVES 4-6

This pasta dish uses meat in a traditionally Mediterranean way: in small amounts as a flavor and texture enhancer.

14 oz (400g) pasta of your choice (penne works well)

2 cups frozen fava (broad) beans, thawed, leathery outer skin removed

4 cups arugula (rocket), stems trimmed, leaves washed, and roughly chopped

4 tablespoons extra virgin olive oil

7 oz (200g) thinly sliced prosciutto, chopped

4 cloves garlic, finely chopped

20 pitted black olives, halved

4 tablespoons chopped fresh flat-leaf parsley

1 teaspoon salt

½ teaspoon freshly ground black pepper

½ cup grated Parmesan cheese

BRING a large pot of water to a boil. ADD the pasta to the boiling water and cook according to package directions, adding the fava beans and arugula to the pot for the final 2 minutes of cooking. WHILE the pasta is cooking, heat the oil in a skillet over medium heat and cook the prosciutto and garlic, stirring occasionally, for 2 minutes. DRAIN the cooked pasta, fava beans, and arugula in a colander, reserving 4 tablespoons of cooking water in the pot. PUT the garlic and prosciutto in the bottom of the pot, and top with the hot pasta, fava beans, and arugula. ADD the olives, parsley, salt, and pepper and toss together gently to combine well and heat through. SERVE the pasta sprinkled with the Parmesan cheese.

Pasta with Tuna, Green Beans, Olives & Romesco Sauce

SERVES 4-6

Freshly cooked pasta and green beans are tossed with chunks of tuna, olives, and a robust sauce made with roasted red peppers and toasted almonds, for a pasta dish with a Spanish twist.

14 oz (400g) pasta of your choice (fusilli or penne works well)

32 green beans, ends trimmed, cut in half

2 cups Romesco Sauce (page 283)

12 ounces (340g) canned light meat tuna in olive oil, drained and broken into chunks

24 pitted black olives, halved

BRING a large pot of water to a boil. ADD the pasta to the boiling water and cook according to package directions, adding the green beans to the pot for the final 6 minutes of cooking. DRAIN the cooked pasta and green beans in a colander, reserving 4 tablespoons of cooking water in the pot. PUT the Romesco Sauce in the bottom of the pot and top with the hot pasta, tuna, green beans, and olives. TOSS together gently to combine well and heat through.

Variation: This dish is also delicious with broccoli instead of green beans.

Creamy Chicken, Mushroom, & Sun-Dried Tomato Pasta

SERVES 4-6

A delightfully creamy pasta dish dotted with bite-size pieces of chicken, sliced mushrooms, and sun-dried tomatoes.

14 oz (400g) pasta (farfalle or penne works well)

24 ounces (700g) boneless skinless chicken breasts, cut into bite-size pieces

3 cups broccoli florets

3 tablespoons extra virgin olive oil

2 cups sliced button mushrooms

4 scallions (white and green parts), thinly sliced

4 cloves garlic, finely chopped

3 cups milk

6 tablespoons finely chopped sun-dried tomatoes in oil

2 teaspoons salt

½ teaspoon freshly ground black pepper

1 teaspoon dried rosemary

3 tablespoons cornstarch (corn flour), mixed to a paste with 3 tablespoons water

1 cup grated Parmesan cheese

BRING a large pot of water to a boil. ADD the pasta to the boiling water and cook according to package directions, adding the chicken and broccoli for the final 6 minutes of cooking. WHILE the pasta is cooking, heat the oil in a skillet over medium heat and cook the mushrooms, scallions, and garlic, stirring occasionally, for 3 minutes. ADD the milk, sun-dried tomatoes, salt, pepper, and rosemary and heat until almost boiling. STIR the cornstarch mixture into the hot milk in the skillet and continue stirring until thickened. STIR in the Parmesan cheese until well combined. DRAIN the pasta, chicken, and broccoli in a colander. PUT the hot pasta, chicken, and broccoli in the bottom of the empty pot, top with the creamy sauce, then toss together gently to combine well.

CHAPTER 13

STIR-FRIES

Shrimp, Bok Choy & Snow Pea Stir-Fry

SERVES 4

We've found that bok choy combines perfectly with snow peas and shrimp. So, not surprisingly, this is one of our favorite stir-fry dishes.

1 cup long-grain white rice

6 tablespoons oyster sauce

4 tablespoons soy sauce

2 tablespoons Chinese rice wine (or dry sherry)

2 tablespoons water

2 teaspoons sesame oil

1 tablespoon brown sugar

4 tablespoons peanut or canola oil

32 large uncooked shrimp (prawns), peeled

2 red bell peppers, cut into thin strips

2 bunches bok choy, roughly chopped

32 snow peas, trimmed and halved on the diagonal

4 cloves garlic, finely chopped

BRING 1½ cups of water to a boil in a saucepan. STIR in the rice and keep stirring until the water returns to a boil. COVER the pot with a tight-fitting lid, reduce the heat to very low, and simmer gently for 15 minutes. WHILE the rice cooks, mix together the oyster sauce, soy sauce, Chinese rice wine, water, sesame oil, and sugar in a small bowl. HEAT a wok or large skillet over high heat, add 2 tablespoons of the peanut oil, and stir-fry the shrimp for 2 minutes. REMOVE the shrimp from the wok and set aside on a plate. Heat the remaining oil in the wok and stir-fry the bell pepper for 2 minutes. ADD the bok choy and snow peas and stir-fry for 4 minutes. ADD the garlic and stir-fry for 1 minute, then return the shrimp to the wok. ADD the sauce mixture and mix to heat through. SERVE with the rice.

Chicken, Broccoli & Mushroom Stir-Fry

SERVES 4

Stir-fried chicken, broccoli and mushrooms coated in a fragrant Chinese inspired sauce.

1 cup long-grain white rice

6 tablespoons soy sauce

4 tablespoons hoisin sauce

2 teaspoons toasted sesame oil

2 cups chicken or vegetable stock

2 tablespoons cornstarch (cornflour), mixed to a paste with 2 tablespoons water

4 tablespoons peanut or canola oil

24 oz (700g) uncooked boneless skinless chicken breasts, cut into bite-size pieces

2 heads broccoli, cut into small florets

20 button mushrooms, wiped clean and quartered

2 tablespoons finely grated fresh ginger

4 garlic cloves, finely chopped

BRING 1½ cups of water to a boil in a saucepan. STIR in the rice and keep stirring until the water returns to a boil. COVER the pot with a tight-fitting lid, reduce the heat to very low, and simmer gently for 15 minutes. WHILE the rice cooks, mix together the soy sauce, hoisin sauce, sesame oil and stock in a small bowl. MIX the cornstarch to a paste with 2 tablespoons of water in another small bowl. HEAT a wok or large frying pan over a high heat, add 2 tablespoons of the oil and stir-fry the chicken for 3 minutes. REMOVE the chicken from the wok and set aside on a plate. HEAT the remaining oil in the wok and stir-fry the broccoli for 4 minutes. ADD the mushrooms and stir-fry for 2 minutes. ADD the ginger and garlic and stir-fry for 1 minute. RETURN the cooked chicken to the wok then, stirring continuously, add the sauce mixture and cornstarch paste until the sauce is heated through. SERVE with the rice.

Variations: You can make this stir-fry with fresh tuna, shrimp, squid or tofu in place of chicken. Add a handful of cashews or almonds, or use green beans or snow peas instead of broccoli.

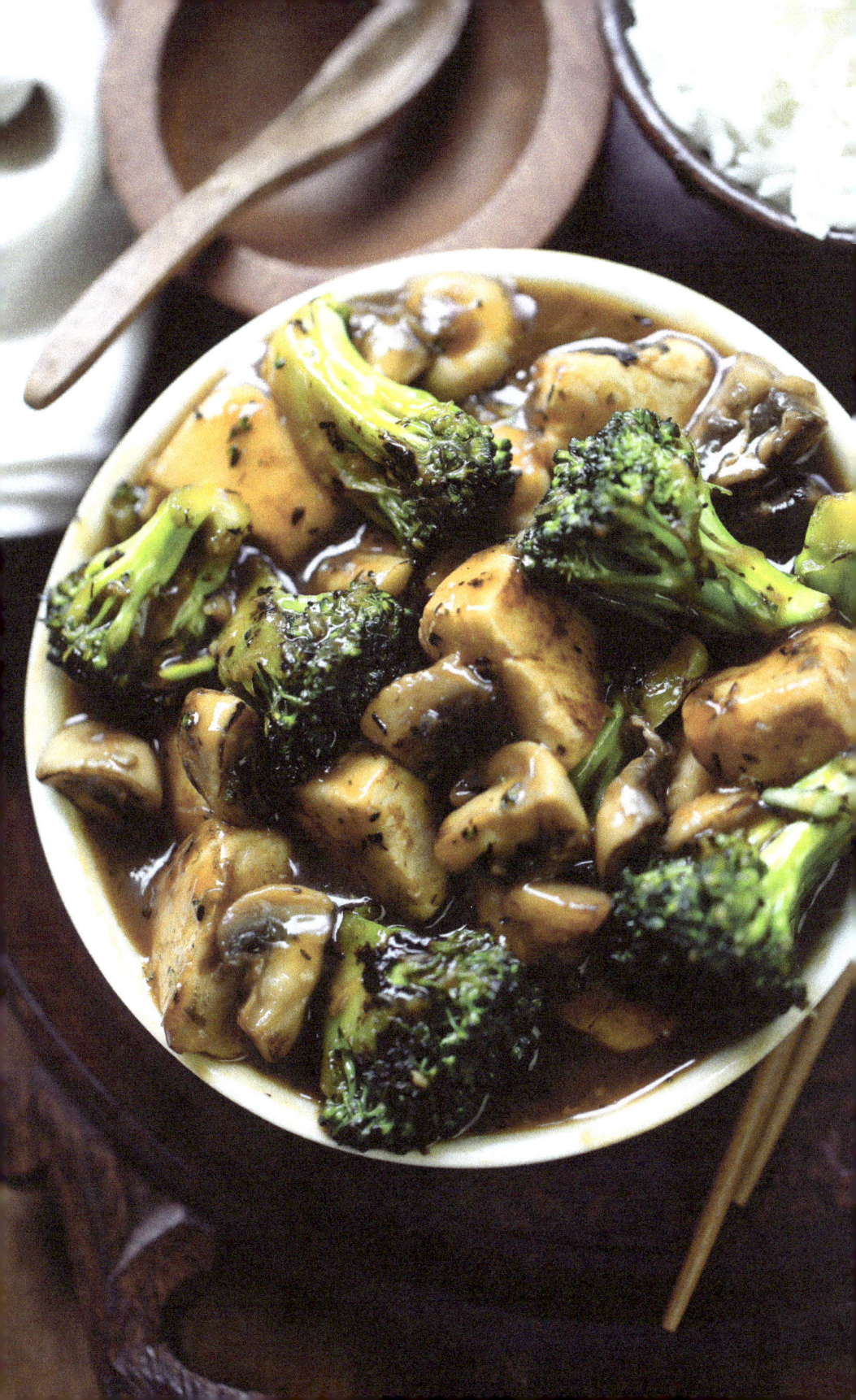

Stir-Fried Scallops & Vegetables with Honey-Ginger Sauce

SERVES 4

Succulent scallops are stir-fried with aromatic ginger and fresh vegetables, then glazed with a Chinese honey-ginger sauce.

1 cup long-grain white rice

4 tablespoons soy sauce

4 tablespoons oyster sauce

2 tablespoons Chinese rice wine (or dry sherry)

4 teaspoons honey

4 tablespoons peanut or canola oil

24 uncooked large scallops

2 carrots, peeled and julienned

2 green bell peppers, cut into thin strips

2 zucchini (courgettes), sliced into ¼-inch rounds

4 cloves garlic, finely chopped

4 teaspoons finely grated fresh ginger

2 cups fish, chicken, or vegetable stock

2 tablespoons cornstarch (corn flour), mixed to a paste with 2 tablespoons water

2 scallions, thinly sliced

BRING 1½ cups of water to a boil in a saucepan. STIR in the rice and keep stirring until the water returns to a boil. COVER the pot with a tight-fitting lid, reduce the heat to very low, and simmer gently for 15 minutes. WHILE the rice cooks, mix together the soy sauce, oyster sauce, Chinese rice wine, and honey in a bowl. HEAT a wok or large skillet over high heat, add 1 tablespoon of the oil, and stir-fry the scallops for 1½ minutes. REMOVE the scallops from the wok and set aside on a plate. HEAT the remaining oil in the wok and stir-fry the carrots and bell peppers for 3 minutes. ADD the zucchini and stir-fry for another 2 minutes. ADD the garlic and ginger and stir-fry for 1 minute, then return the scallops to the wok. ADD the sauce mixture and stock. ADD the cornstarch paste and cook until thickened and thoroughly combined, then toss with the scallions. SERVE on a bed of the rice.

Variations: Use chicken or shrimp instead of scallops.

Stir-Fried Tofu, Vegetables & Water Chestnuts in Oyster Sauce

SERVES 4

This stir-fry features tofu, assorted vegetables, and crunchy water chestnuts in a thick and flavorful Chinese stir-fry sauce.

8 ounces (230g) dried wheat noodles

6 tablespoons oyster sauce

4 tablespoons soy sauce

4 tablespoons water

4 tablespoons of peanut or canola oil

30 green beans, ends trimmed, halved

2 red bell peppers, cut into thin strips

12 ounces (340g) firm tofu, cut into small cubes

1 cup canned water chestnuts, rinsed and drained

2 scallions, thinly sliced

4 cloves garlic, finely chopped

4 teaspoons finely grated fresh ginger

ADD the dried noodles to a saucepan of boiling water and cook for 5 minutes. WHILE the noodles cook, mix together the oyster sauce, soy sauce, and water in a small bowl. HEAT a wok or large skillet over high heat; add the oil and stir-fry the beans for 2 minutes. ADD the bell peppers and stir-fry for 2 minutes. ADD the tofu and stir-fry for 3 minutes. ADD the water chestnuts, scallions, garlic, and ginger and stir-fry for 1 minute. ADD the sauce mixture and mix to heat through. SERVE on a bed of the noodles.

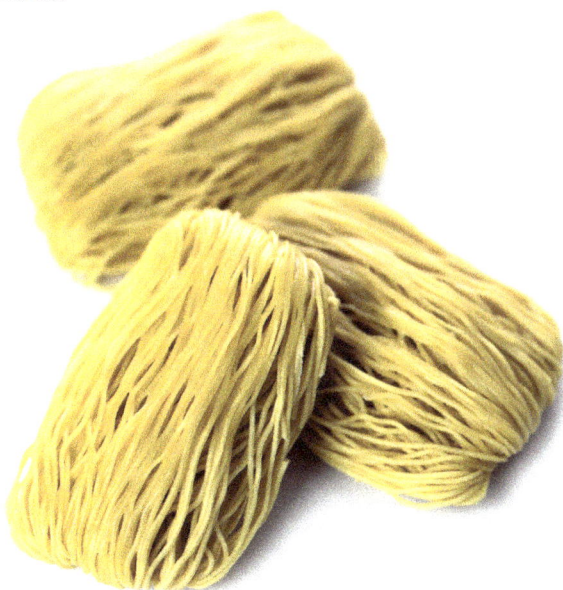

Thai Chicken Stir-Fry

SERVES 4

Strips of chicken and a selection of tasty vegetables are stir-fried with Thai seasonings and accented with crunchy crushed peanuts.

1 cup jasmine rice

6 tablespoons fish sauce

4 tablespoons freshly squeezed lemon juice

2 teaspoons brown sugar

4 teaspoons sesame oil

5 tablespoons peanut or canola oil

24 ounces (700g) boneless skinless chicken breasts, cut into thin strips

2 green bell peppers, cut into thin strips

4 cloves garlic, finely chopped

4 teaspoons Thai red curry paste

4 ripe tomatoes, diced

1 cup frozen peas, thawed

4 scallions, thinly sliced on the diagonal; reserve a little for garnish

A handful of cilantro (fresh coriander) leaves; reserve a little for garnish

4 tablespoons crushed roasted peanuts

BRING 1½ cups of water to a boil in a saucepan. STIR in the rice and keep stirring until the water returns to a boil. COVER the pot with a tight-fitting lid, reduce the heat to very low, and simmer gently for 15 minutes. WHILE the rice cooks, mix together the fish sauce, lemon juice, sugar, and sesame oil in a small bowl. HEAT a wok or large skillet over high heat, add 2 tablespoons of the peanut oil, and stir-fry the chicken for 3 minutes; remove from the wok and set aside on a plate. ADD the remaining oil to the hot wok and stir-fry the bell pepper for 3 minutes. ADD the garlic and curry paste and stir-fry for 30 seconds until the curry paste has dissolved. ADD the tomatoes and peas and stir-fry for 1 minute. ADD the sauce mixture, scallions, and chicken and heat through. STIR through the cilantro and peanuts and serve over rice garnished with the reserved scallions and cilantro.

Honey-Lemon Chicken with Almonds

SERVES 4

In this tasty Chinese dish, a mixture of soy sauce, hoisin sauce, lemon juice, and honey coats succulent chicken pieces and vegetables with a sweet and savory glaze.

8 ounces (230g) dried wheat noodles

6 tablespoons freshly squeezed lemon juice

6 tablespoons soy sauce

3 tablespoons honey

2 tablespoons hoisin sauce

4 tablespoons peanut or canola oil

24 ounces (700g) uncooked boneless skinless chicken breasts, cut into bite-size pieces

4 cups broccoli florets

2 red bell peppers, cut into thin strips

1 stick celery, finely sliced on the diagonal

4 tablespoons sliced almonds

4 cloves garlic, finely chopped

4 teaspoons finely grated fresh ginger

2 cups chicken stock

2 tablespoons cornstarch (corn flour), mixed to a paste with 2 tablespoons water

BRING a saucepan of water to a boil. ADD the dried noodles to the boiling water and cook for 5 minutes. WHILE the noodles cook, mix together the lemon juice, soy sauce, honey, and hoisin sauce in a bowl. HEAT a wok or large skillet over high heat, add 2 tablespoons of the oil, and stir-fry the chicken for 3 minutes. REMOVE the chicken from the wok and set aside on a plate. HEAT the remaining oil in the wok and stir-fry the broccoli, bell pepper, and celery for 6 minutes. ADD the sliced almonds and stir-fry for another minute. ADD the garlic and ginger and stir-fry for 1 minute, then return the chicken to the wok. ADD the sauce mixture and stock, then add the cornstarch paste and cook, stirring continuously, until thickened. SERVE on a bed of the noodles.

Variations: Replace the chicken with shrimp, scallops, or fish.

Fragrant Shrimp & Vegetable Stir-Fry

SERVES 4

Stir-fried shrimp and tender vegetables combined with a rich and aromatic Chinese sauce.

1 cup long-grain white rice

6 tablespoons oyster sauce

4 tablespoons soy sauce

¼ cup water

2 teaspoons sesame oil

1 teaspoon five-spice powder

1 tablespoon brown sugar

3 tablespoons peanut or canola oil

32 green beans, ends trimmed, and cut in half

2 red bell peppers, cut into thin strips

3 scallions, thinly sliced on diagonal

4 cups bean sprouts

4 cloves garlic, finely chopped

32 large cooked peeled shrimp

BRING 1½ cups of water to a boil in a saucepan. STIR in the rice and keep stirring until the water returns to a boil. COVER the pot with a tight-fitting lid, reduce the heat to very low, and simmer gently for 15 minutes. WHILE the rice cooks, mix together the oyster sauce, soy sauce, water, sesame oil, five-spice powder and sugar in a small bowl. HEAT a wok or large skillet over a high heat, add the oil and stir-fry the green beans and red pepper for 4 minutes. ADD the garlic and stir-fry for a minute. ADD the scallions, bean sprouts and cooked shrimp and stir-fry for a minute. ADD the sauce mixture and cook for 30 seconds to heat through. SERVE with the rice.

Variations: Use chicken, squid, scallops or cubed firm tofu in place of shrimp. Serve with noodles instead of rice.

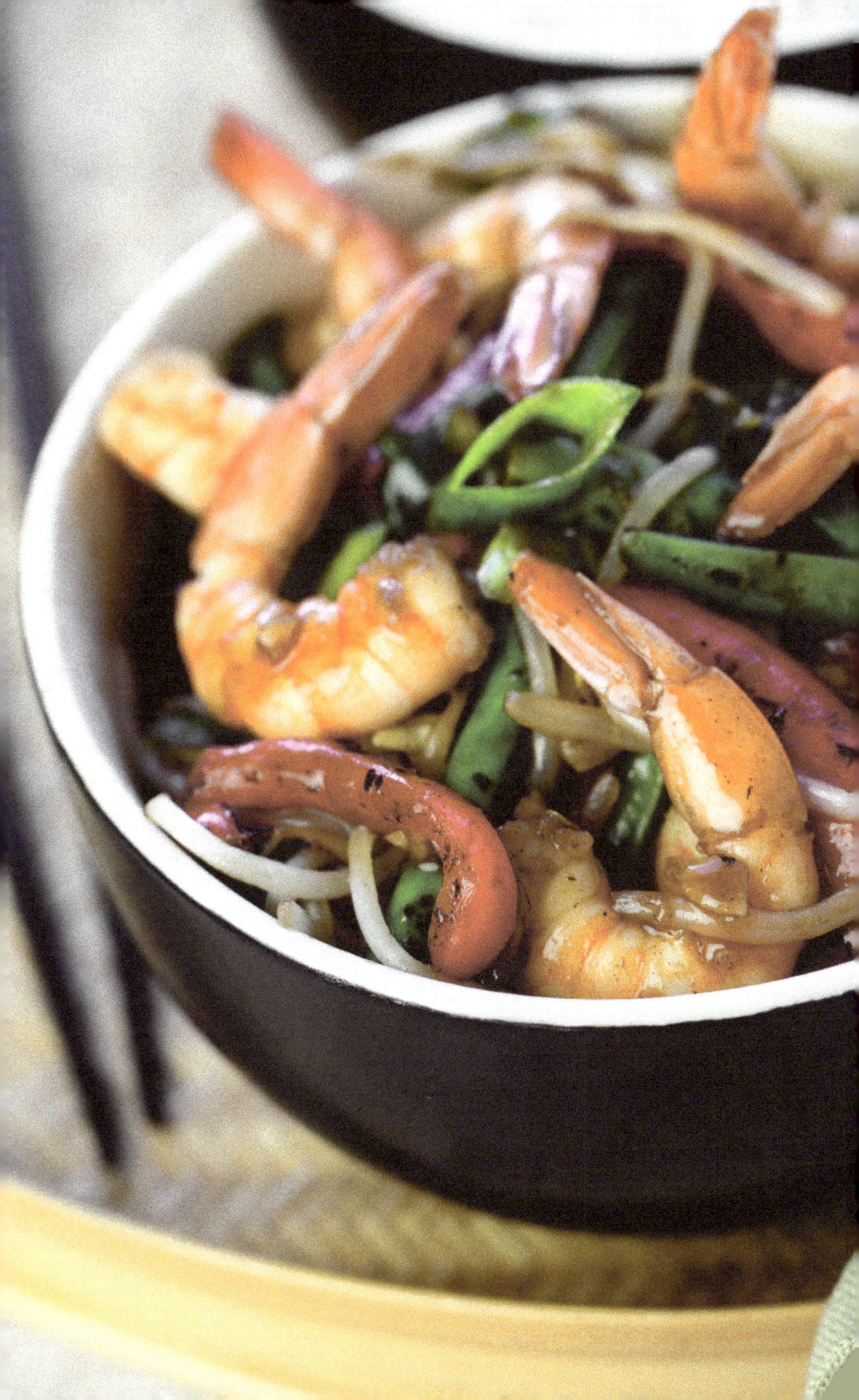

Stir-Fried Beef in Black Bean Sauce

SERVES 4

Tender beef strips and vegetables in a rich black bean sauce. Stir-frying is a great way to make a little red meat stretch a long way.

1 cup long-grain white rice

6 tablespoons black bean sauce

4 tablespoons soy sauce

2 tablespoons Chinese rice wine (or dry sherry)

4 teaspoons brown sugar

1 teaspoon ground black pepper

4 tablespoons peanut or canola oil

24 oz (700g) lean beef, cut into thin strips along the grain

24 green beans, ends trimmed, cut in half on the diagonal

2 red bell peppers, cut into thin strips

2 onions, each cut into 8 wedges and separated into pieces

6 cloves garlic, finely chopped

4 teaspoons finely grated fresh ginger

2 cups beef stock

2 tablespoons cornstarch (corn flour), mixed to a paste with 2 tablespoons water

BRING 1½ cups of water to a boil in a saucepan. STIR in the rice and keep stirring until the water returns to a boil. COVER the pot with a tight-fitting lid, reduce the heat to very low, and simmer gently for 15 minutes. WHILE the rice cooks, mix together the black bean sauce, soy sauce, Chinese rice wine, sugar, and black pepper in a bowl. HEAT a wok or large skillet over high heat, add 2 tablespoons of the oil, and stir-fry the beef for 5 minutes. REMOVE the beef from the wok and set aside on a plate. HEAT the remaining oil in the wok and stir-fry the green beans, bell peppers, and onions for 6 minutes. ADD the garlic and ginger and stir-fry for another minute, then return the beef to the wok. ADD the sauce mixture and stock, then add the cornstarch paste and cook, stirring continuously, until thickened. SERVE on a bed of the rice.

Variations: This black bean sauce also goes well with chicken, lean pork, squid, shrimp, or bite-sized pieces of firm white fish.

Indonesian Stir-fried Tempeh & Vegetables

SERVES 4

Made from fermented soybeans, tempeh has a nutty flavor and a firm, meaty texture. Here it's combined with red pepper and snow peas to make a simple and satisfying Indonesian-style stir-fry.

1 cup long-grain white rice

4 tablespoons kecap manis (Indonesian sweet soy sauce)

4 tablespoons soy sauce

4 tablespoons water

2 teaspoons tamarind puree

4 tablespoons peanut or canola oil

14 ounces (400g) tempeh, cut into small cubes

2 red bell peppers, cut into thin strips

32 snow peas, ends trimmed

4 cloves garlic, finely chopped

2 tablespoons finely grated fresh ginger

2 scallions, thinly sliced on the diagonal

4 tablespoons roughly torn cilantro (fresh coriander) leaves

BRING 1½ cups of water to a boil in a saucepan. STIR in the rice and keep stirring until the water returns to a boil. COVER the pot with a tight-fitting lid, reduce the heat to very low, and simmer gently for 15 minutes. WHILE the rice cooks, mix together the kecap manis, soy sauce, water, and tamarind puree in a small bowl. HEAT the oil in a wok or large skillet over high heat, add the tempeh, bell pepper, and snow peas and stir-fry for 5 minutes. ADD the garlic and ginger and stir-fry for 1 minute. ADD the sauce mix, scallions, and cilantro and stir-fry for 30 seconds. SERVE with the rice.

Five-Spice Squid

SERVES 4

This dish combines quick-cooking squid and vegetables with a rich sauce laced with fragrant Chinese five-spice powder. Scoring the squid makes the pieces curl up when cooked, but feel free to omit this step.

4 tablespoons hoisin sauce

4 tablespoons soy sauce

2 tablespoons Chinese rice wine (or dry sherry)

2 teaspoons brown sugar

1 teaspoon five-spice powder

2 teaspoons sesame oil

6 tablespoons peanut or canola oil

4 cleaned squid hoods, each cut in half, scored on the inside in a crisscross pattern, and cut into large pieces

2 red bell peppers, cut into thin strips

2 bunches Asian greens (such as bok choy or choy sum), roughly chopped

4 cloves garlic, minced

2 teaspoons finely grated fresh ginger

2 small red chilies, deseeded and finely chopped

2 cups fish, chicken, or vegetable stock

2 tablespoons cornstarch (corn flour), mixed to a paste with 2 tablespoons water

Cooked rice or noodles, to serve

MIX together the hoisin sauce, soy sauce, Chinese rice wine, sugar, five-spice powder, and sesame oil in a bowl. HEAT a wok or large skillet over high heat, add 2 tablespoons of the peanut oil, and stir-fry the squid for 40 seconds. REMOVE the squid from the wok and set aside on a plate. HEAT the remaining oil in the wok over high heat and stir-fry the bell peppers for 2 minutes. ADD the Asian greens and stir-fry for another 4 minutes. ADD the garlic, ginger, and chilies and stir-fry for 1 minute. ADD the sauce mixture and stock, then add the cornstarch paste and cook, stirring continuously, until thickened. RETURN the squid to the wok and thoroughly combine. SERVE with cooked rice or noodles.

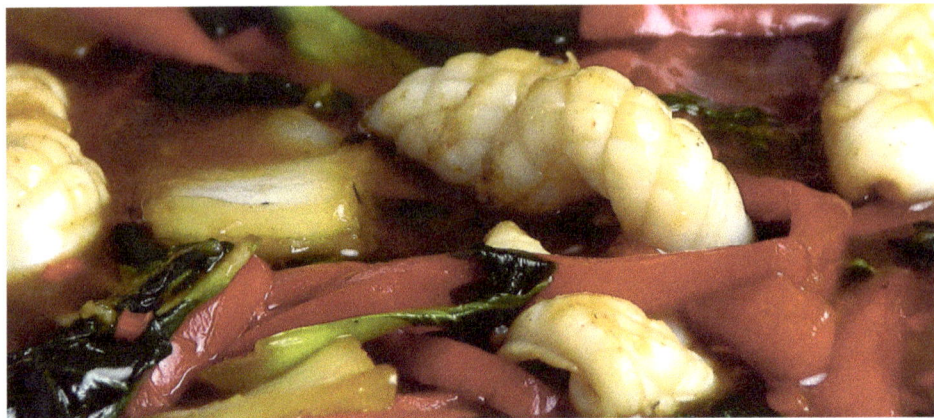

CHAPTER 14

PIZZA

raditional Italian pizza is markedly different from a typical Western pizza. For a start, a thick doughy crust isn't traditional. Instead, a thin crust— which contains far fewer calories—is the usual choice. Meaty toppings certainly aren't traditional either. Instead, popular toppings include fresh herbs (like torn basil), anchovies, olives, bell peppers, and mushrooms. And traditional pizza isn't smothered in cheese; only a moderate amount is used, simply to accent the flavors of the toppings. So pizza made the Italian way ends up containing far fewer calories and bad fats than typical Western pizza, which means you can enjoy it without guilt (especially if you enjoy it with a fresh salad on the side). Below is a "master recipe" for pizza, followed by a number of variations.

Basic Pizza Recipe

SERVES 2

3 tablespoons canned chopped tomatoes

1 tablespoon tomato paste

½ clove garlic, minced

1 teaspoon extra virgin olive oil

¼ teaspoon freshly ground black pepper

1 store-bought prebaked pizza crust (about 12-inches in diameter and preferably thin crust, or a large whole-grain pita bread)

Toppings (topping variations follow)

2½ ounces (70g) mozzarella cheese, cut into small cubes or grated

PREHEAT the oven to 450°F (230°C). IN a small bowl, mix together the tomatoes, tomato paste, garlic, olive oil, and pepper. SPREAD a thin layer evenly over the pizza crust. ARRANGE the toppings evenly over the pizza crust. PLACE the cubed cheese evenly on top. PLACE the pizza on a baking tray and cook for 10 minutes. CUT into 6 slices to serve.

Smoked Salmon & Feta Pizza

Pizza Toppings

Sicilian Tuna & Basil Pizza

5 large fresh basil leaves, roughly torn

½ green bell pepper, finely sliced

6 ounces (170g) canned light tuna in olive oil, drained and broken into small chunks

Broccoli, Tuna, Blue Cheese & Walnut Pizza

6 ounces (170g) canned tuna in olive oil, drained and broken into chunks

⅓ cup lightly crushed walnuts

1½ cups small broccoli florets, steamed over simmering water for 3 minutes

1½ ounces (45g) crumbled blue cheese, such as Gorgonzola

Earth & Sea Pizza

8 peeled uncooked large shrimp

8 large scallops

6 thinly sliced red onion rings

½ red bell pepper, finely diced

5 black olives, sliced

Greek Pizza with Chicken, Artichokes & Feta

1 cup shredded, precooked skinless chicken breast

1 handful fresh spinach leaves, roughly chopped

2 jarred marinated artichoke hearts, quartered

¼ red bell pepper, diced

6 pitted kalamata olives, thinly sliced

2½ ounces (70g) feta cheese, crumbled (used in place of the mozzarella cheese)

Anchovy, Olive, and Basil Pizza

5 large fresh basil leaves, roughly torn

5 anchovy fillets, chopped

8 pitted black olives, halved

Ham, Mushroom & Tomato Pizza

2 tomatoes, thinly sliced

3 white button mushrooms, sliced

2 thin slices ham, diced

Pesto Chicken Pizza

3 tablespoons Pesto (page 285) or store-bought pesto spread over the crust instead of the tomato sauce mix

2 tomatoes, thinly sliced

1 cup shredded, precooked skinless chicken breast

6 thinly sliced red onion rings

8 pitted black olives, thinly sliced

Thai Shrimp Pizza

4 tablespoons sweet chili sauce spread over the crust instead of the tomato sauce mix

12 peeled uncooked large shrimp (prawns)

¼ red bell pepper, diced

¼ green bell pepper, diced

1 scallion, thinly sliced

Smoked Salmon & Feta Pizza

½ zucchini, finely diced

2 tablespoons finely diced red onion

3½ oz (100g) thinly sliced smoked salmon, cut into pieces

Fresh dill, for garnishing

Lemon juice, for squeezing

2½ ounces (70g) feta cheese, crumbled (used in place of the mozzarella cheese)

CHAPTER 15

CURRIES, STEWS & BAKES

Thai Red Chicken Curry

SERVES 4

Thai red curry made with a subtle blend of hot, salty, sweet, and sour flavors to get the taste buds tingling. You can make your own curry paste from scratch, but to save time we recommend you buy a good-quality premade Thai curry paste.

4 tablespoons peanut or canola oil

2 onions, finely chopped

2 tablespoons Thai red curry paste

4 cloves garlic, finely chopped

2 cups coconut milk

2 cups chicken stock

4 tablespoons fish sauce

2 tablespoons brown sugar

1 teaspoon salt

2 zucchini (courgettes), sliced into thin rounds

2 red bell peppers, cut into thin strips

1 cup jasmine rice

24 oz (700g) uncooked skinless chicken breast fillets, cut into bite-sized pieces

3 tablespoons cornstarch (corn flour), mixed to a paste with 3 tablespoons water

3 tablespoons freshly squeezed lemon juice

10 large fresh basil leaves, finely sliced

HEAT the oil in a large saucepan over medium heat and cook the onions, stirring occasionally, for 8 minutes. ADD the curry paste and garlic and cook, stirring, for 1 minute. ADD the coconut milk, stock, fish sauce, sugar, and salt, then bring to a boil. ADD the zucchini and bell peppers, reduce the heat to medium, and simmer for 12 minutes. WHILE the curry simmers, bring 1½ cups of water to a boil in a saucepan. STIR in the rice and keep stirring until the water returns to a boil. COVER the pot with a tight-fitting lid, reduce the heat to very low, and simmer gently for 15 minutes. ADD the chicken to the curry and simmer for another 8 minutes. ADD the cornstarch paste and stir continuously until the curry thickens, then stir in the lemon juice and basil. SERVE on a bed of the rice.

Variations: This curry tastes equally delicious using any selection of seafood, such as shrimp, scallops, or pieces of firm fish, or cubed firm tofu. You can also use a variety of different vegetables with this curry including shredded cabbage, thinly sliced carrots, or green beans. Be flexible and adapt the recipe to make the most of seasonal produce.

Greek-Style Lentil & Eggplant Bake

SERVES 4

A delicious and comforting layered casserole dish with herb-infused lentil and tomato sauce, slices of grilled eggplant, and cheesy béchamel sauce. To make this dish even more substantial, add layers of cooked potato, cooked rice, or cooked pasta (macaroni is ideal) before baking.

2 eggplants — cut lengthwise into ½-inch slices

6 tablespoons extra virgin olive oil (plus extra for greasing the baking dish)

1 onion — finely chopped

3 garlic cloves — finely chopped

14 oz (400g) canned chopped tomatoes

2 tablespoons tomato paste

1½ teaspoons salt

1 teaspoon dried oregano

½ teaspoon ground cinnamon

½ teaspoon freshly ground black pepper

14 oz (400g) canned brown lentils — rinsed and drained

2 tablespoons finely chopped fresh flat-leaf parsley

3 tablespoons plain flour

2 cups milk

½ cup finely grated Parmesan cheese

½ cup crumbled feta cheese

PREHEAT the oven broiler (grill) to high. BRUSH the eggplant slices on both sides with 2 tablespoons of olive oil. PLACE on a large baking tray and cook directly under the broiler for 5 minutes on each side. WHILE the eggplant cooks make the lentil sauce. HEAT 2 tablespoons of olive oil in a pan and cook the onion for 5 minutes, stirring occasionally. ADD the garlic and cook 2 minutes. ADD the canned tomatoes, tomato paste, salt, oregano, cinnamon and pepper and bring to a boil. REDUCE the heat to low and simmer, uncovered, for 10 minutes. STIR in the lentils and parsley to combine. REMOVE the eggplant slices from the broiler once cooked and preheat the oven to 400°F/200°C. MAKE the cheese sauce by heating 2 tablespoons olive oil in a saucepan. STIR in the flour to combine and cook 1 minute. ADD the milk gradually, stirring continuously, and cook until the sauce thickens. STIR in the grated Parmesan and crumbled feta until well combined and melted. SPOON a few tablespoons of the lentil sauce in the bottom of a lightly greased baking dish. TOP with half the eggplant slices, then layer with half the lentil sauce, and half the cheese sauce. REPEAT the layers of eggplant slices, lentil sauce, and cheese sauce. BAKE for 35 minutes, then remove from the oven and allow to stand for at least 10 minutes to firm up before cutting into pieces and serving.

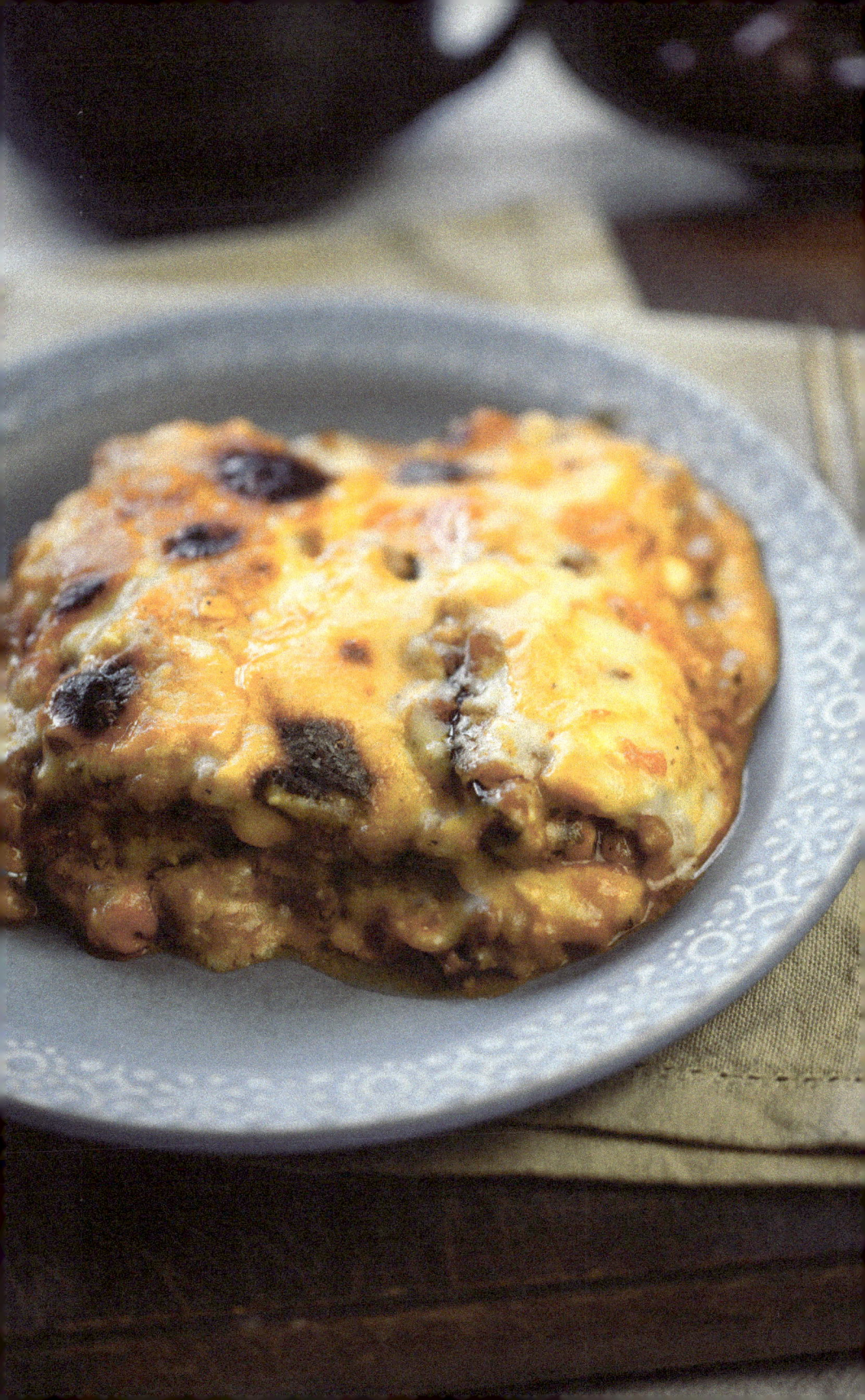

Dahl with Carrot & Cauliflower

SERVES 4

A traditional Indian dahl (lentil curry) with carrots and cauliflower, served on a bed of basmati rice. Lentils are a good source of protein and fiber, and cook quickly into a thick and creamy puree. Dahl is usually eaten with rice or Indian breads, like naan or chapati, to soak up the delicious and nutritious gravy.

3 tablespoons peanut or canola oil

2 onions, finely chopped

2 carrots, diced

4 cloves garlic, finely chopped

1 tablespoon finely grated fresh ginger

1½ teaspoons ground coriander

1½ teaspoons ground cumin

1 teaspoon turmeric

¾ teaspoon cinnamon

¾ teaspoon chili powder

2 cups cauliflower florets

1½ cups red lentils

14 oz (400g) canned chopped tomatoes

1½ cups coconut milk

1½ cups vegetable or chicken stock

1½ teaspoons salt

1 cup basmati rice

2 tablespoons freshly squeezed lemon juice

HEAT the oil in a large saucepan over medium heat and cook the onions and carrots, stirring occasionally, until softened, about 8 minutes. ADD the garlic, ginger, coriander, cumin, turmeric, cinnamon, and chili powder and cook, stirring, for 1 minute. ADD the cauliflower and red lentils and stir to coat them with the spice mixture. ADD the tomatoes, coconut milk, stock, and salt, bring to a boil, and cover with a lid. Reduce the heat to medium and simmer for 20 minutes, stirring occasionally. WHILE the dahl simmers, bring 1½ cups of water to a boil in a saucepan. STIR in the rice and keep stirring until the water returns to a boil. COVER the pot with a tight-fitting lid, reduce the heat to very low, and simmer gently for 15 minutes. REMOVE the dahl from the heat and stir in the lemon juice. SERVE on a bed of the basmati rice.

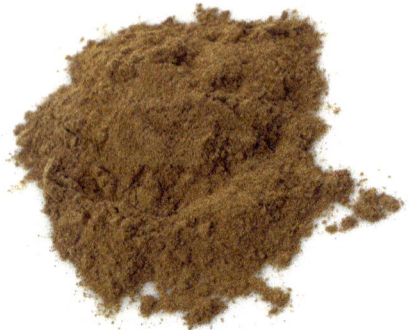

Chicken Cacciatore

SERVES 4

In this classic Italian dish, tender chicken breast fillets are coated with a flavorful sauce made with tomatoes, anchovies, olives and wine, and seasoned with oregano and balsamic vinegar.

1 cup long-grain white rice

6 tablespoons extra virgin olive oil

Four 6-ounce (170g) uncooked skinless chicken breast fillets

2 onions, chopped

1 red bell pepper, cut into thin strips

4 cloves garlic, finely chopped

4 anchovy fillets, finely chopped

14 oz (400g) canned chopped tomatoes

1 cup white wine

2 tablespoons tomato paste

2 tablespoons balsamic vinegar

16 black pitted olives, quartered

1 teaspoon dried oregano

1 teaspoon salt

½ teaspoon freshly ground black pepper

4 teaspoons finely chopped fresh flat-leaf parsley

BRING 1½ cups of water to a boil in a saucepan. STIR in the rice and keep stirring until the water returns to a boil. COVER the pot with a tight-fitting lid, reduce the heat to very low, and simmer gently for 15 minutes. WHILE the rice is cooking, heat 2 tablespoons of the olive oil in a large skillet over medium-high heat. COOK the chicken for 3 minutes each side, then remove from the pan and set aside on a plate. HEAT the reserved oil in the same pan and cook the onions and bell pepper, stirring occasionally, until softened, about 7 minutes. ADD the garlic and anchovies and cook 1 minute more, stirring to break up the anchovies. ADD the tomatoes, white wine, tomato paste, vinegar, olives, oregano, salt, and pepper and simmer over medium heat, covered, for 10 minutes. RETURN the chicken fillets to the pan and cook for 3 minutes. SERVE on a bed of the rice, garnished with the parsley.

South Indian Shrimp & Chickpea Curry

SERVES 4

Plump, juicy shrimp combine wonderfully with the nutty flavor and creamy texture of chickpeas in this comforting and fragrant Indian curry.

2 tablespoons peanut or canola oil

2 onions, finely chopped

4 cloves garlic, finely chopped

2 teaspoons finely grated fresh ginger

½ cup of canned chickpeas

4 teaspoons ground cumin

3 teaspoons ground turmeric

2 teaspoons paprika

1 teaspoon chili powder

28 oz (800g) canned chopped tomatoes

2 cups coconut milk

2 teaspoons salt

1 cup basmati rice

32 large uncooked shrimp, peeled and deveined

3 tablespoons finely chopped fresh cilantro (fresh coriander)

2 tablespoons lemon juice

HEAT the oil in a large saucepan over a medium heat and cook the onion for 8 minutes, stirring occasionally. ADD the garlic and ginger, and cook for two minutes. ADD the cumin, turmeric, garam masala and chili powder and cook, stirring, for a minute. ADD the tomatoes, coconut milk and salt and bring to a boil. REDUCE the heat and simmer, uncovered, for 10 minutes. WHILE the curry simmers, bring 1½ cups of water to a boil in a saucepan. STIR in the rice and keep stirring until the water returns to a boil. COVER the pot with a tight-fitting lid, reduce the heat to very low, and simmer gently for 15 minutes. ADD the shrimp and chickpeas to the curry and simmer for another 4 minutes, then stir in the chopped cilantro and lemon juice. SERVE on a bed of basmati rice.

Variations: Use scallops or cubed pieces of fish or chicken instead of the shrimp. Use fresh mint instead of cilantro.

Tip: If you're vegan or vegetarian, simply omit the shrimp and double the amount of chickpeas.

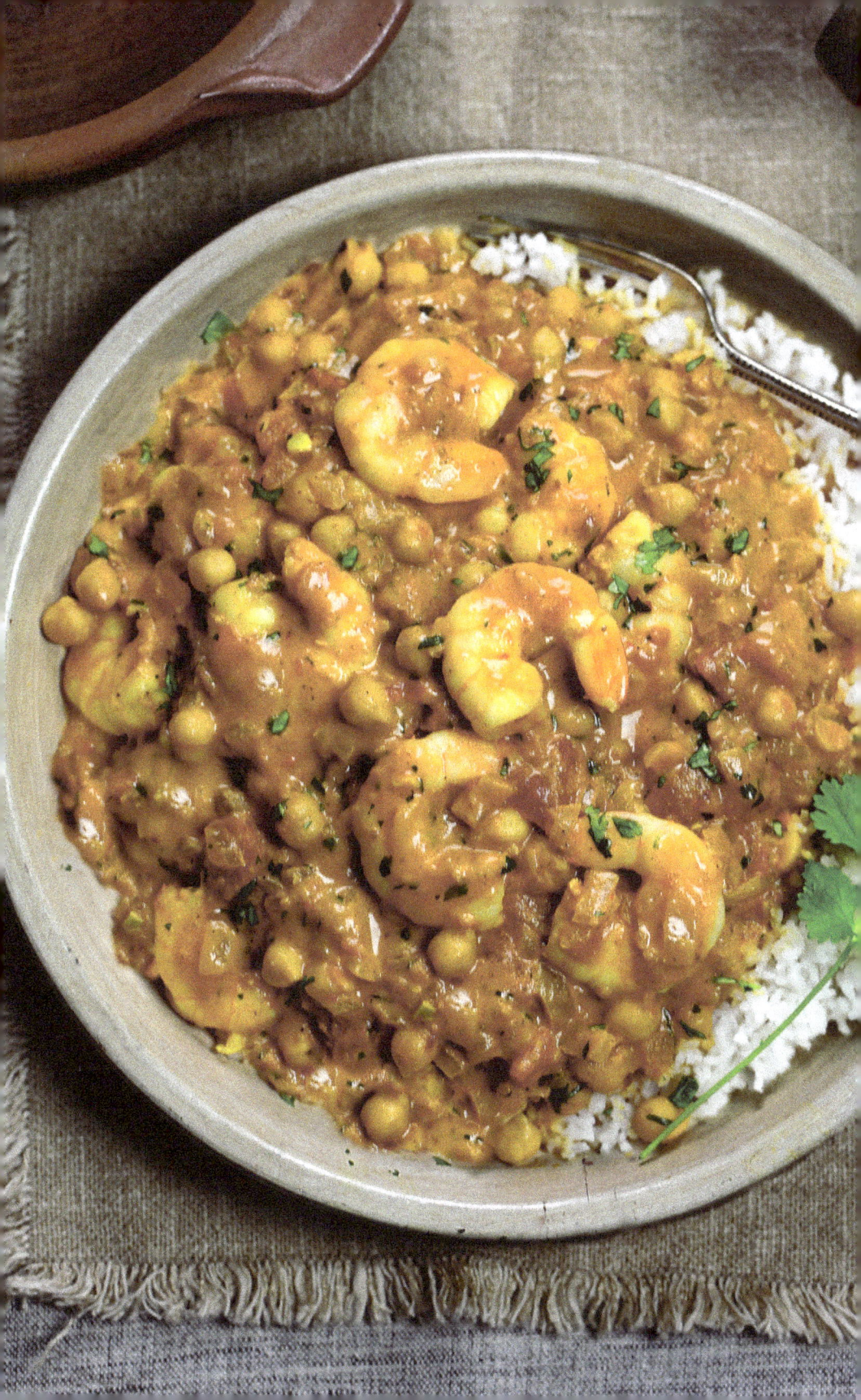

Thai Fish Curry

SERVES 4

An aromatic and richly flavored Thai fish curry with green beans and red pepper and served with jasmine rice.

4 tablespoons peanut or canola oil

1 red bell pepper, cut into thin strips

32 green beans, trimmed and halved

4 cloves garlic, finely chopped

2 teaspoons finely chopped lemongrass

2 teaspoons finely grated fresh ginger

2 teaspoons turmeric

2 cups coconut milk

1 cup water

4 tablespoons fish sauce

1 tablespoon brown sugar

1 teaspoon chili powder

1 cup jasmine rice

Four 6-ounce (170g) firm white fish fillets (such as snapper, cod, or haddock), each cut into thirds

2 tablespoons freshly squeezed lemon juice

2 tablespoons finely chopped fresh basil

HEAT the oil in a large skillet over medium heat and cook the bell pepper and green beans, stirring occasionally, until the pepper is softened, about 4 minutes. ADD the garlic, lemongrass, ginger, and turmeric and cook, stirring constantly, for 1 minute. ADD the coconut milk, water, fish sauce, sugar, and chili powder and bring to a boil. REDUCE the heat to medium and simmer for 8 minutes. WHILE the curry simmers, bring 1½ cups of water to a boil in a saucepan. Stir in the rice and keep stirring until the water returns to a boil. COVER the pot with a tight-fitting lid, reduce the heat to very low, and simmer gently for 15 minutes. ADD the fish, spooning the curry sauce over the fish to coat, and simmer, covered, for 8 minutes. REMOVE from the heat and stir in the lemon juice and basil. SERVE with the rice.

Fragrant Chicken Curry

SERVES 4

With a few key ingredients stocked in your pantry (such as spices, canned tomatoes, and coconut milk) and a selection of vegetables, it's easy to produce authentic Indian curries in your own kitchen. Like most curries, this recipe is simple, doesn't involve a lot of steps, and simmers away with no effort required, filling the kitchen with mouthwatering aromas.

4 tablespoons peanut or canola oil

2 onions, finely chopped

4 cloves garlic, finely chopped

2 teaspoons finely grated fresh ginger

2 teaspoons turmeric

2 teaspoons ground cumin

1 teaspoon chili powder

2 cups canned chopped tomatoes

2 cups coconut milk

3 teaspoons garam masala

2 teaspoons salt

1 cup basmati rice

24 oz (700g) uncooked skinless chicken breast fillets, cut into bite-sized pieces

1 cup frozen green peas, thawed

2 tablespoons freshly squeezed lemon juice

3 tablespoons finely chopped fresh cilantro (fresh coriander)

HEAT the oil in a frying pan over medium heat and cook the onions, stirring occasionally, until golden, about 8 minutes. ADD the garlic and cook, stirring, for 2 minutes. ADD the ginger, turmeric, cumin, and chili powder and cook, stirring, for 1 minute. ADD the tomatoes, coconut milk, garam masala, and salt and bring to a boil. REDUCE the heat to medium and simmer for 8 minutes. WHILE the curry simmers, bring 1½ cups of water to a boil in a saucepan. STIR in the rice and keep stirring until the water returns to a boil. COVER the pot with a tight-fitting lid, reduce the heat to very low, and simmer gently for 15 minutes. ADD the chicken and peas to the curry, cover with a lid, and simmer for another 8 minutes, then stir in the lemon juice and cilantro. SERVE on a bed of the rice.

Variation: Replace the chicken with seafood such as shrimp or scallops.

Greek Shrimp with Feta

SERVES 4

This highly appetizing shrimp dish echoes the traditional flavors of Greek cuisine.

6 tablespoons extra virgin olive oil

2 onions, finely chopped

2 green bell peppers, diced

4 scallions, thinly sliced

6 cloves garlic, finely chopped

28 oz (800g) canned chopped tomatoes

1 cup white wine

1 teaspoon dried oregano

2 teaspoons salt

1 teaspoon freshly ground black pepper

1 cup long-grain white rice

24 large uncooked shrimp, peeled and deveined

4 tablespoons chopped fresh flat-leaf parsley

5 oz (140g) crumbled feta cheese

HEAT 4 tablespoons of the oil in an ovenproof skillet over medium heat and cook the onions and bell peppers, stirring occasionally, until softened, about 7 minutes. ADD the scallions and garlic and cook, stirring, for another 2 minutes. ADD the tomatoes, wine, oregano, salt, and pepper and bring to a boil. REDUCE the heat to medium and simmer for 10 minutes. BRING 1½ cups of water to a boil in a saucepan. STIR in the rice and keep stirring until the water returns to a boil. COVER the pot with a tight-fitting lid, reduce the heat to very low, and simmer gently for 15 minutes. ADD the shrimp, parsley, and reserved oil to the stew and simmer, covered, for another 3 minutes. SPRINKLE the feta cheese on top and place the skillet under a hot oven broiler to brown the feta, about 2 minutes. SERVE with the rice.

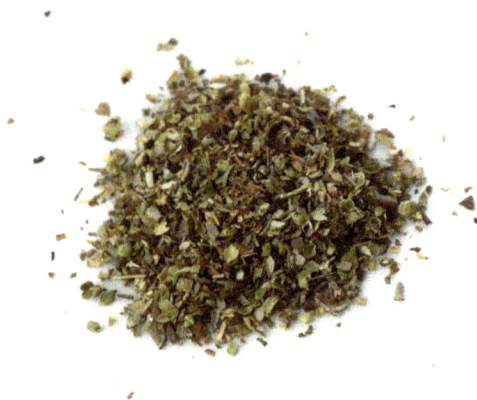

Spanish Tuna & Vegetable Stew

SERVES 4

Spanish cuisine makes the most of foods from the land and the sea, and this traditional recipe combines the best of both.

6 tablespoons extra virgin olive oil

2 red onions, finely chopped

1 red bell pepper, cut into thin strips

1 green bell pepper, cut into thin strips

28 oz (800g) canned chopped tomatoes

2 small potatoes, peeled and cut into small cubes

6 cloves garlic, finely chopped

3 cups fish, vegetable, or chicken stock

1 cup white wine

2 tablespoons tomato paste

4 teaspoons paprika

2 teaspoons salt

1 teaspoon freshly ground black pepper

1 cup long-grain white rice

12 oz (340g) canned light tuna, drained and broken into small chunks

2 tablespoons finely chopped fresh flat-leaf parsley

HEAT 4 tablespoons of the oil in a large saucepan over medium heat and cook the onions and bell peppers, stirring occasionally, until softened, about 8 minutes. ADD the tomatoes, potatoes, and garlic and cook, stirring, for 2 minutes. ADD the stock, wine, tomato paste, paprika, salt, and pepper and bring to a boil. REDUCE the heat to medium-high and simmer, stirring occasionally, for 25 minutes. WHILE the stew simmers, bring 1½ cups of water to a boil in a saucepan. STIR in the rice and keep stirring until the water returns to a boil. COVER the pot with a tight-fitting lid, reduce the heat to very low, and simmer gently for 15 minutes. STIR the tuna, parsley, and reserved oil into the stew and serve over the rice.

Variation: Instead of rice, you can serve this stew with good-quality crusty bread.

Mediterranean Fish & Vegetable Parcels

SERVES 4

Baked fish in parcels with sliced tomatoes, fresh basil, green beans, red onion and olives.

6 tablespoons extra virgin olive oil

4 tablespoons white wine

2 cloves garlic, finely chopped

4 tablespoons finely chopped fresh basil

1 teaspoon salt

½ teaspoon fresh ground black pepper

four 12-inch pieces of baking parchment paper (or aluminum foil)

32 green beans, ends trimmed

4 x 6 oz (170g) firm white fish fillets (such as cod or snapper)

4 tomatoes, thickly sliced

20 thinly sliced red onion rings

12 black olives, pitted and halved

PREHEAT the oven to 440°F (225°C). MIX together the olive oil, lemon juice, garlic, basil, salt and pepper until well combined. PLACE equal amounts of green beans in the center of each piece of paper. PLACE a fish fillet on top of each bed of beans. ARRANGE the tomato slices overlapping over the fish, then place equal amounts of the red onion rings and olives on top. SPOON the oil mixture evenly over each. FOLD the baking parchment paper (or foil) over the fish and vegetables and wrap up the parcels tightly. PLACE the parcels on a baking tray and cook in a preheated oven for 16 minutes. REMOVE the parcels from the oven and open (be careful, the steam is hot).

Variations: Use sliced zucchini instead of green beans. Replace the basil with fresh parsley. Substitute lemon juice for the white wine.

Serving suggestions: Serve with a fresh salad and crusty bread on the side, or with steamed or boiled potatoes.

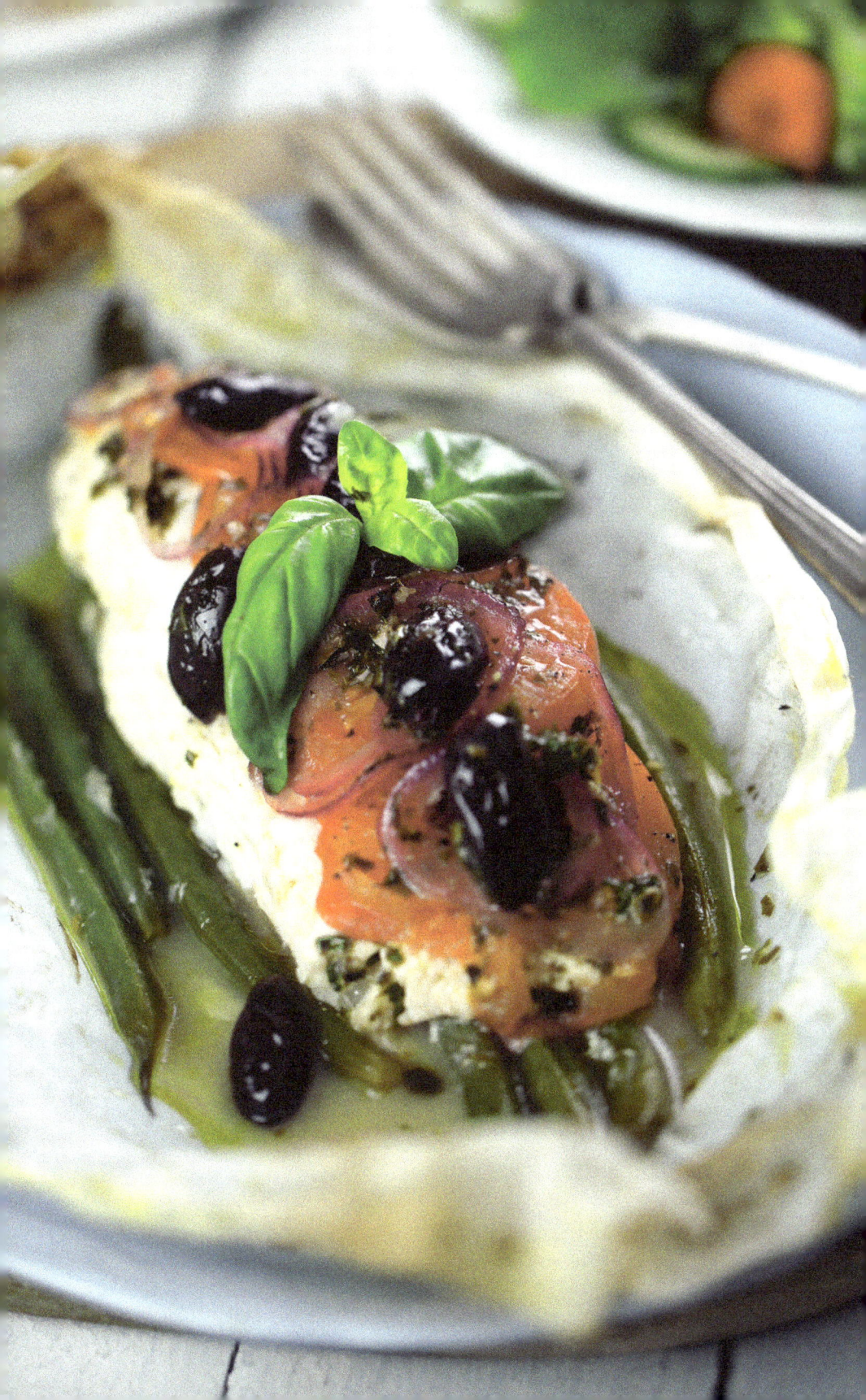

Moroccan Stew with Couscous

SERVES 4

An abundance of nourishing ingredients including chickpeas, cabbage, sweet potatoes, and green beans are simmered in a delicately spiced tomato-peanut sauce and served with fluffy couscous.

3 tablespoons extra virgin olive oil

2 onions, finely chopped

3 cloves garlic, finely chopped

2 teaspoons finely grated fresh ginger

½ teaspoon chili powder

1½ cups of green beans, ends trimmed and cut in half

2 sweet potatoes, peeled and cut into bite-size cubes

3 cups shredded cabbage

2 cups canned chopped tomatoes

4 tablespoons natural peanut butter

2 cups vegetable or chicken stock

2 teaspoons salt

1½ cups canned chickpeas, rinsed and drained

1 cup couscous

3 tablespoons freshly squeezed lemon juice

3 tablespoons chopped cilantro (fresh coriander)

HEAT the oil in a large saucepan over medium heat and cook the onions, stirring occasionally, until softened, about 8 minutes. ADD the garlic, ginger, and chili powder and cook, stirring, for 1 minute. ADD the green beans, sweet potatoes, cabbage, tomatoes, peanut butter, stock, and salt and bring to a boil. REDUCE the heat to medium and simmer for 15 minutes. ADD the chickpeas and simmer for 10 minutes. WHILE the stew simmers, mix 1¼ cups of boiling water with the couscous in a bowl. Cover with a dish towel or plate to seal in the steam and let sit for 5 minutes. FLUFF with a fork to separate the grains. Stir the lemon juice and cilantro into the stew and serve with the couscous.

Variations: Garnish with sliced hard-boiled eggs. Replace the sweet potato with pumpkin. Use spinach instead of cabbage.

Greek Fava Bean, Eggplant & Olive Stew with Feta

SERVES 4

A delicately flavored Greek stew with fava beans, eggplant, zucchini, red pepper, potatoes, and kalamata olives, served with crumbled feta cheese.

6 tablespoons extra virgin olive oil

2 red onions, diced

1 eggplant (aubergine), cut into small cubes

1 red bell pepper, diced

1 zucchini (courgette), diced

1 potato, cut into small cubes

6 cloves garlic, minced

1 teaspoon dried oregano

28 oz (800g) canned chopped tomatoes

2 cups chicken or vegetable stock

2 teaspoons salt

1 teaspoon freshly ground black pepper

1 cup bulgur

8 oz (230g) frozen fava (broad) beans, cooked in boiling water for 5 minutes, rinsed under cold water, skins removed.

4 tablespoons finely chopped fresh flat-leaf parsley

24 pitted kalamata olives, halved

4 oz (115g) feta cheese

HEAT 4 tablespoons of the oil in a large saucepan and cook the onions, stirring occasionally, until lightly browned, about 8 minutes. ADD the eggplant, bell pepper, and zucchini and cook, stirring, for 5 minutes. ADD the potato, garlic, and oregano and cook, stirring, for 1 minute. ADD the tomatoes, stock, salt, and pepper; stir well to combine and bring to a boil. REDUCE the heat to medium and cook, stirring occasionally, for 20 minutes. WHILE the stew simmers, mix the bulgur with 1½ cups of water in a saucepan. Bring to a boil, cover, then turn the heat on very low and cook for 15 minutes. FLUFF with a fork to separate the grains. ADD the cooked, peeled fava beans, parsley, and olives to the stew and cook for 10 minutes. Remove from the heat and stir in the reserved 2 tablespoons of olive oil. SERVE over the bulgur with crumbled feta cheese on top.

Variation: Instead of bulgur, serve the stew with rice or crusty bread.

Vietnamese Baked Fish

SERVES 4

Tender fillets of fish combined with chopped tomatoes, fresh mint, and Vietnamese-style seasonings, then baked in foil to infuse the flavors.

4 tomatoes, diced

4 tablespoons fish sauce

2 tablespoons freshly squeezed lemon juice

2 teaspoons sesame oil

4 teaspoons finely grated fresh ginger

2 cloves garlic, finely chopped

2 tablespoons finely chopped fresh mint

1 teaspoon sugar

½ teaspoon black pepper

Four 6-ounce (170g) fillets firm white fish (such as snapper, cod, or haddock)

2 carrots, peeled and julienned

1 cup long-grain white rice

PREHEAT the oven to 440°F (225°C). IN a bowl, mix together the tomatoes, fish sauce, lemon juice, sesame oil, ginger, garlic, mint, sugar, and pepper until well combined. PLACE a fish fillet in the center of each of four 12-inch pieces of foil and arrange the carrots on top. SPOON equal amounts of the tomato mixture over each. FOLD the foil over the fish and vegetables and seal the foil packets tightly (fold the edges together so no steam can escape). PLACE the packets on a baking sheet and bake in the oven for 16 minutes. While the fish cooks, bring 1½ cups of water to a boil in a saucepan. Stir in the rice and keep stirring until the water returns to a boil. COVER the pot with a tight-fitting lid, reduce the heat to very low, and simmer gently for 15 minutes. REMOVE the packets from the oven and open (be careful—the steam is very hot). TRANSFER the fish, vegetables, and sauce from the foil packets to serving plates and accompany with the rice.

Tip: These foil packets can be prepared in advance and left to marinate in the fridge until you're ready to cook.

CHAPTER 16

RICE & GRAIN DISHES

Turkish Bulgur Pilaf with Chickpeas & Tomatoes

SERVES 4-6

This simple, tasty and nutritious Turkish pilaf recipe only takes around 30 minutes to cook, and it's made in just one pot. Traditionally it's eaten with thick plain yogurt (Greek yogurt is ideal), but it's also delicious served with crumbled feta cheese on top.

4 tablespoons extra virgin olive oil

2 red onions, finely chopped

2 red peppers, diced

4 garlic cloves, minced

2 teaspoons ground cumin

½ teaspoon ground cinnamon

½ teaspoon dried chili flakes

2 tablespoons tomato paste

2 cups bulgur (coarse bulgur is ideal)

28 oz (800g) canned chopped tomatoes

1½ cups vegetable or chicken stock

2 cups canned chickpeas, rinsed and drained

2 teaspoons salt

½ teaspoon ground black pepper

2 tablespoons finely chopped fresh flat-leaf parsley

2 tablespoons finely chopped fresh mint

HEAT the oil in a saucepan over medium heat. ADD the onion and red pepper and cook for 10 minutes, stirring occasionally. ADD the garlic, cumin, cinnamon, chili flakes and tomato paste and cook for 1 minute, then add the bulgur and stir to coat for 1 minute. ADD the tomatoes, stock, chickpeas, salt and pepper, increase the heat to high and bring to a boil. COVER with a lid, reduce the heat to low, and cook for 15 minutes. REMOVE the pan from the heat and let stand, with the lid on, for 5 minutes. STIR in the parsley and mint, then serve the pilaf with a dollop of Greek yogurt (optional).

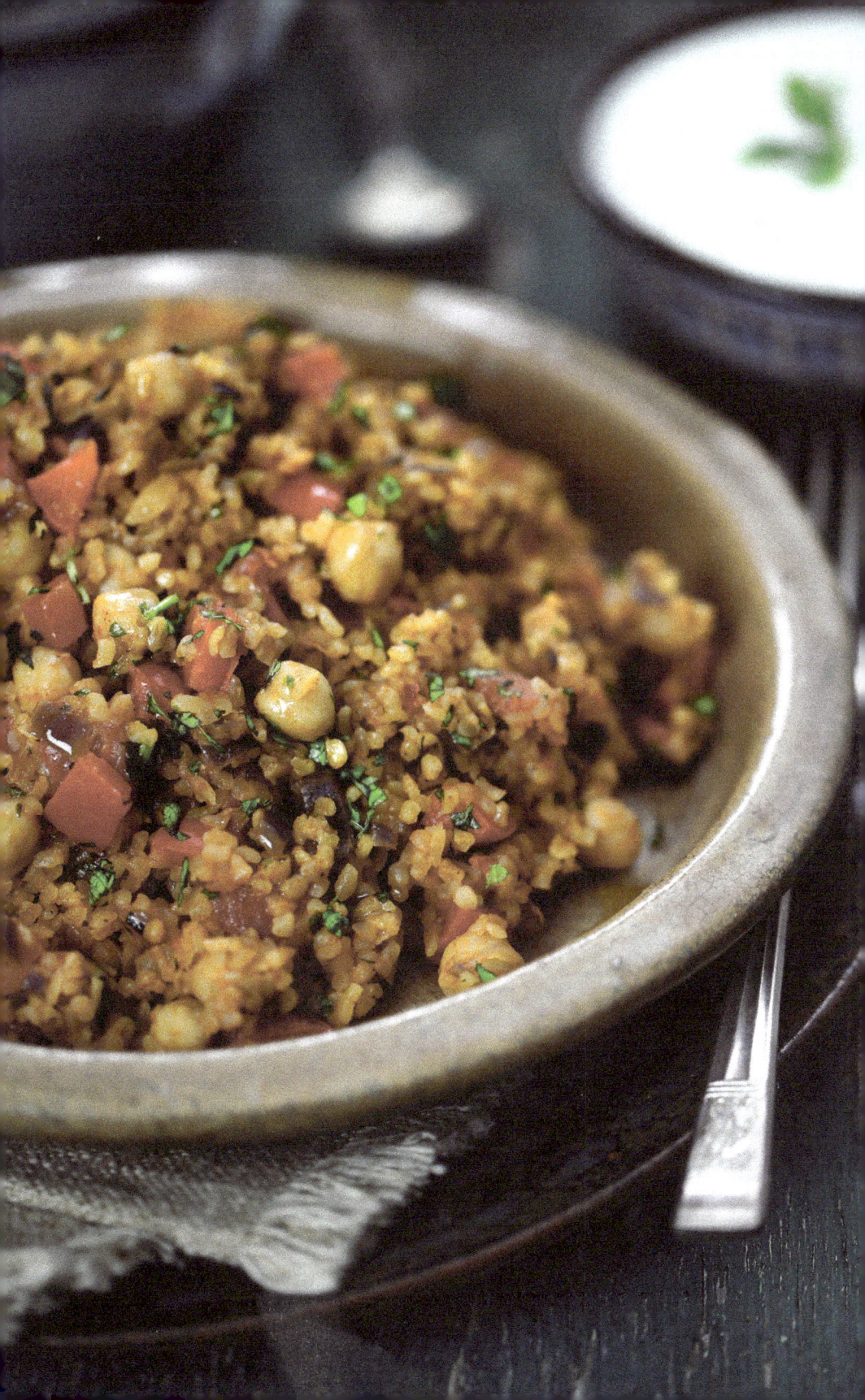

Shrimp, Tomato, Pea & Basil Risotto

SERVES 4-6

Risottos are usually quite time-consuming to make because you have to stand over the cooking pot and stir constantly while regularly adding small amounts of stock. But we've discovered that you don't have to go to such trouble in order to end up with a delicious creamy risotto. By simply adding all the ingredients to the pot, then covering with a lid, the risotto will cook by itself without the need to stir at all. In this risotto, tangy tomatoes and flavorful basil combine exquisitely with shrimp and peas.

5 tablespoons extra virgin olive oil

2 onions, finely chopped

4 cloves garlic, finely chopped

2 cups arborio rice

4 tomatoes, diced

½ cup frozen green peas, thawed

1 cup white wine

4 cups fish, chicken, or vegetable stock

1 teaspoon salt

½ teaspoon freshly ground black pepper

32 large uncooked shrimp (prawns), peeled

2 tablespoons finely chopped fresh basil

⅔ cup grated Parmesan cheese

HEAT 3 tablespoons of the olive oil in a large saucepan over medium heat and cook the onions, stirring occasionally, until softened, about 8 minutes. ADD the garlic and rice and cook for 1 minute, stirring to coat the rice with oil. ADD the tomatoes, peas, wine, stock, salt, and pepper, bring to a boil, cover with a lid, and reduce the heat to low. SIMMER gently for 15 minutes without lifting the lid. REMOVE the lid, quickly place the shrimp on top of the rice, cover and cook for 5 minutes. STIR the basil, cheese, and reserved olive oil through the rice and serve.

Mushroom, Bacon & Walnut Risotto

SERVES 4-6

This rustic risotto is one of our favorites. The mushrooms, walnuts, and creamy arborio rice make a wonderful combination, and the bacon is used in small amounts as a flavor and texture enhancer.

5 tablespoons extra virgin olive oil

2 onions, finely chopped

4 bacon slices, diced

2 cups arborio rice

14 oz (400g) white button mushrooms, cleaned and thickly sliced

4 cloves garlic, finely chopped

½ cup roughly chopped walnuts

4 cups chicken stock

1 cup white wine

1 teaspoon salt

½ teaspoon freshly ground black pepper

2 tablespoons finely chopped fresh flat-leaf parsley

⅔ cup grated Parmesan cheese

HEAT 3 tablespoons of the olive oil in a large saucepan over medium heat and cook the onions, stirring occasionally, for 6 minutes. ADD the bacon and cook, stirring regularly, for 2 minutes. ADD the rice, mushrooms, garlic, and walnuts and cook, stirring to coat the rice with oil, for 1 minute. ADD the stock, wine, salt, and pepper, bring to a boil, cover with a lid, and reduce the heat to low. SIMMER gently for 20 minutes without lifting the lid. STIR the parsley, cheese, and reserved olive oil through the rice and serve.

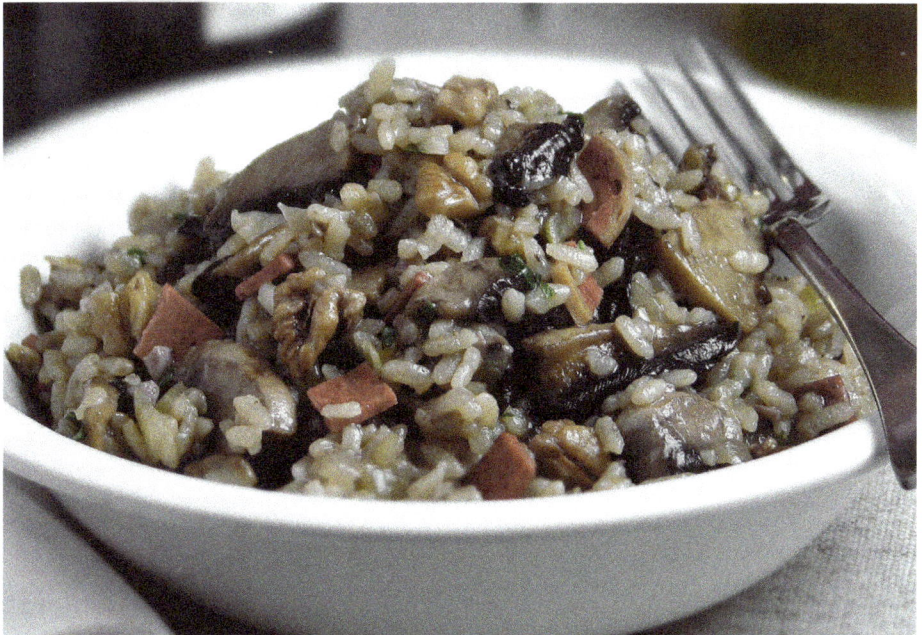

Risotto Primavera

Primavera is Italian for spring, and this colorful risotto is a great way of celebrating the arrival of tender spring vegetables.

½ cup pine nuts

5 tablespoons extra virgin olive oil

2 onions, finely chopped

4 cloves garlic, finely chopped

2 cups arborio rice

16 fresh asparagus spears, ends trimmed, cut into 1-inch pieces

16 cherry tomatoes, halved

8 white button mushrooms, thickly sliced

½ cup frozen green peas, thawed

1 cup white wine

4 cups vegetable or chicken stock

1 teaspoon salt

½ teaspoon freshly ground black pepper

4 tablespoons chopped fresh basil

⅔ cup grated Parmesan cheese

TOAST the pine nuts in a large saucepan over medium heat for 1 minute, then set aside. HEAT 3 tablespoons of the olive oil in the same saucepan over medium heat and cook the onions, stirring occasionally, until softened, about 8 minutes. ADD the garlic and rice and cook for 1 minute, stirring to coat the grains with oil. ADD the asparagus, tomatoes, and mushrooms and cook for another minute. ADD the peas, wine, stock, salt, and pepper, bring to a boil, then cover with a lid and reduce the heat to low. SIMMER gently for 20 minutes without lifting the lid. STIR the basil, cheese, pine nuts, and reserved olive oil through the rice and serve.

Variations: Lots of vegetables work well—green beans, broccoli florets, corn kernels, zucchini, celery, or carrots—choose a variety of colors and textures. You can also jazz up this risotto by adding some chopped canned artichoke hearts or sun-dried tomatoes.

Chicken Risotto with Red Pepper, Arugula & Olives

SERVES 4-6

The delicate peppery flavor of the arugula and the heat of the chili are highlighted by the sweetness of the red pepper.

5 tablespoons extra virgin olive oil

2 onions, finely chopped

4 cloves garlic, finely chopped

2 red bell peppers, finely diced

2 small red chilies, deseeded and finely chopped

2 cups arborio rice

1 cup white wine

4 cups chicken stock

1 teaspoon salt

½ teaspoon freshly ground black pepper

24 oz (680g) uncooked skinless chicken breast fillets, cut into bite-size pieces

4 cups arugula (rocket), stems trimmed, and leaves washed and roughly chopped

⅔ cup grated Parmesan cheese

16 pitted black olives, sliced

HEAT 3 tablespoons of the olive oil in a large saucepan over medium heat and cook the onions, stirring occasionally, until softened, about 8 minutes. ADD the garlic, bell peppers, and chilies and cook for 1 minute. ADD the rice and cook for another minute, stirring to coat the grains with oil. ADD the wine, stock, salt, and pepper, bring to a boil, cover with a lid, and reduce the heat to low. SIMMER gently for 12 minutes without lifting the lid. REMOVE the lid, quickly place the chicken and arugula on top of the rice, cover, and cook for 8 minutes. STIR the cheese, olives, and reserved olive oil through the rice and serve.

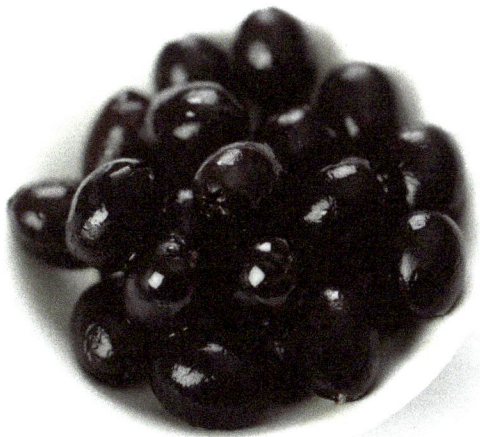

Risotto with Pumpkin, Spinach, Cannellini Beans & Walnuts

SERVES 4-6

In some parts of Italy, such as Venice, they prefer a slightly liquid risotto, where the rice ripples like a wave if the plate is tilted. In other parts of Italy the rice is cooked to a creamier consistency—and that's the way we prefer it. In this risotto the sweet pumpkin, creamy cannellini beans, and crunchy walnuts perfectly accent the delicate spinach. And when the Parmesan and fresh basil are mixed in at the end of cooking, some of the edges of the pumpkin break off and disintegrate into the rice, adding a unique and heavenly texture.

5 tablespoons extra virgin olive oil

2 onions, finely chopped

4 garlic cloves, finely chopped

2 cups arborio rice

4 cups vegetable or chicken stock

1 cup white wine

2 teaspoons salt

1 teaspoon freshly ground black pepper

4 cups peeled and cubed pumpkin or winter squash (cut into half inch cubes)

4 cups firmly-packed fresh spinach, roughly chopped

1 cup canned cannellini beans, rinsed well and drained

½ cup roughly chopped toasted walnuts

⅔ cup finely grated Parmesan cheese

2 tablespoons finely chopped fresh basil

HEAT 3 tablespoons of the oil in a large saucepan and cook the onion for 6 minutes, stirring occasionally. ADD the garlic and rice, stirring to coat the grains in oil and cook for 1 minute. ADD the wine, stock, salt, black pepper, pumpkin and spinach, stir to combine and bring to a boil. COVER with a lid, reduce the heat to low and cook for 20 minutes without lifting the lid. STIR in the cannellini beans, walnuts, Parmesan, basil and remaining 2 tablespoons of oil to combine.

Variations: Use toasted pine nuts instead of the walnuts. Use chickpeas instead of the cannellini beans.

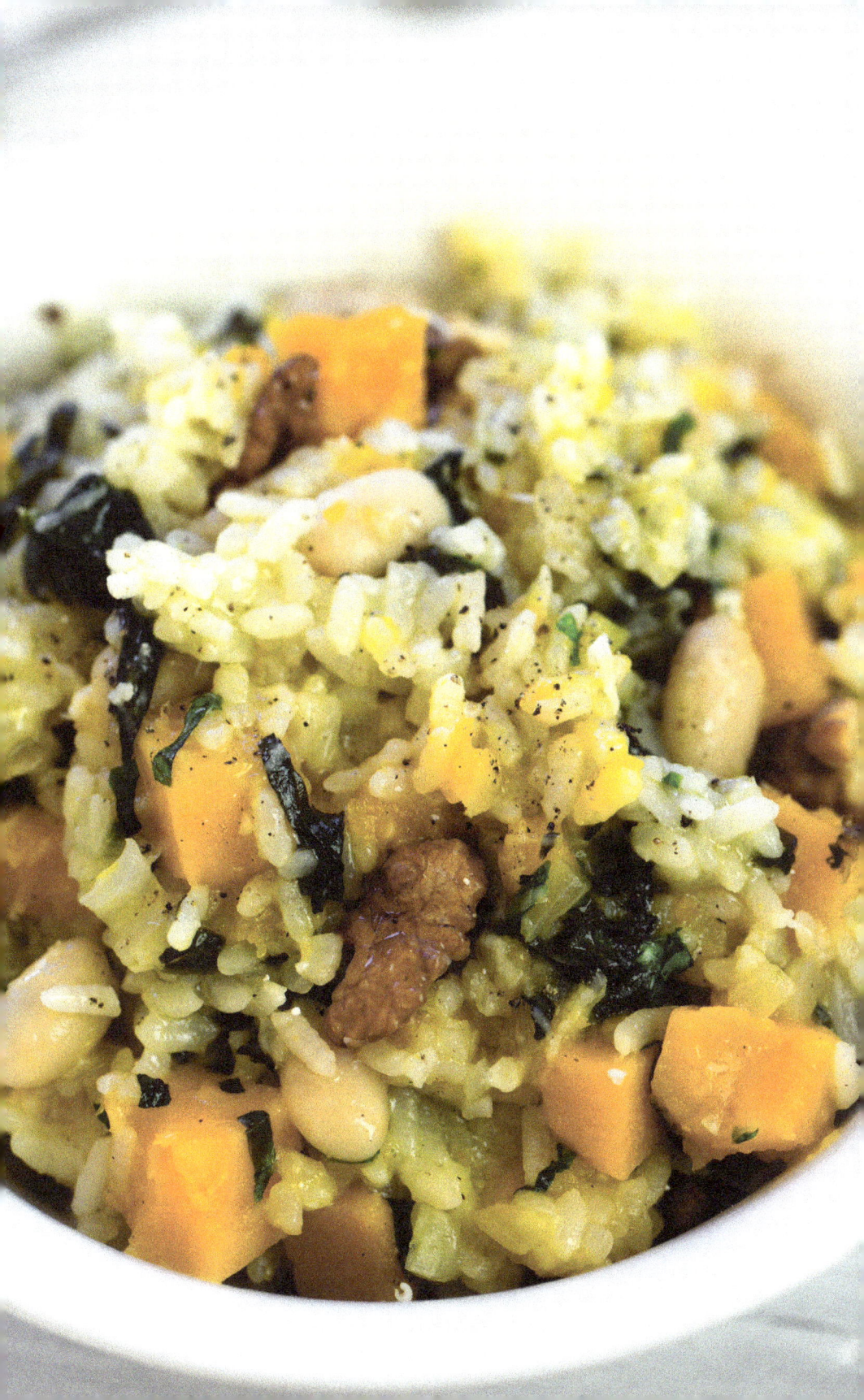

Salmon Kedgeree

SERVES 4-6

Kedgeree is based on a traditional Indian rice and lentil dish called *kitchri*, which was adapted by the British to be a breakfast dish containing fish. This hearty kedgeree makes an ideal leisurely weekend breakfast, or can turn up just as easily on the lunch or dinner table.

4 teaspoons peanut or canola oil

4 teaspoons butter

2 onions, finely chopped

2 carrots, peeled and diced

4 cloves garlic, minced

6 teaspoons good-quality curry powder

1½ cups basmati or long-grain white rice

3 cups fish or vegetable stock

2 teaspoons brown sugar

2 teaspoons salt

4 large eggs

14 oz (400g) canned Alaskan red salmon, drained, bones removed, broken into chunks

½ cup frozen green peas, thawed

2 tablespoons freshly squeezed lemon juice

2 tablespoons finely chopped cilantro (fresh coriander)

HEAT the oil and butter in a large saucepan over medium heat and cook the onions and carrots, stirring occasionally, until softened, about 8 minutes. ADD the garlic and curry powder and cook, stirring, for 1 minute. ADD the rice and cook, stirring to coat the grains, for another minute. ADD the stock, sugar, and salt; stir to combine, bring to a boil, and cover with a lid. REDUCE the heat to low and simmer gently for 15 minutes without lifting the lid. WHILE the rice cooks, place the eggs in a pot of boiling water and cook until hard-boiled, about 6 minutes. REMOVE the eggs from pot, peel, cut into quarters and set aside. REMOVE the saucepan lid, quickly place the salmon and peas on top of the rice, replace the lid, and cook for another 5 minutes. ADD the lemon juice and cilantro and fluff up the rice gently with a fork to combine the ingredients. SERVE the kedgeree on plates with the quartered eggs on top.

Variation: Replace the salmon with canned tuna or use sliced smoked salmon for a lavish alternative.

Tunisian Chicken and Almond Couscous

SERVES 4-6

Couscous, a staple food of North Africa, is one of the most ancient convenience foods and is ready to eat in five minutes. In this dish, couscous is steamed in stock with chicken, vegetables, and spices, becoming light and fluffy as it soaks up the delicious Tunisian-inspired flavors.

⅓ cup sliced almonds

5 tablespoons extra virgin olive oil

24 oz (680g) uncooked skinless chicken breast fillets, cut into bite-size pieces

1 red bell pepper, cut into thin strips

1 green bell pepper, cut into thin strips

2 scallions, thinly sliced

4 cloves garlic, finely chopped

2 teaspoons ground cumin

2 teaspoons paprika

2 teaspoons salt

1½ teaspoons ground black pepper

1 teaspoon cinnamon

2 cups couscous

4 cups chicken stock

2 tablespoons freshly squeezed lemon juice

4 tablespoons chopped fresh flat-leaf parsley

TOAST the almonds in a large saucepan over medium heat for 1 minute, then set aside. HEAT 3 tablespoons of the oil in the same saucepan over medium heat and cook the chicken, stirring occasionally, for about 2 minutes. ADD the bell peppers and cook, stirring occasionally, for 4 minutes. ADD the scallions, garlic, cumin, paprika, salt, pepper, and cinnamon and cook, stirring, for another minute. ADD the couscous and stock, bring to a boil, cover with a lid, then remove the saucepan from the heat. ALLOW to stand for 5 minutes, without lifting the lid, so the couscous absorbs the stock. FLUFF up the couscous with a fork, and stir in the lemon juice, parsley, reserved olive oil, and almonds, and serve.

Variation: Canned chickpeas (rinsed and drained) are a good alternative to chicken.

Serving Idea: This dish can be served with a dollop of plain Greek yogurt.

Ham & Egg Fried Rice

SERVES 4-6

Ham and eggs not only make a good breakfast combination, they also taste great together in this fried rice dish. In fact, you could even eat this dish as a breakfast.

2 cups long-grain white rice

6 tablespoons soy sauce

2 tablespoons oyster sauce

2 teaspoons sesame oil

4 tablespoons peanut or canola oil

1 red bell pepper, diced

2 zucchini (courgette), diced

1 cup frozen green peas, thawed

4 cloves garlic, finely chopped

4 thin ham slices, finely chopped

4 large eggs

BRING 3 cups of water to a boil in a saucepan. Stir in the rice and keep stirring until the water returns to a boil. COVER the pot with a tight-fitting lid, reduce the heat to very low, and simmer gently for 15 minutes. LEAVE the rice to cool (preferably in the fridge overnight). MIX together the soy sauce, oyster sauce, and sesame oil in a small bowl and set aside. HEAT a wok or large skillet over high heat and add the peanut oil. ADD the bell pepper and cook, stirring, for 2 minutes. ADD the zucchini and cook, stirring, for 2 minutes. ADD the peas and garlic and stir for 30 seconds, then add the ham and eggs and stir for another minute. ADD the rice and stir, tossing to separate the grains and combine well, for a minute. ADD the sauce mixture; cook, stirring, for 2 minutes and serve.

Shrimp Fried Rice

SERVES 4-6

A traditional Chinese fried rice dish with fresh succulent shrimp, red pepper, zucchini, and green peas.

2 cups long-grain white rice

6 tablespoons soy sauce

2 tablespoons oyster sauce

4 teaspoons sesame oil

6 tablespoons peanut or canola oil

32 large uncooked shrimp (prawns)

1 red bell pepper, diced

2 zucchini (courgette), diced

1 cup frozen green peas, thawed

4 cloves garlic, finely chopped

BRING 3 cups of water to a boil in a saucepan. STIR in the rice and keep stirring until the water returns to a boil. COVER the pot with a tight-fitting lid, reduce the heat to very low, and simmer gently for 15 minutes. LEAVE the rice to cool (preferably in the fridge overnight). MIX together the soy sauce, oyster sauce, and sesame oil in a small bowl and set aside. HEAT a wok or large skillet over high heat, then add 2 tablespoons of the peanut oil. ADD the shrimp and cook, stirring, for 2 minutes. REMOVE the shrimp from the wok and set aside on a plate. HEAT the remaining 4 tablespoons of oil in the same pan, add the bell peppers and cook, stirring, for 1 minute. ADD the zucchini and cook, stirring, for 2 minutes. ADD the peas and garlic and cook, stirring, for 30 seconds. ADD the rice and stir for another minute, tossing to separate the grains and combine well. ADD the sauce mixture and cook, stirring, for 2 minutes. ADD the cooked shrimp, toss to mix and heat through, and serve.

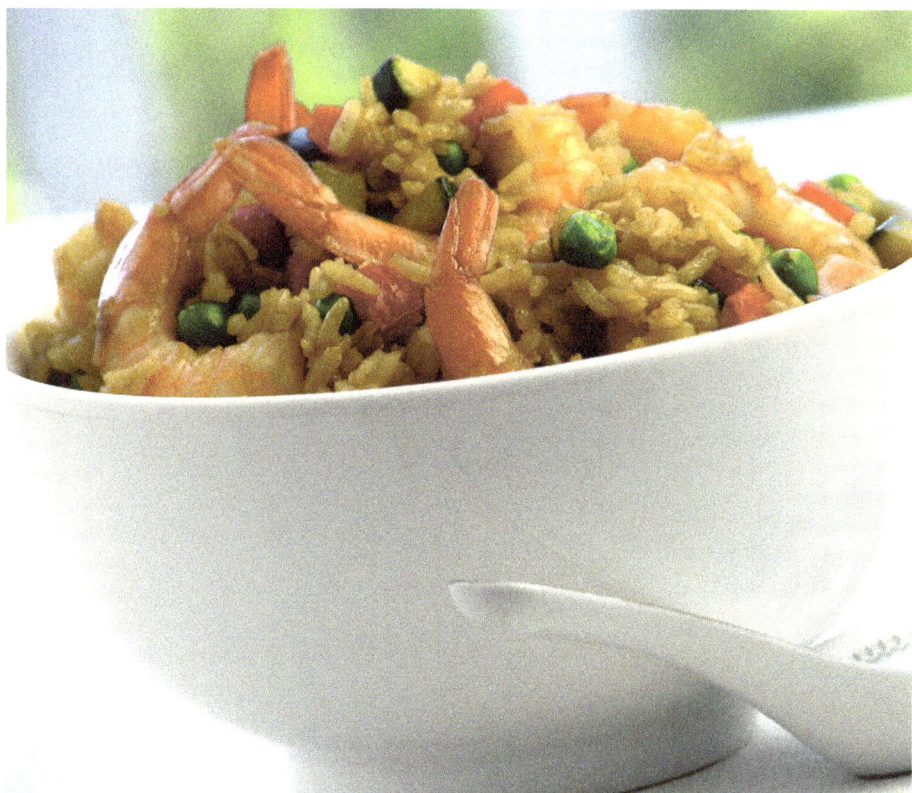

CHAPTER 17

NOODLE DISHES

Seafood Chow Mein

SERVES 4

Chow mein is Chinese for "fried noodles." Cooking your own chow mein at home is quick and simple, and it's a great way to use up whatever spare ingredients you have on hand. In this version we combine noodles with fresh seafood, colorful vegetables, and a flavorful Chinese-style sauce.

8 oz (230g) dried Chinese wheat noodles

4 tablespoons soy sauce

2 tablespoons black bean sauce

4 tablespoons oyster sauce

2 tablespoons Chinese rice wine (or dry sherry)

1 tablespoon brown sugar

6 tablespoons peanut or canola oil

12 large uncooked shrimp (prawns), peeled

12 uncooked large scallops

2 squid tubes, cut into bite-size pieces

2 red bell peppers, cut into thin strips

20 snow peas, ends trimmed, cut in half on the diagonal

2 bunches bok choy or choy sum, washed and roughly chopped

4 cloves garlic, finely chopped

4 teaspoons finely grated fresh ginger

ADD the dried noodles to a saucepan of boiling water and cook for 5 minutes, then rinse under cold water and set aside. MIX together the soy sauce, black bean sauce, oyster sauce, Chinese rice wine, and sugar in a bowl and set aside. HEAT a wok or large skillet over high heat, add 2 tablespoons of the oil and cook the shrimp and scallops, stirring, for 1½ minutes. ADD the squid and cook, stirring, for 1 minute, then remove the seafood from the wok and set aside on a plate. ADD the remaining oil to the wok and cook the bell peppers, stirring, for 3 minutes. ADD the snow peas and bok choy or choy sum and cook, stirring, for another 4 minutes. ADD the garlic and ginger, stir for 1 minute, then return the seafood to the wok. ADD the noodles to the wok and stir to combine. ADD the sauce mixture and cook, stirring, until thoroughly combined, and serve.

Thai Lime-Pepper Chicken Noodles

SERVES 4

Long before chilies (a New World food) were introduced to Thailand, pepper was the favored way to add heat and pungency to food. And although chilies have now become an integral part of Thai cuisine, pepper is still used in many Thai dishes. This tasty Thai noodle dish combines chicken and a selection of colorful vegetables with black pepper, lime, basil and other traditional seasonings. It's simple to put together, so it makes a great weeknight meal—especially if you're in the mood for something a bit more exotic.

2 tablespoons soy sauce

2 tablespoons fish sauce

6 tablespoons oyster sauce

4 tablespoons water

2 teaspoons freshly ground black pepper

7 oz (200g) dried rice stick noodles

5 tablespoons peanut or canola oil

24 oz (700g) uncooked skinless chicken breast fillets, cut into bite size pieces

2 red peppers, cut into thin strips

10 button mushrooms, quartered

24 snow peas, ends trimmed, and left whole

2 garlic cloves, finely chopped

2 teaspoons finely chopped lime zest

2 scallions, thinly sliced on the diagonal

2 tablespoons finely chopped fresh basil

2 tablespoons fresh lime juice

MIX together the soy sauce, fish sauce, oyster sauce, water and pepper in a small bowl until combined. PLACE the rice stick noodles in a large bowl, cover with boiling water and soak for 8 minutes, then rinse under cold water, drain, and set aside. HEAT a wok or large frying pan over a high heat then add 2 tablespoons of the oil. STIR-FRY the chicken for 4 minutes then remove from the wok and set aside on a plate. ADD the remaining 3 tablespoons of oil to the hot wok and stir-fry the pepper for 3 minutes. ADD the mushrooms and snow peas and cook for 2 minutes. ADD the garlic and lime zest and cook a minute. ADD the cooked chicken, noodles and sauce mixture, and stir-fry until thoroughly combined and heated through. STIR through the scallion, basil and lime juice and serve.

Variations: Instead of chicken you can use shrimp, scallops, squid, or tofu. Other vegetables that go well with this dish include green beans, bean sprouts, broccoli, canned bamboo shoots, or carrots. And if you want to add some extra crunch, cashews or chopped peanuts are ideal.

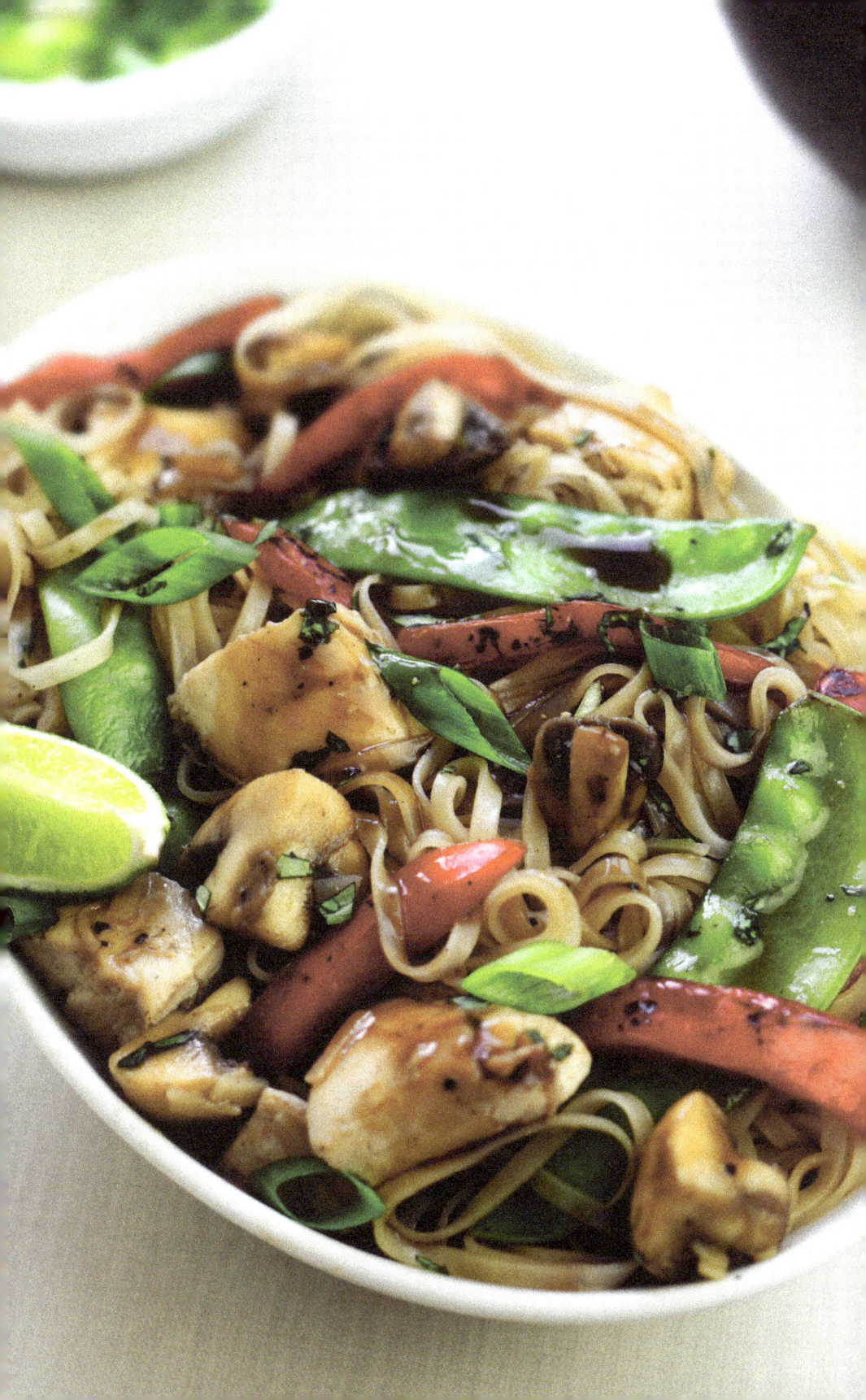

Teriyaki Chicken Noodles

SERVES 4

The savory-sweet teriyaki sauce combines perfectly with the tender chicken and vegetables in this quick and flavorful noodle dish.

7 oz (200g) dried somen noodles

½ cup water

8 tablespoons soy sauce

6 tablespoons mirin (rice wine)

4 teaspoons brown sugar

4 tablespoons peanut or canola oil

24 oz (680g) uncooked skinless chicken breast fillets, cut into bite-size pieces

2 carrots, peeled and julienned

Small bunch of bok choy, washed and roughly chopped

4 teaspoons finely grated fresh ginger

2 scallions, thinly sliced on the diagonal

4 teaspoons cornstarch (corn flour), mixed to a paste with 4 teaspoons water

COOK the noodles in a pot of boiling water for 3 minutes, then drain under cold water and set aside. MIX together the water, soy sauce, mirin, and brown sugar in a bowl and set aside. HEAT a wok or large skillet over high heat, add 2 tablespoons of the oil, and cook the chicken, stirring, for 5 minutes. REMOVE the chicken from the pan and set aside on a plate. SCRAPE the wok or skillet clean. ADD the remaining oil to the wok and cook the carrots and bok choy, stirring, until softened, for 7 minutes. ADD the cooked somen noodles and stir for 30 seconds. ADD the ginger, scallions, and chicken and cook, stirring, for 1 minute. ADD the sauce and stir to combine. WHILE stirring constantly, add the cornstarch paste, cook until the sauce thickens, and serve.

Variation: This dish can easily be transformed into Teriyaki Scallop Noodles by replacing the chicken with 24 oz (680g) of uncooked large scallops, which you need to stir-fry for only 2 minutes.

Chicken & Ham Chow Mein

SERVES 4

An assortment of crisp vegetables, chicken, and ham are tossed with soft noodles in a delicate Peking-style sauce.

8 oz (230g) dried Chinese wheat noodles

4 tablespoons soy sauce

6 tablespoons hoisin sauce

2 tablespoons Chinese rice wine (or dry sherry)

2 teaspoons sesame oil

4 tablespoons peanut or canola oil

12 oz (340g) uncooked skinless chicken breast fillet, cut into bite-size pieces

2 carrots, peeled and julienned

2 cups broccoli florets

4 cups shredded Chinese (Napa) cabbage

4 thin ham slices, chopped

4 cloves garlic, minced

1 tablespoon finely grated fresh ginger

2 scallions, thinly sliced

ADD the dried noodles to a saucepan of boiling water and cook for 5 minutes, then rinse under cold water and set aside. MIX together the soy sauce, hoisin sauce, Chinese rice wine, and sesame oil in a bowl and set aside. HEAT a wok or large skillet over high heat, add 2 tablespoons of the oil, and cook the chicken, stirring, for 4 minutes. REMOVE the chicken from the wok and set aside on a plate. ADD the remaining oil to the wok and cook the carrots and broccoli, stirring, for 4 minutes. ADD the cabbage and cook, stirring, for another 2 minutes. ADD the ham, garlic, and ginger, stir for 1 minute, then return the chicken to the wok. ADD the noodles and stir to combine. ADD the sauce mixture and scallions, mix to heat through, and serve.

Variation: Use whatever you have on hand to create your own combination chow mein: replace the chicken and ham with tofu, shrimp, or scallops; add other vegetables like green beans, snow peas, red and green bell peppers, or mushrooms (fresh or dried).

Tofu & Cashew Chow Mein

SERVES 4

Crunchy cashews and vegetables complement the soft texture of the noodles and tofu in this quick and satisfying dish.

20 oz (550g) precooked thick Chinese wheat noodles

6 tablespoons soy sauce

4 tablespoons oyster sauce

4 teaspoons sesame oil

4 tablespoons water

4 tablespoons peanut or canola oil

2 carrots, peeled and julienned

4 cups small broccoli florets

12 oz (340g) firm tofu, cut into cubes

4 cloves garlic, finely chopped

4 teaspoons finely grated fresh ginger

1 cup roasted cashew nuts

LOOSEN the precooked noodles by soaking in a bowl of hot water for 2 to 3 minutes, then drain and set aside. MIX together the soy sauce, oyster sauce, sesame oil, and water in a bowl and set aside. HEAT a wok or large skillet over high heat, add the oil, and cook the carrots and broccoli, stirring, for 2 minutes. ADD the tofu and cook, stirring, for 4 minutes. ADD the garlic and ginger and stir for 1 minute. ADD the noodles and stir to combine. ADD the sauce mixture and cashews, mix until thoroughly combined and heated through, and serve.

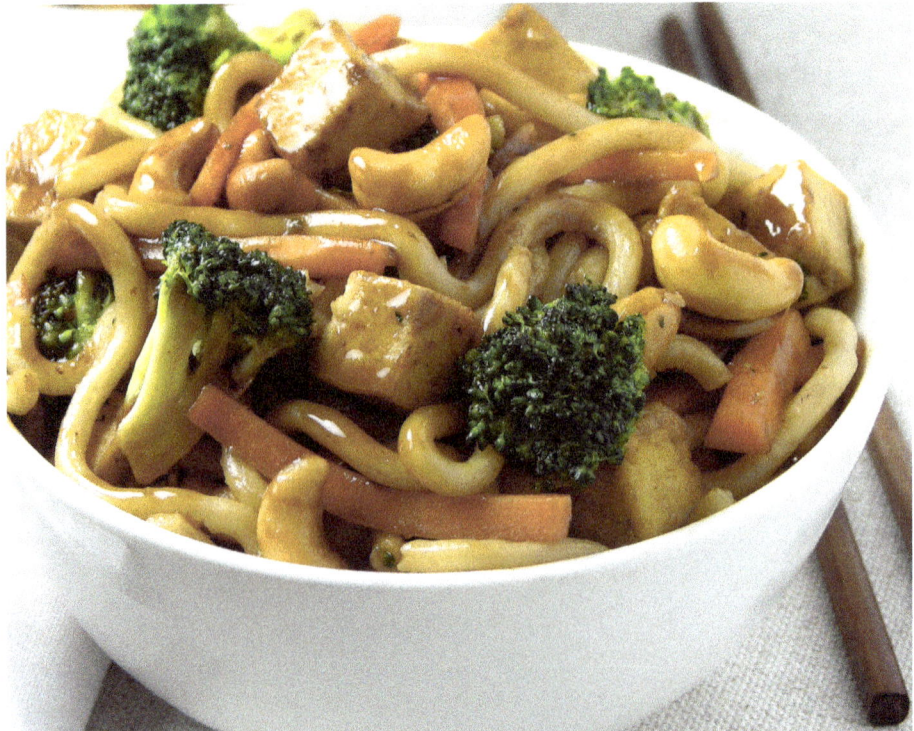

Peanut Chicken Noodles

SERVES 4

Long, slippery rice noodles with strips of stir-fried chicken and vegetables in a rich and spicy Indonesian peanut sauce.

10 oz (280g) dried rice stick noodles

4 tablespoons peanut or canola oil

24 oz (680g) uncooked skinless chicken breast fillets, cut into strips

2 carrots, cut into thin rounds

2 zucchini, cut into thin strips

1 cup Indonesian Peanut Sauce (page 284), hot

SOAK the rice stick noodles in boiling water for 10 minutes, then rinse under cold water and set aside. HEAT a wok or large skillet over high heat then add 2 tablespoons of the oil. COOK the chicken, stirring, for 3 minutes, then remove from the wok and set aside on a plate. ADD the remaining oil to the hot wok and cook the carrots, stirring, for 1 minute. ADD the zucchini and cook, stirring, for another 4 minutes. ADD the cooked noodles and chicken and toss to combine and heat through. POUR in the hot peanut sauce, thoroughly mix all the ingredients together, and serve.

Soba Noodle Scallops

SERVES 4

This delicate Japanese broth with soba noodles and tender scallops is simple to prepare and highly satisfying.

8 cups dashi stock (dashi stock powder is available at Asian food stores)

4 tablespoons Japanese soy sauce

2 carrots, cut into thin rounds

4 teaspoons finely grated fresh ginger

6 oz (170g) soba noodles

24 uncooked large scallops

2 scallions, thinly sliced on the diagonal

BRING 8 cups of dashi stock to a boil in a saucepan. ADD the soy sauce, carrots, and ginger and simmer, covered, for 6 minutes. WHILE the broth simmers, cook the noodles in boiling water in a separate saucepan for 5 minutes, then drain. ADD the scallops to the broth, simmer for 2 minutes, remove from the heat, and add the noodles. SERVE in bowls with scallions scattered on top.

Japanese Tuna & Vegetable Udon Noodle Pot

SERVES 4

In this one-pot meal, tuna and vegetables are simmered in a flavorsome stock, then served over soft and slippery udon noodles.

4 oz (115g) dried udon noodles

8 cups chicken stock

24 oz (680g) fresh tuna steak, cut into bite-size pieces

4 cups shredded green cabbage

2 carrots, peeled and julienned

20 snow peas, ends trimmed and cut in half on the diagonal

16 fresh shiitake mushrooms, stems removed and sliced into halves

2 teaspoons finely grated fresh ginger

4 tablespoons Japanese soy sauce

2 tablespoons freshly squeezed lemon juice

2 scallions, thinly sliced

Add the dried udon noodles to a saucepan of boiling water and cook for 7 minutes. PLACE the stock in a large saucepan and bring to a boil. ADD the tuna, cabbage, carrots, snow peas, mushrooms, and ginger and return to a boil. COVER the pot, reduce the heat and simmer for 6 minutes. REMOVE from the heat and stir in the soy sauce and lemon juice. DRAIN the noodles and put equal amounts into soup bowls and scatter scallions on top. POUR over the boiling tuna-vegetable broth to cover and allow to stand for 1 minute. SERVE with chopsticks and a soup spoon.

Variations: Replace the tuna with chicken, shrimp, or scallops. Cubes of firm tofu also make a tasty addition (tofu soaks up flavors well). Dried rice or cellophane noodles that have been soaked until soft can replace the udon noodles.

Mie Goreng (Indonesian Fried Noodles

SERVES 4

An Indonesian fried noodle dish with shrimp, pork, and vegetables, flavored with a spicy sauce mixture, and topped with fresh cilantro and crisp cucumber.

8 oz (230g) dried Chinese wheat noodles

4 tablespoons soy sauce

4 tablespoons kecap manis (Indonesian sweet soy sauce, which is available at Asian food stores)

3 tablespoons fish sauce

2 teaspoons sambal oelek (Indonesian chili sauce)

4 tablespoons peanut or canola oil

10 oz (280g) lean pork, finely diced

4 cups shredded green cabbage

4 scallions (spring onions), thinly sliced

6 cloves garlic, finely chopped

10 oz (280g) small peeled cooked shrimp

Finely chopped cilantro (fresh coriander), for garnish

Thin strips of cucumber, for garnish

ADD the dried noodles to a saucepan of boiling water and cook for 5 minutes, then rinse under cold water and set aside. MIX together the soy sauce, kecap manis, fish sauce, and sambal oelek in a bowl and set aside. HEAT the oil in a wok or large skillet over high heat and cook the pork, stirring, for 3 minutes. ADD the cabbage and cook, stirring, for 2 minutes. ADD the scallions and garlic and cook, stirring, for 2 minutes. ADD the noodles, shrimp, and sauce mixture and stir for 1 minute to combine well and heat through. SERVE in bowls garnished with cilantro and cucumber strips on top.

Variation: Replace the pork with lean bacon or ham.

Malaysian Fish Ball Curry Laksa

SERVES 4

There's nothing more comforting than slurping down a bowl of tasty *laksa* (a spicy Malaysian coconut-based noodle soup). The star of this laksa is the fish balls, which develop a tender texture as they cook. When you bite into them they break apart releasing the beautiful flavor of fresh, lightly seasoned fish.

7 oz (200g) dried rice stick noodles

4 cups bean sprouts

4 scallions, thinly sliced

A handful of cilantro (fresh coriander) leaves

20 oz (550g) uncooked firm white fish fillets (such as cod or snapper), roughly chopped

2 tablespoons soy sauce

1 tablespoon cornstarch (cornflour)

2 tablespoons peanut or canola oil

2 tablespoons green curry paste

4 garlic cloves, finely chopped

1 teaspoon finely grated lime zest

28 oz (800g) coconut milk

4 cups fish, chicken or vegetable stock

5 tablespoons fish sauce

2 tablespoons brown sugar

2 yellow or red peppers, cut into thin strips

2 carrots, thinly sliced into rounds

2 tablespoons lime juice

SOAK the noodles in boiling water for 10 minutes, then drain and rinse under cold water. PLACE equal amounts of noodles in the bottom of four large bowls. PLACE even amounts of bean sprouts, the green part of the scallions and cilantro on top of each (reserve a little scallion and cilantro for garnish). PLACE the fish, soy sauce and cornstarch in a food processor and process until the fish is minced. FORM the mixture into walnut-size balls and set aside on a plate. HEAT the oil over a medium heat and cook the curry paste, garlic and lime zest for 1 minute. ADD the coconut milk, stock, fish sauce and brown sugar, increase the heat and bring to a rolling simmer. COOK for 2 minutes, uncovered, then add the yellow peppers, carrots and white parts of the scallions and cook for 2 minutes, uncovered. ADD the fish balls, cover with a lid, and cook for 5 minutes. REMOVE from the heat and stir in the lime juice. LADLE equal amounts of the fish ball-vegetable soup into each bowl over the noodles, and garnish with extra scallion and cilantro to serve.

Variations: Replace the fish balls with bite-size pieces of white fish or salmon. Or add chicken, shrimp, scallops, squid, mussels, tofu, or use a combination. Use other vegetables such as cabbage, broccoli, mushrooms and red pepper.

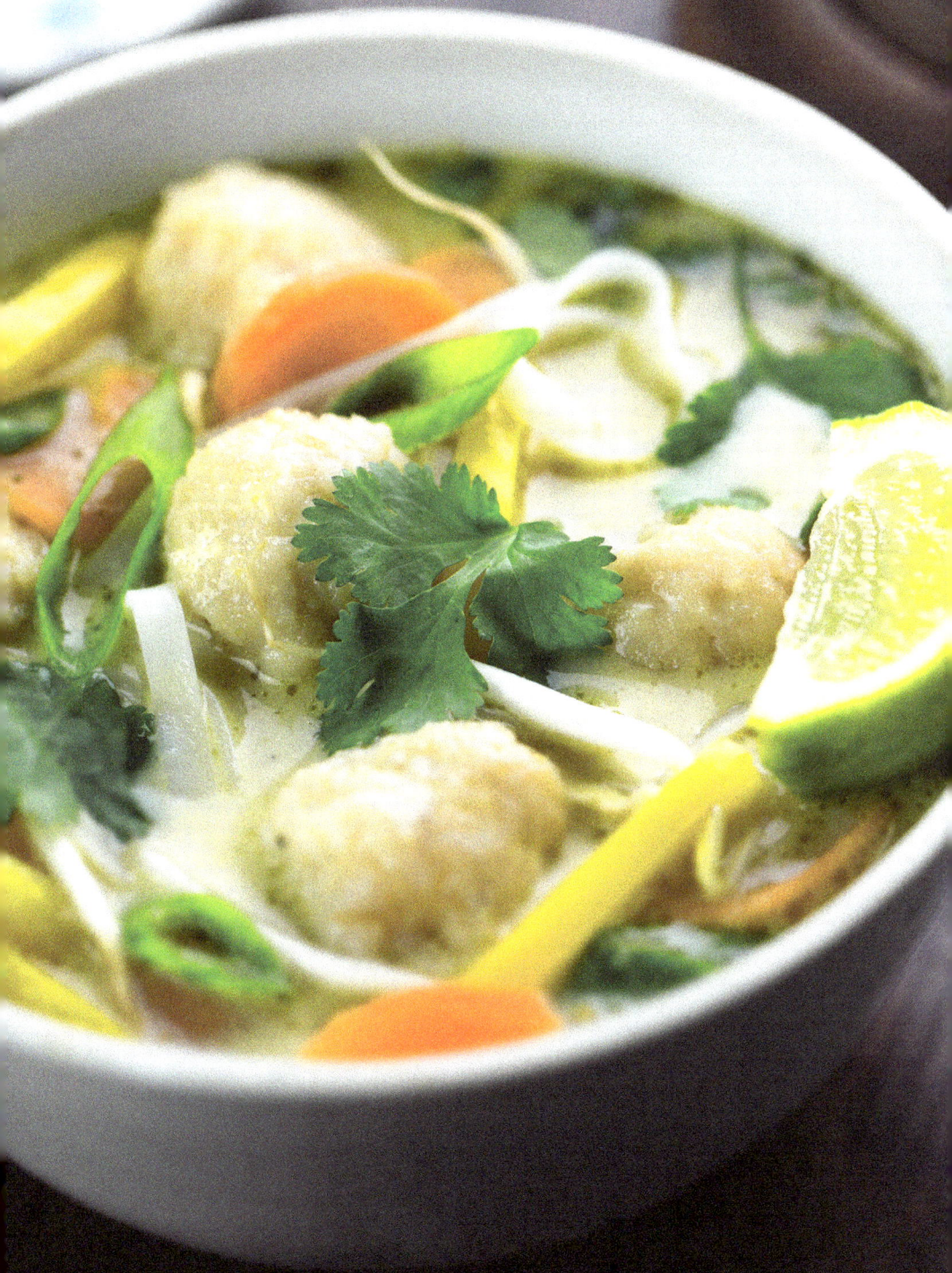

Asian Cilantro-Peanut Pesto Noodles with Chicken, Broccoli & Red Pepper

SERVES 4

This recipe combines rice noodles with chicken, lightly steamed vegetables, and an Asian-inspired pesto.

8 oz (230g) dried rice stick noodles

2 red bell peppers, cut into thin strips

4 cups broccoli florets

1½ cups Asian Cilantro-Peanut Pesto (page 287)

24 oz (680g) cooked skinless chicken breast, shredded

SOAK the noodles in boiling water for 10 minutes. WHILE the noodles are soaking, cook the red peppers and broccoli in a saucepan of rapidly boiling water for 6 minutes. DRAIN the noodles, toss with the pesto, cooked vegetables, and chicken until thoroughly combined and serve.

Variation: Replace the chicken with cooked seafood or cubes of firm tofu.

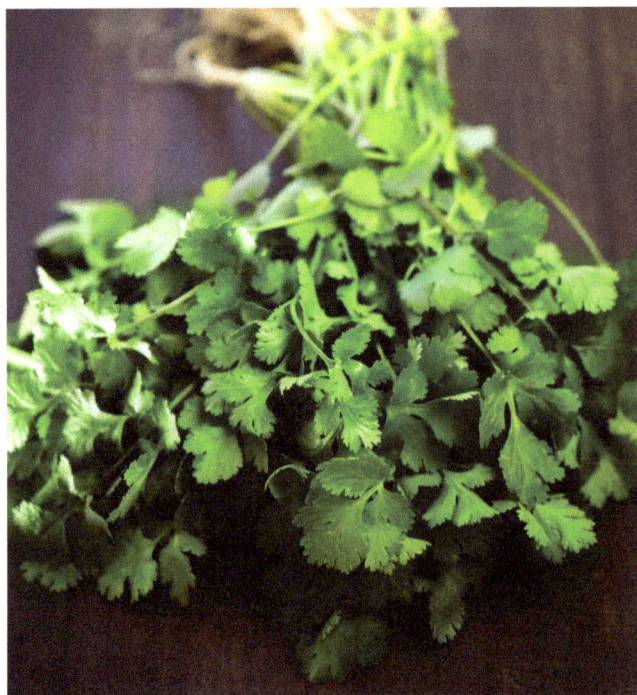

CHAPTER 18

SUSHI & RICE PAPER ROLLS

Sushi Rolls

SERVES 4-6

There are two main types of sushi, *nigiri* sushi, which is vinegared rice, hand-formed into oval shapes and topped with various raw and cooked seafood, and *maki* sushi which is vinegared rice, combined with seafood and vegetables then wrapped in an edible seaweed called nori and sliced into rounds. Nigiri sushi is quite finicky to make at home and we tend to eat this type of sushi at Japanese restaurants and sushi bars. Maki sushi, on the other hand, is far easier to prepare in your own kitchen and the taste of these delightful morsels has left many (including us) with an addiction for life! This sushi recipe requires a sushi mat for rolling.

2½ cups Japanese short-grain white rice (like Koshihikari rice)

2½ cups cold water

4 tablespoons rice vinegar

3 tablespoons sugar

2 teaspoons salt

Your choice of fillings (Sushi Roll Variations, page 220)

6 sheets nori

Wasabi paste, for serving

Japanese soy sauce, for serving

Pickled ginger (gari), for serving

PLACE the rice in a colander and rinse thoroughly under the tap until the water runs clear, then drain well. PLACE the rice and the cold water in a medium saucepan and bring to a boil. COVER the saucepan, turn the heat down to very low, and cook for 15 minutes without lifting the lid. TURN off the heat, allow to stand for 10 minutes, still covered, then spoon the rice into a large bowl. MIX together the vinegar, sugar and salt in a small bowl until the sugar dissolves, then drizzle over the rice. MIX together gently to coat the rice with the sushi vinegar, then set aside to cool to room temperature. TO fill and roll the sushi rolls, see the diagram on page 219.

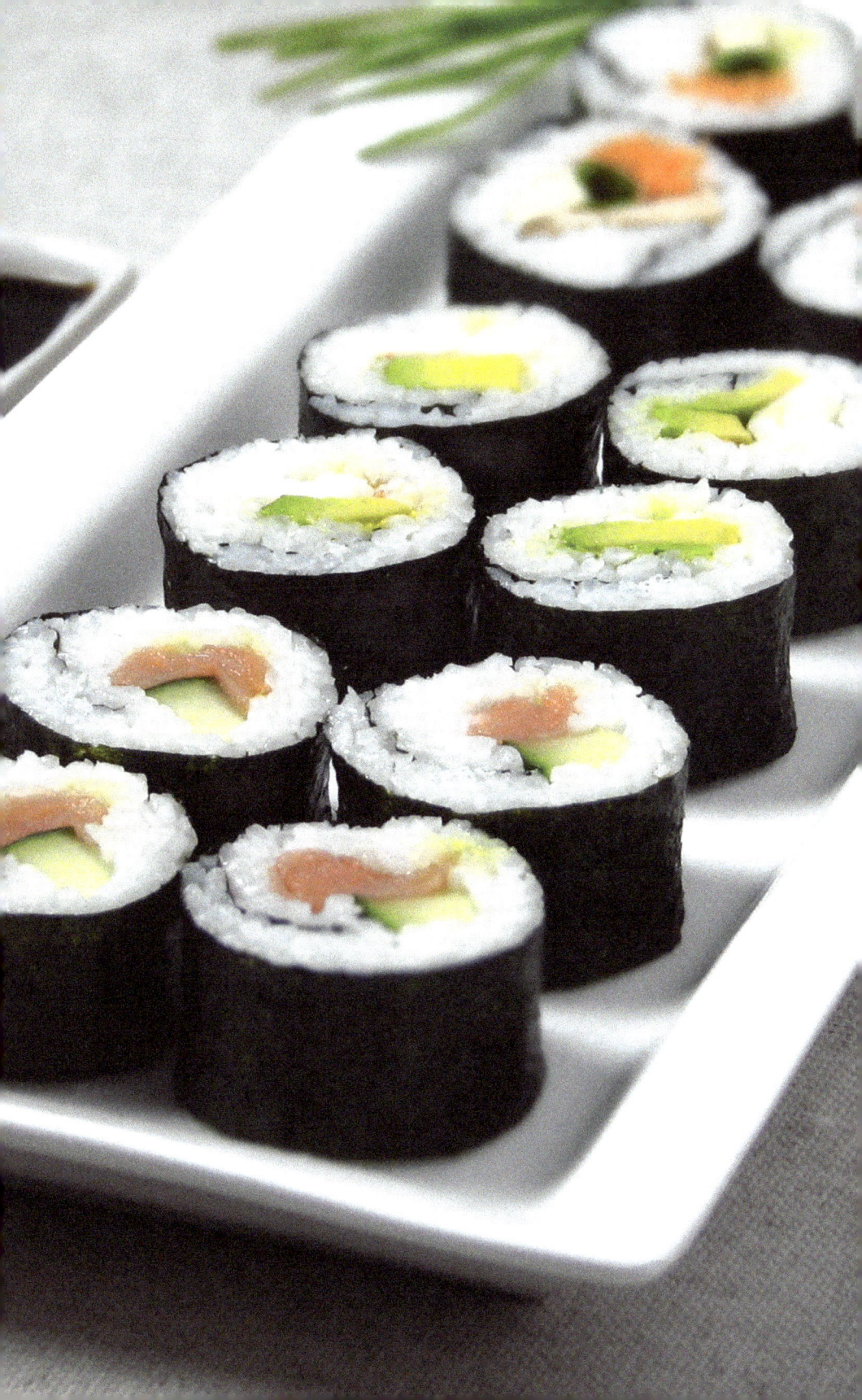

HOW TO ROLL SUSHI

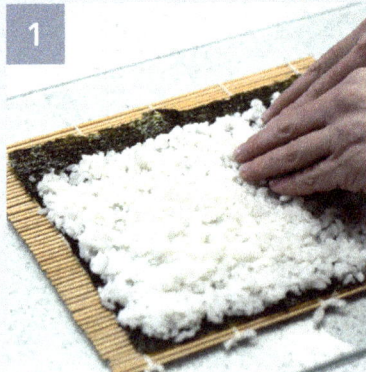

1 PLACE a nori sheet on your rolling mat (shiny side down) and spread cooked sushi rice evenly over the nori by pressing with wet fingertips, leaving a 1-inch border at the far edge.

ARRANGE small portions of your chosen fillings (in this case, smoked salmon slices and avocado) in a horizontal line down the center of the rice.

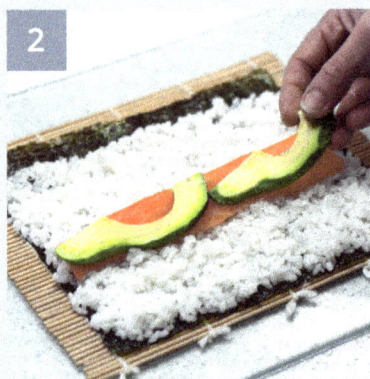

2

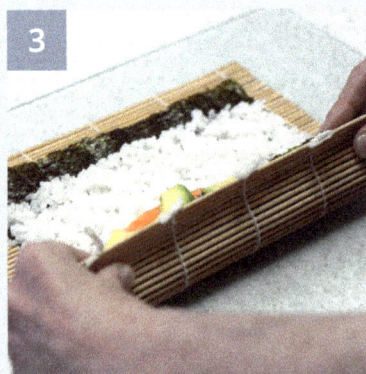

3 ROLL up the sushi tightly with the sushi mat to form a neatly packed cylinder (like a fat cigar).

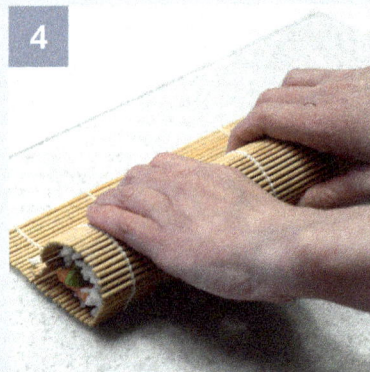

4

SQUEEZE firmly to make sure the sushi roll is tightly packed.

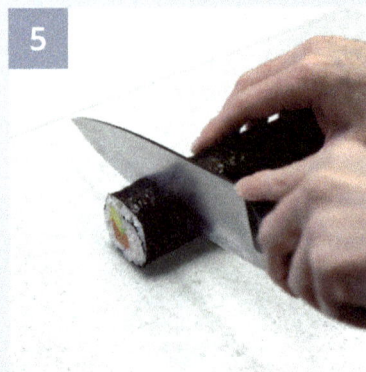

5 CUT each sushi roll into 1½-inch rounds using a sharp, damp knife. SERVE the sushi with a small bowl of shoyu (soy sauce) and wasabi (Japanese horseradish) for dipping, and slices of gari (Japanese pickled ginger) for cleansing the palate between sushi pieces.

Variations: The range of possible fillings for sushi rolls is enormous. By mixing and matching various ingredients you can create many different varieties. Here are some popular sushi roll fillings.

- Smoked salmon
- Cooked shrimp (prawns)
- Crab (or surimi)
- Very fresh raw tuna and salmon
- Tofu (firm or silken)
- Eggs (made into an omelet and cut into strips)
- Toasted sesame seeds

- Cucumber
- Avocado
- Scallions
- Mushrooms
- Snow peas
- Snow pea sprouts
- Asparagus (lightly steamed)
- Carrot

Our Favorite Sushi Rolls

Each of the following sushi recipes makes 6 sushi rolls (or approximately 36 sushi rounds)

Smoked Salmon and Avocado Sushi Rolls. CUT 6 ounces (170g) of sliced smoked salmon into thin strips. PEEL an avocado and cut the flesh into strips. ARRANGE equal amounts of salmon and avocado across the middle of each rice-topped nori sheet. ROLL the sushi up and cut into 1½-inch rounds to serve.

Tuna and Cucumber Sushi Rolls. CUT a 10-ounce (280g) piece of very fresh raw tuna into thin strips. PEEL and remove the seeds from half a small cucumber and cut the flesh into thin strips. ARRANGE equal amounts of tuna and cucumber across the middle of each rice-topped nori sheet. ROLL the sushi up and cut into 1½-inch rounds to serve.

Shrimp and Vegetable Sushi Rolls. CUT 12 large peeled, cooked shrimp (prawns) in half lengthways. PEEL and remove the seeds from half a small cucumber and cut the flesh into thin strips. TRIM and cut 2 scallions (white and green parts) into thin diagonal slices and thinly slice the flesh of ½ avocado. ARRANGE equal amounts of the filling across the middle of each rice-topped nori sheet. ROLL the sushi up and cut into 1½-inch rounds to serve.

Tofu, Sesame, and Mixed Vegetable Sushi Rolls. LIGHTLY toast 3 teaspoons of sesame seeds in a frying pan. CUT 6½ ounces (185g) of firm tofu into thin strips. PEEL and grate a small carrot. REMOVE the stems from 6 fresh shitake mushrooms (or use soaked, dried mushrooms or regular mushrooms) and thinly slice. WASH and drain ½ cup snow pea sprouts. ARRANGE equal amounts of the filling across the middle of each rice-topped nori sheet. ROLL the sushi up and cut into 1½-inch rounds to serve.

Crab and Avocado Sushi Rolls. CUT 10 ounces (280g) of crab (or imitation crab, surimi) into thin strips and mix with 2 tablespoons of Japanese or regular mayonnaise. PEEL an avocado and cut the flesh into strips. PEEL and remove the seeds from half a small cucumber and cut the flesh into thin strips. ARRANGE equal amounts of the filling across the middle of each rice-topped nori sheet. ROLL the sushi up and cut into 1½-inch rounds to serve. AS a variation, replace the crab with cooked shrimp.

Egg and Vegetable Sushi Rolls. COOK an ordinary omelet using 2 eggs seasoned with salt and pepper, then slice it into thin strips. CUT 12 snow peas into thin strips and grate a small carrot. ARRANGE equal amounts of the filling across the middle of each rice-topped nori sheet. ROLL the sushi up and cut into 1½-inch rounds to serve.

Smoked Salmon and Asparagus Sushi Rolls. CUT 6 ounces (170g) of sliced smoked salmon into strips. LIGHTLY steam 12 trimmed asparagus spears, then cool them in cold water. ARRANGE equal amounts of the filling across the middle of each rice-topped nori sheet. ROLL the sushi up and cut into 1½-inch rounds to serve.

Rice Paper Rolls

SERVES 4-6

These soft, uncooked rolls—which are popular in Vietnam and parts of China—make a refreshing change to deep-fried spring rolls. Nutritious fillings including noodles, seafood, chicken, fresh vegetables, and aromatic herbs are wrapped in delicate rice paper sheets and served cold with the dipping sauces of your choice. You can prepare these rolls up to 4 hours ahead and chill them in the refrigerator, covered with a clean dampened dish towel to keep them moist, until you're ready to serve.

1 ounce (30g) dried rice vermicelli noodles

1 tablespoon rice vinegar

1 tablespoon water

1 teaspoon sugar

½ teaspoon salt

1 clove garlic, minced

Your choice of fillings (Rice Paper Roll Variations follow)

8 rice paper sheets

Your choice of Nuoc Cham Dipping Sauce (page 289), Chinese-Style Dipping Sauce (page 292), Sesame-Hoisin Dipping Sauce (page 292), or sweet chili sauce, for serving

PREPARE the noodles by placing them in a large bowl and pouring boiling water over them to cover. LET soak until noodles soften and separate when stirred, about 5 minutes. WHILE the noodles are soaking, mix together the vinegar, water, sugar, salt, and garlic in a small bowl until the sugar dissolves. RINSE the noodles under cold water, drain well, then cut into 3-inch lengths. MIX together the noodles and the dressing gently to coat. MIX together the dressed noodles with your choice of filling ingredients in a bowl until well combined. TO fill and roll the rice paper rolls, see the diagram on page 224.

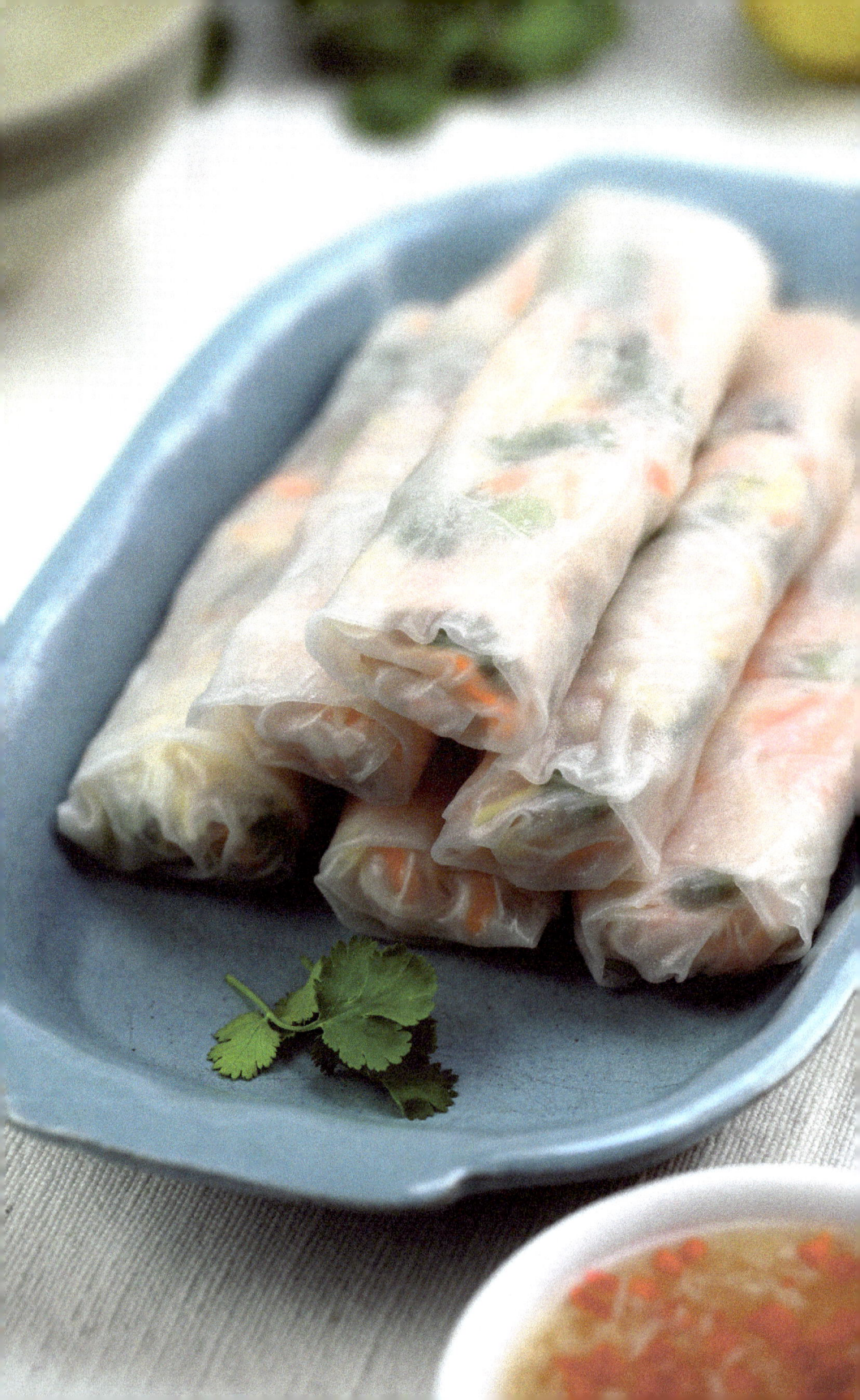

HOW TO ROLL RICE PAPER ROLLS

1

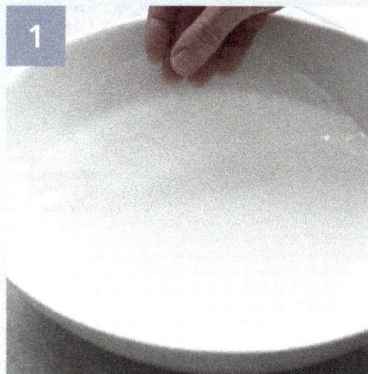

SOAK a sheet of rice paper in a large dish of warm water for about 20 seconds, then drain well.

2

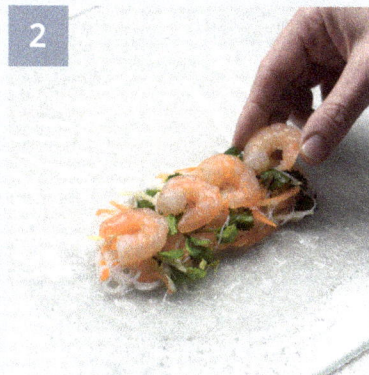

DELICATELY place the sheet of rice paper out on top of a clean chopping board, then place the filling ingredients toward the lower edge of the rice paper.

3

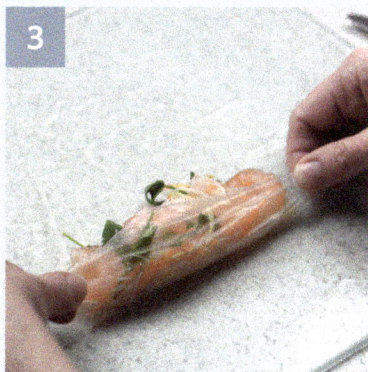

NEATLY fold the bottom edge of the rice paper over the filling.

4

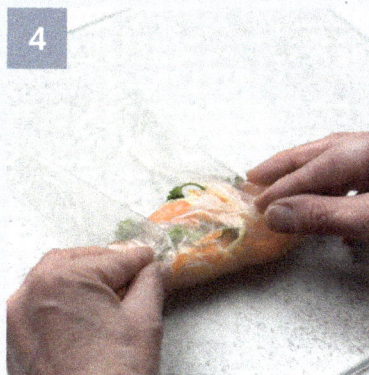

FOLD in the side edges of the rice paper.

5

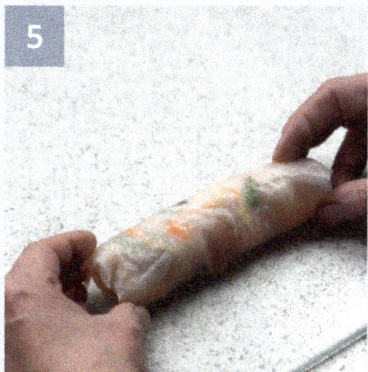

ROLL up the rice paper roll to form a neatly packed cylinder, then arrange the rice paper rolls on a plate with your choice of dipping sauce to serve.

Variations: There are lots of fillings you can wrap in rice paper sheets. Feel free to come up with your own varieties or use the following suggestions. Here are some popular rice paper roll fillings.

- Chicken breast
- Cooked salmon and tuna
- Cooked shrimp
- Crab (or surimi)
- Tofu (firm or silken)
- Bean sprouts
- Red and green bell peppers
- Chinese (Napa) cabbage
- Cucumber
- Scallions
- Mushrooms
- Snow peas

- Zucchini
- Carrot
- Water chestnuts
- Mint
- Cilantro (fresh coriander)
- Basil
- Garlic
- Chili
- Ginger
- Roasted peanuts
- Toasted sesame seeds

Our Favorite Rice Paper Rolls

Each of the following variations makes 8 rice paper rolls.

Vietnamese Shrimp and Vegetable Rolls. MIX together the dressed noodles with ½ cup bean sprouts, 1 peeled and grated carrot, ½ cup finely diced red bell pepper, ½ cup finely diced cucumber, 2 tablespoons of finely chopped fresh mint, 12 ounces (340g) cooked peeled shrimp, and 2 tablespoons chopped roasted peanuts in a bowl until well combined. ROLL up in rice paper sheets and serve with the dipping sauces of your choice—Nuoc Cham Dipping Sauce (page 289) or sweet chili sauce are ideal with these rolls.

Chinese-Style Chicken and Vegetable Rolls. MIX together the dressed noodles with 1 peeled and grated carrot, 8 thinly sliced snow peas, ½ cup finely chopped canned water chestnuts (rinsed and drained), 1 teaspoon finely grated fresh ginger, 2 trimmed and finely sliced scallions (white and green parts), 2 tablespoons finely chopped cilantro (fresh coriander) and 12 ounces (340g) shredded cooked skinless chicken breast in a bowl until well combined. ROLL up in rice paper sheets and serve with the dipping sauces of your choice—Chinese-Style Dipping Sauce (page 292) is particularly good with these rolls.

Combination Seafood Rolls. MIX together the dressed noodles with 1 cup finely shredded Chinese (Napa) cabbage, ½ cup finely chopped red bell pepper, 1 teaspoon finely grated fresh ginger, 2 tablespoons finely chopped cilantro (fresh coriander), and 6 ounces (170g) each of shredded crab (or imitation crab, surimi) and cooked shrimp in a bowl until well combined. ROLL up in rice paper sheets and serve with the dipping sauces of your choice—these rolls are ideal with Sesame-Hoisin Dipping Sauce (page 292).

Mushroom, Tofu, and Sesame Rolls. MIX together the dressed noodles with 1 cup finely diced mushrooms, 1 cup cubed tofu, 1 peeled and grated carrot, 2 trimmed and thinly sliced scallions (white and green parts), and 2 tablespoons of lightly toasted sesame seeds in a bowl until well combined. ROLL up in rice paper sheets and serve with the dipping sauces of your choice—these rolls are particularly good with Chinese-Style Dipping Sauce (page 292).

Fresh Tuna and Vegetable Rolls. CUT 12 ounces (340g) of raw tuna into 3-inch strips. Poach the tuna in simmering water for 4 minutes and set aside to cool. Mix the dressed noodles with 1 cup shredded Chinese (Napa) cabbage, 1 peeled and grated carrot, ½ stick finely chopped celery, 2 trimmed and thinly sliced scallions (white and green parts), 1 teaspoon finely grated fresh ginger, and the cooled poached tuna in a bowl until well combined. ROLL up in the rice paper sheets and serve with the dipping sauces of your choice—Chinese-Style Dipping Sauce (page 292) and Sesame-Hoisin Dipping Sauce (page 292) are ideal with these rolls. Good-quality canned tuna (rinsed and drained) makes a reasonable substitute for fresh.

Thai Chicken and Basil Rice Paper Rolls. MIX together the dressed noodles with ½ cup finely diced red bell pepper, ½ cup finely diced zucchini, 1 small seeded and finely chopped red chili, 2 tablespoons finely chopped fresh basil and 12 ounces (340g) shredded cooked skinless chicken breast in a bowl until well combined. ROLL up in rice paper sheets and serve with the dipping sauces of your choice—sweet chili sauce or Nuoc Cham Dipping Sauce (page 289) are particularly good with these rolls.

CHAPTER 19

GRILLED DISHES

Mediterranean Tuna & Vegetable Skewers

SERVES 4

Fresh tuna is threaded onto skewers with cherry tomatoes, zucchini, red onion, and green bell pepper, then marinated in a Mediterranean-style dressing and grilled until tender.

12 metal or wooden skewers (soak wooden skewers in water before use)

24 oz (680g) fresh tuna, cut into bite-size cubes

24 cherry tomatoes

2 zucchini (courgettes), cut into ½-inch rounds

1 red onion, cut in wedges and separated into pieces

2 green bell peppers, cut into bite-size pieces

5 tablespoons extra virgin olive oil

3 tablespoons freshly squeezed lemon juice

2 tablespoons finely chopped fresh flat-leaf parsley

3 cloves garlic, minced

1 teaspoon salt

½ teaspoon freshly ground black pepper

Lemon wedges, for serving

THREAD the tuna, cherry tomatoes, zucchini, red onions, and bell peppers alternately onto each skewer. MIX together the oil, lemon juice, parsley, garlic, salt, and pepper in a small bowl until well combined and brush over the prepared tuna and vegetable skewers. MARINATE, covered, in the refrigerator for at least 30 minutes, turning the skewers halfway through marinating time. COOK the skewers on a hot grill for 10 minutes, turning and brushing regularly with the marinade. SERVE the skewers with lemon wedges for squeezing.

Honey-Soy Chicken & Vegetable Skewers

SERVES 4

These mouthwatering chicken and vegetable skewers are coated in a sweet and savory Chinese marinade then grilled outdoors to bring out the most flavor. The mixture of honey, soy sauce, and hoisin sauce creates a delicious marinade that goes beautifully with chicken. It also complements the natural sweetness of the peppers, zucchini and red onion.

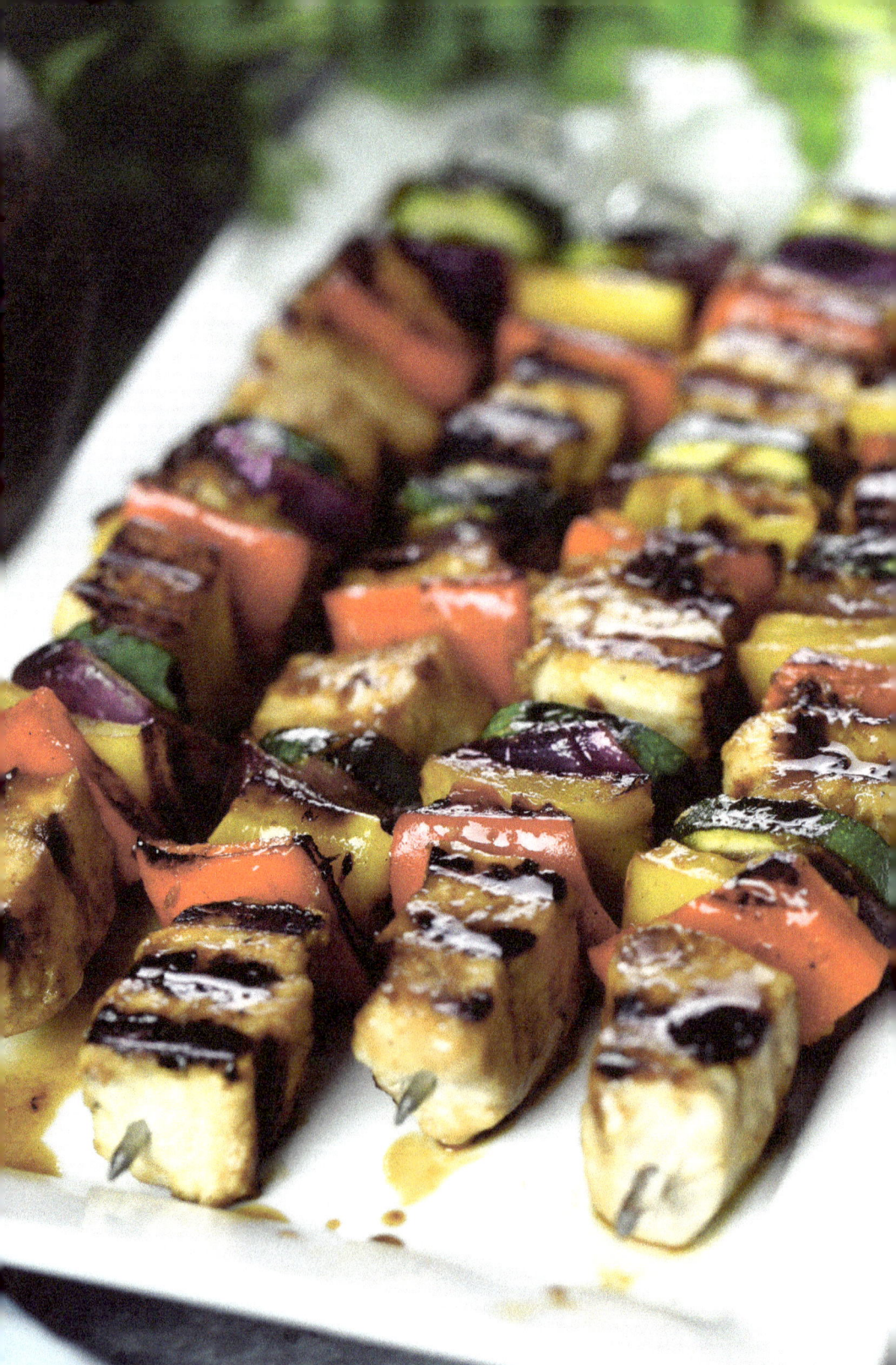
Honey-Soy Chicken & Vegetable Skewers

12 metal or wooden skewers (soak wooden skewers in water before use to prevent burning)

24 oz (680g) uncooked skinless chicken breast fillets, cut into bite-size pieces

2 zucchini (courgettes), cut into ½-inch rounds

2 red bell peppers, cut into bite-size pieces

2 yellow bell peppers, cut into bite-size pieces

1 red onion, cut in wedges and separated into pieces

¼ cup soy sauce

4 tablespoons hoisin sauce

¼ cup liquid honey

1 tablespoon rice vinegar

2 teaspoons sesame oil

3 garlic cloves, minced

2 tablespoons finely grated fresh ginger

THREAD the chicken, zucchini, peppers and red onion alternately onto each skewer. MIX together the remaining ingredients in a small bowl until well combined. BRUSH the marinade over the prepared chicken and vegetable skewers to coat evenly. MARINATE, covered, in the refrigerator for at least 30 minutes, turning the skewers halfway through marination. COOK the skewers on a hot grill for 10 minutes, turning and brushing regularly with the marinade.

Asian Shrimp & Vegetable Skewers

SERVES 4

A selection of Asian-style vegetables and shrimp are threaded onto skewers, marinated, and grilled until melt-in-the-mouth tender.

12 metal or wooden skewers (soak wooden skewers in water before use)

2 dozen large uncooked shrimp (prawns), peeled

12 buttom mushrooms, halved

12 snow peas, ends trimmed and cut in half on the diagonal

2 red bell peppers, cut into bite-size pieces

2 cloves garlic, minced

4 tablespoons peanut or canola oil

6 tablespoons soy sauce

3 tablespoons freshly squeezed lime juice

4 teaspoons brown sugar

2 tablespoons finely chopped cilantro (fresh coriander)

MIX together the garlic, oil, soy sauce, lemon juice, cilantro, and brown sugar in a bowl until well combined. THREAD alternating shrimp, mushrooms, snow peas, and bell peppers onto the skewers. MARINATE them in the mixture, covered, in the refrigerator for at least 30 minutes, turning the skewers halfway through marinating time. COOK the skewers on a hot grill for 10 minutes, turning and brushing regularly with the marinade.

Variation: You can replace the shrimp with scallops, or use a combination of shrimp and scallops.

Grilled Tuscan Chicken with Asparagus & Red Pepper

SERVES 4

This is a great way to enjoy chicken, asparagus, and red pepper—marinated in a blend of olive oil, lemon juice, garlic, oregano, and rosemary, then grilled and served with a green salad and crusty bread.

6 tablespoons extra virgin olive oil

4 tablespoons freshly squeezed lemon juice

4 cloves garlic, minced

1 teaspoon dried oregano

½ teaspoon dried rosemary

1 teaspoon salt

½ teaspoon freshly ground black pepper

Four 6-ounce (170g) uncooked skinless chicken breast fillets

2 red bell peppers, deseeded and cut into quarters lengthways

16 fresh asparagus spears, bottoms trimmed

MIX together the oil, lemon juice, garlic, oregano, rosemary, salt, and pepper in a bowl until well combined. MARINATE the chicken, bell peppers, and asparagus in the mixture, covered, in the refrigerator for at least 30 minutes. COOK the chicken on a hot grill for 4 minutes on each side, brushing with the marinade. Cook the vegetables on the grill at the same time, turning and brushing regularly with the marinade. SERVE immediately.

Mediterranean Grilled Salmon

SERVES 4

Serve these simple and stylish salmon steaks with a crisp salad and fresh crusty bread.

5 tablespoons extra virgin olive oil

3 tablespoons freshly squeezed lemon juice

2 tablespoons finely chopped fresh flat-leaf parsley

2 tablespoons finely chopped fresh basil

1 teaspoon salt

¼ teaspoon freshly ground black pepper

Four 6-ounce (170g) uncooked salmon steaks

MIX together the olive oil, lemon juice, parsley, basil, salt, and pepper in a bowl until well combined. MARINATE the salmon steaks in the mixture, covered, in the refrigerator for at least 30 minutes. COOK the salmon on a hot grill for 3 minutes on each side, brushing with the marinade.

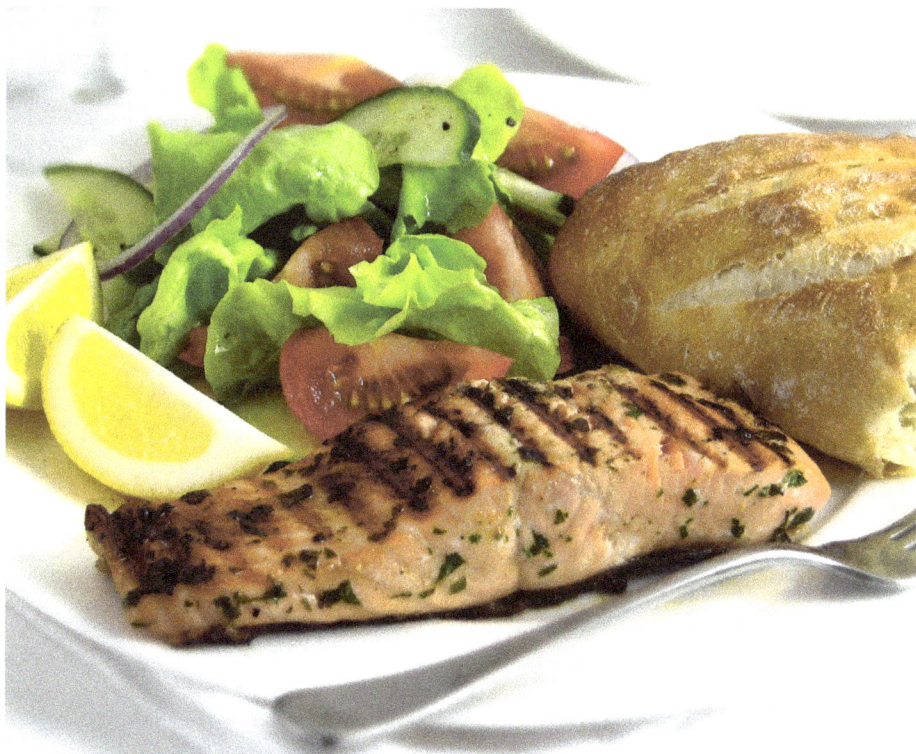

Marinated Mixed Seafood Grill

There's something very special about the taste of freshly grilled seafood like shrimp, squid, and scallops. This simple olive oil and white wine marinade adds flavor and depth, and also helps keep the seafood tender as it cooks.

6 tablespoons extra virgin olive oil

6 tablespoons white wine

2 cloves garlic, minced

2 tablespoons finely chopped fresh flat-leaf parsley

1 teaspoon finely grated lemon zest

1 teaspoon salt

½ teaspoon freshly ground black pepper

½ teaspoon dried rosemary

10 ounces (280g) uncooked shrimp, peeled

10 ounces (280g) uncooked scallops

10 ounces (280g) uncooked squid, cut into rings or bite-sized pieces

Lemon wedges, for serving

MIX together the oil, white wine, garlic, parsley, lemon zest, salt, pepper, and rosemary in a bowl until well combined. MARINATE the shrimp, scallops, and squid in the mixture, covered, in the refrigerator for at least 30 minutes. COOK the shrimp and scallops on a hot grill for 3 minutes, turning and brushing regularly with the marinade. ADD the squid and cook for 1 minute more, turning once. SERVE immediately with lemon wedges for squeezing.

Thai Fish Parcels

SERVES 4

Fish and red and green bell peppers are cooked in parcels with a simple infusion of Thai flavors.

2 tablespoons finely chopped cilantro (fresh coriander)

2 cloves garlic, minced

2 small red chilies, deseeded and finely chopped

2 teaspoons finely chopped lemongrass (or 1 teaspoon lemon zest)

2 teaspoons brown sugar

4 tablespoons fish sauce

2 tablespoons freshly squeezed lime juice

Four 6-ounce (170g) uncooked firm white fish fillets (such as snapper, cod, or haddock)

2 red bell peppers, cut into thin strips

2 green bell peppers, cut into thin strips

MIX together the cilantro, garlic, chilies, lemongrass or zest, sugar, fish sauce, and lime juice in a small bowl. PLACE each fish fillet in the center of a 12-inch piece of foil and spoon equal amounts of the dressing over each. ARRANGE the bell peppers on top of the fish. FOLD the foil over the fish and vegetables and seal the parcels tightly. COOK the parcels on a hot grill, on one side only, for 12 minutes. TRANSFER the fish, vegetables, and sauce from the foil packets to serving plates.

Variations: Use skinless chicken breast fillets (and cook for 15 minutes) or seafood such as scallops or shrimp in place of the fish.

Grilled Sweet Chili Scallops

SERVES 4

These succulent scallops are coated in a flavorful Thai-inspired marinade and seared quickly on a hot grill so they stay plump and tender.

4 tablespoons sweet chili sauce

2 tablespoons peanut or canola oil

2 tablespoons fish sauce

2 tablespoons freshly squeezed lemon or lime juice

2 tablespoons finely chopped fresh basil

2 cloves garlic, minced

1 teaspoon salt

24 large uncooked scallops

8 metal or wooden skewers (soak wooden skewers in water before use)

MIX together the chili sauce, oil, fish sauce, lemon or lime juice, basil, garlic and salt in a small bowl. MARINATE the scallops in the mixture, covered, in the refrigerator for at least 30 minutes. THREAD the scallops evenly onto each skewer. GRILL the scallops on a hot grill for 1 minute on each side, brushing with the marinade. REMOVE the scallops from the skewers and serve immediately.

Mediterranean Grilled Vegetables

SERVES 4

These grilled vegetables are so simple to prepare yet taste absolutely wonderful. Adjust the amount of marinade and vegetables used to the number of mouths to feed.

6 tablespoons extra virgin olive oil

3 tablespoons balsamic vinegar

4 cloves garlic, minced

1 teaspoon dried oregano

1 teaspoon dried rosemary

1 teaspoon salt

½ teaspoon freshly ground black pepper

VEGETABLES FOR THE GRILL (Choose about 8 cups of any combination)

- Asparagus, bottoms trimmed, left whole
- Mushrooms, peeled or wiped clean, stems removed, caps left whole (button mushrooms or portobellos)
- Tomatoes, sliced thickly, or whole cherry tomatoes
- Red, green, and yellow bell peppers, sliced into strips
- Zucchini, cut in half lengthways
- Eggplant, cut into ¼-inch rounds
- Onions (red are particularly sweet), sliced and separated into rings
- Fennel, cut in half lengthways and sliced
- Sweet potato, peeled and cut into ¼-inch slices
- Potatoes, scrubbed and cut into ¼-inch slices

MIX together the oil, balsamic vinegar, garlic, oregano, rosemary, salt, and pepper in a bowl until well combined. COOK the vegetables of your choice on a hot grill for 10 minutes, turning and brushing regularly with the marinade.

Serving Ideas: Serve a selection of grilled vegetables with grilled fish, chicken, or seafood and crusty bread (like baguette or ciabatta, or make bruschetta) accompanied by spreads like aioli, tapenade, or pesto. Leftover grilled vegetables make a delicious pizza topping or frittata filling, or can be served as part of an antipasto platter.

Japanese-Style Grilled Tuna

SERVES 4

Fish like tuna and swordfish are ideal for barbecuing because they have a firm and "meaty" texture. These tuna fillets are marinated and basted with a mouthwatering combination of Japanese flavors.

4 teaspoons finely grated fresh ginger

4 tablespoons Japanese soy sauce

2 tablespoons mirin (rice wine)

2 teaspoons sesame oil

Four 6-ounce (170g) uncooked tuna steaks

MIX together the ginger, soy sauce, mirin, and sesame oil in a bowl until well combined. Marinate the tuna in the mixture, covered, in the refrigerator for at least 30 minutes. COOK the fish on a hot grill for 3 minutes on each side, brushing with the marinade, and serve immediately.

Serving Idea: This dish is ideal served on a bed of Japanese Soba Noodle Salad (page 261).

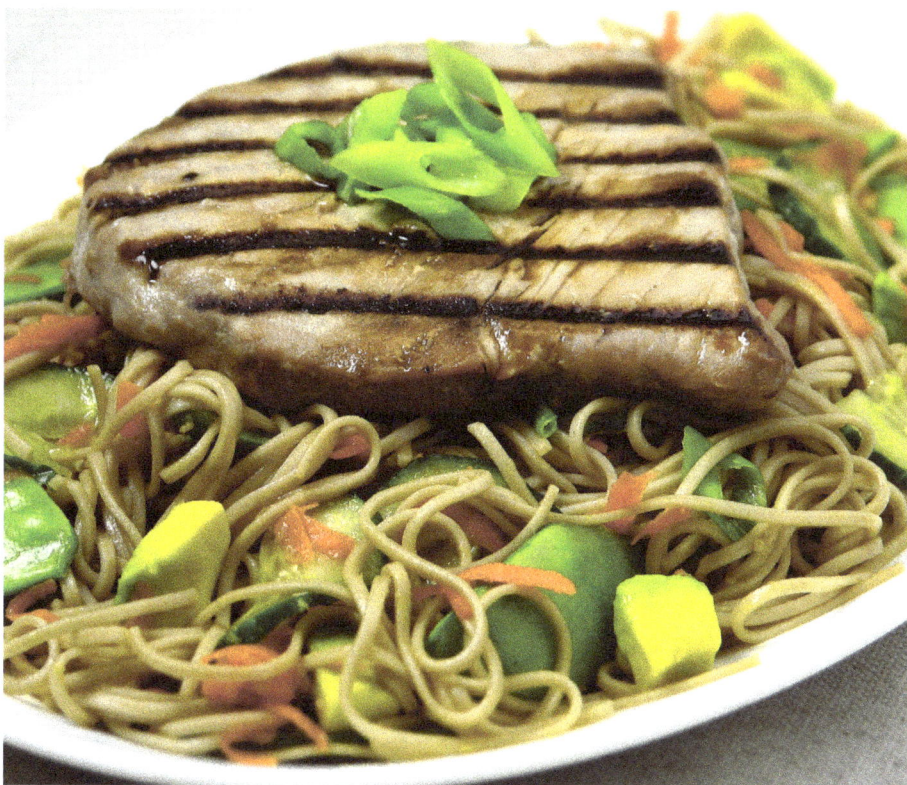

CHAPTER 20

SANDWICHES & WRAPS

Pan Bagnat

SERVES 4

Literally meaning "bathed bread," this sandwich, which originates from the Provence region of southern France, makes great picnic fare and can be made up the night before to allow the flavors to mingle.

5 tablespoons extra virgin olive oil

1½ tablespoons white wine vinegar

1 teaspoon Dijon mustard

1 clove garlic, minced

1 teaspoon salt

½ teaspoon freshly ground black pepper

1 large baguette

12 oz (340g) canned tuna in olive oil, drained and broken into chunks

½ green bell pepper, diced

2 tomatoes, sliced

3 eggs, hard-boiled, peeled and sliced

12 half rings of red onion

10 pitted black olives, sliced

PLACE the oil, vinegar, mustard, garlic, salt, and pepper in a jar with screw-top lid and shake until well combined. WARM the baguette in the oven to lightly crisp the outside, then cut in half lengthwise and remove some of the soft bread from the center of each half to hollow out a little. ARRANGE the tuna, bell pepper, tomatoes, eggs, onions, and olives on the bottom half, then drizzle with the dressing. TOP with the other baguette half, and cut into quarters to serve.

Banh Mi Sandwich

SERVES 4

Vietnam was a French colony from 1885 to 1954, and over that time certain French foods became integrated into the Vietnamese diet. Remnants of French colonization can still be seen in Vietnamese cuisine today, and the tastiest example of this is *banh mi* (pronounced 'bun me'), a Vietnamese sandwich with a distinctly French influence. This recipe is our take on banh mi, using staples that we always have in our pantry and fridge.

- 2 tablespoons rice vinegar
- 1 teaspoon superfine (caster) sugar
- ¼ teaspoon salt
- ½ carrot, peeled and grated
- ¼ cup peeled, deseeded and diced cucumber
- 1 cup bean sprouts
- 6 oz (170g) canned tuna in oil, drained

- 1 scallion, finely chopped
- 2 teaspoons fish sauce
- 1 tablespoon mayonnaise
- 1 large baguette
- 2 tablespoons jarred pickled jalapeño slices
- A handful of cilantro (fresh coriander) leaves

MIX the vinegar, sugar and salt together in a bowl. ADD the carrot, cucumber and bean sprouts, toss well to combine, then let stand for at least 20 minutes while you prepare the remaining ingredients. MASH the tuna thoroughly with a fork, then stir through the mayo, scallion and fish sauce to combine. WARM the baguette in the oven to lightly crisp the outside, then cut in half lengthwise and remove some of the soft bread from the center of each half to hollow out a little. SPREAD the tuna mix evenly on the base of the baguette, then place the lightly-pickled carrot, cucumber and bean sprout mixture over the top. PLACE the sliced jalapeño peppers then the cilantro on top. TOP with the other baguette half, and cut into quarters to serve.

Serving ideas: Banh mi makes an exotic flavor-packed lunch, (it's particularly excellent picnic fare in summer), and it can also be sliced into small portions and served as finger food.

Italian-Style Chicken Sandwich

SERVES 4

Italian breads, like focaccia and ciabatta, are tasty alternatives to ordinary sliced bread. In this sandwich, the bread is split, spread with pesto-flavored mayonnaise, and filled with roast chicken, arugula, sun-dried tomatoes, and olives.

- 4 tablespoons mayonnaise
- 2 tablespoons pesto, homemade (page 285) or store-bought
- 1 Italian-style bread loaf such as ciabatta or focaccia, cut in half lengthways

- 1 cup arugula (rocket), stems trimmed and leaves washed
- 12 oz (340g) shredded roast chicken breast
- 8 sun-dried tomatoes, sliced
- 8 pitted black olives, sliced

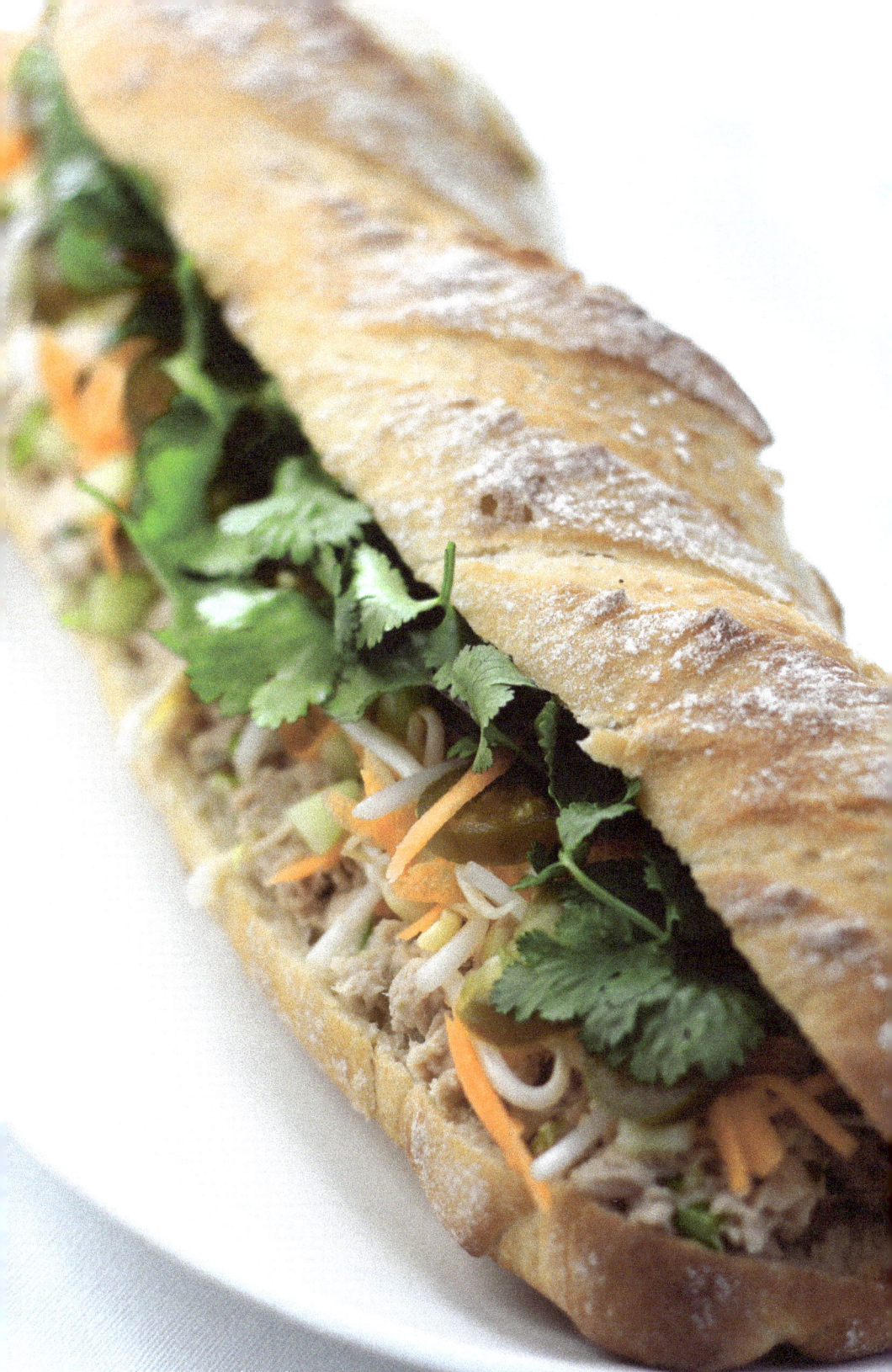

Banh Mi Sandwich

MIX together the mayonnaise and pesto in a small bowl. SPREAD the pesto-mayonnaise mixture over the base of the ciabatta or focaccia loaf. TOP with the arugula leaves, chicken, sun-dried tomatoes, and black olives. COVER with the top half of the loaf and cut into quarters to serve.

Variation: Replace the arugula with mixed salad leaves, and use strips of roasted red pepper instead of sun-dried tomatoes.

Focaccia with Smoked Salmon & Avocado

SERVES 4

Focaccia stuffed with delicate smoked salmon slices, creamy avocado, and crisp salad vegetables.

7 ounces (200g) sliced smoked salmon

1 focaccia bread, cut in half lengthways

4 tomatoes, sliced

1 avocado, sliced

12 thinly sliced rings of red onion

1 cup green mignonette or butter lettuce leaves

2 tablespoons freshly squeezed lemon juice

2 tablespoons extra virgin olive oil

½ clove garlic, minced

½ teaspoon salt

½ teaspoon freshly ground black pepper

ARRANGE equal amounts of the smoked salmon on the base of the focaccia. TOP with the tomato, avocado, red onions, and lettuce. IN a small bowl, mix together the lemon juice, oil, garlic, salt, and pepper. DRIZZLE the dressing over the top, cover with the top half of the focaccia, and cut into quarters to serve.

Tuna & Sweet Chili Wraps

SERVES 4

This simple and healthy wrap embraces the exotic flavors of Thailand.

2 tablespoons mayonnaise

2 tablespoons sweet chili sauce

1 teaspoon fish sauce

1 tablespoon finely chopped cilantro (fresh coriander)

12 ounces (340g) canned tuna in vegetable oil, drained and flaked

4 whole grain flat breads (such as lavash, pocketless pita bread, or tortilla)

2 cups shredded iceberg lettuce

2 carrots, peeled and grated

1 cup finely diced cucumber

MIX together the mayonnaise, sweet chili sauce, fish sauce, and cilantro in a bowl and stir in the tuna. SPREAD the tuna mixture in a horizontal line down the middle of each flat bread. ARRANGE equal amounts of lettuce, carrots, and cucumber on top of the tuna mixture. ROLL up firmly and cut each in half to serve.

Variation: Replace the tuna with 2 cups of shredded skinless cooked chicken breast.

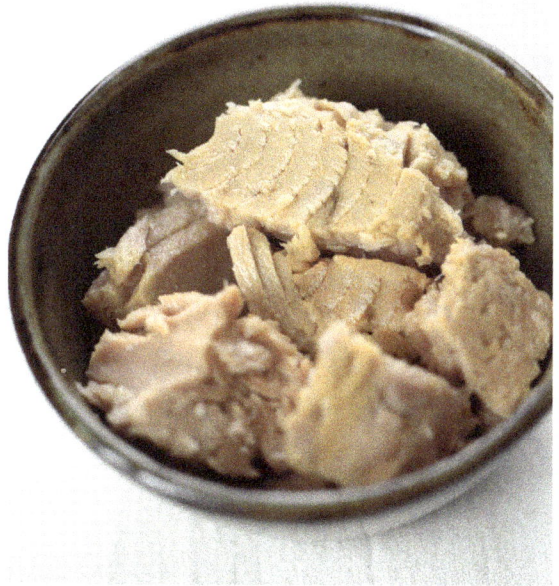

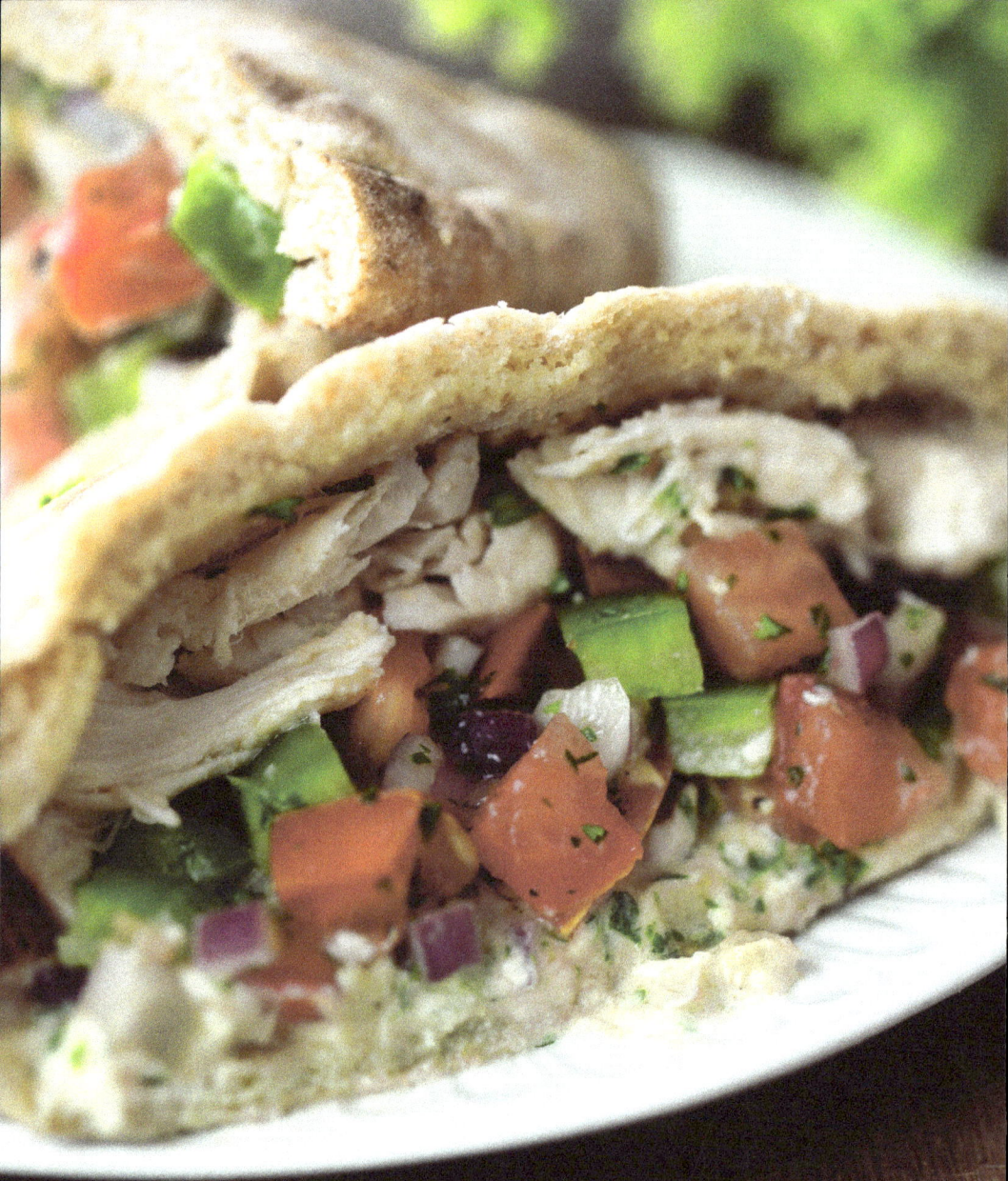

Whole Wheat Pita Pockets

Whole Wheat Pita Pockets with Chicken, Hummus & Mediterranean Salsa

SERVES 4

Here's a recipe for a filling hand-held lunch that's quick to prepare and combines some of the best ingredients of the Mediterranean diet. Hummus, made from wholesome chickpeas and tahini (sesame seed paste), adds creamy, salty and lemony elements. The salsa—with crunchy diced vegetables, fresh herbs and olive oil—accents the natural creaminess of the hummus.

4 tomatoes, diced

½ green bell pepper, diced

½ red onion, finely diced

2 tablespoons finely chopped fresh flat-leaf parsley

2 tablespoons extra virgin olive oil

1 teaspoon salt

½ teaspoon freshly ground black pepper

4 medium-size whole wheat pita breads, halved, opened into pockets

½ cup hummus

2 cups shredded skinless rotisserie chicken

MIX together the tomatoes, green pepper, red onion, parsley, olive oil, salt and pepper in a bowl until well combined. SPREAD 1 tablespoon of hummus in each pita pocket and fill with equal amounts of salsa and shredded chicken to serve.

Variation: Replace the chicken with chunks of good-quality canned tuna.

Turkish Chickpea Salad Wrap

SERVES 4

There are three parts to this easy-to-assemble Middle Eastern wrap: the flat bread, the hummus, and the chickpea salad. The combination of all three makes a healthy and substantial no-cook feast you can hold in your hands.

2 cups canned chickpeas, rinsed and drained

½ small red onion, finely chopped

1 red bell pepper, diced

2 tablespoons finely chopped cilantro (fresh coriander)

1 teaspoon finely grated lemon zest

2 tablespoons extra virgin olive oil

4 whole grain flat breads (such as lavash, pocketless pita bread, or tortilla)

8 tablespoons hummus, homemade (page 288) or store-bought

2 handfuls torn romaine (cos) lettuce

MIX together the chickpeas, onion, bell pepper, cilantro, lemon zest, and oil in a bowl. SPREAD the hummus in a horizontal line down the middle of each flat bread. ARRANGE the lettuce over the hummus and top with the chickpea mixture. ROLL up firmly and cut each in half to serve.

Bruschetta with Tomato, Mozzarella & Anchovy

SERVES 4

Bruschetta is sliced toasted bread, rubbed with garlic and drizzled or brushed with olive oil. It makes the perfect base for this classic Mediterranean combination of juicy tomatoes, fresh basil, creamy mozzarella, and salty anchovies.

8 thick slices of crusty bread such as ciabatta or baguette (sliced on the diagonal)

1 clove garlic, peeled and cut in half

2 tablespoons extra virgin olive oil

4 tomatoes, finely diced

6 anchovy fillets, chopped

¼ teaspoon salt

¼ teaspoon freshly ground black pepper

4 oz (115g) fresh mozzarella cheese, thinly sliced

8 large fresh basil leaves, finely chopped

PREHEAT the oven broiler (griller). TOAST bread on both sides under the broiler. Rub the surface of each slice with the cut side of the garlic. BRUSH or drizzle each slice, on one side only, with a little extra virgin olive oil. IN a bowl, mix together the tomatoes, anchovies, salt, and pepper and place on top of the toasts. TOP with cheese, place under the broiler, and cook until the cheese is bubbly and golden. SPRINKLE with basil and serve immediately.

Mushroom Bruschetta

SERVES 4

Bruschetta topped with pan-fried mushrooms seasoned with salt, freshly ground black pepper, and flat-leaf parsley.

3 tablespoons extra virgin olive oil plus 4 teaspoons for drizzling

4 cups sliced portobello mushrooms

8 thick slices of ciabatta (Italian crusty bread), or use baguette sliced on the diagonal instead

1 clove garlic, peeled and cut in half

2 tablespoons finely chopped flat-leaf parsley

1 teaspoon salt

½ teaspoon freshly ground black pepper

PREHEAT the oven broiler (griller). HEAT 2 tablespoons of the oil in a skillet over medium heat. ADD the mushrooms and cook, stirring regularly, until softened, 4 to 5 minutes. WHILE the mushrooms are cooking, toast the ciabatta slices under the broiler until golden on both sides. RUB one side of each slice of ciabatta with the cut side of garlic. BRUSH or drizzle each slice, on one side only, with half a teaspoon of oil. OFF the heat, add the reserved tablespoon of oil, the parsley, salt, and pepper to the skillet with the mushrooms and stir. SPOON equal amounts on top of each bruschetta and serve immediately.

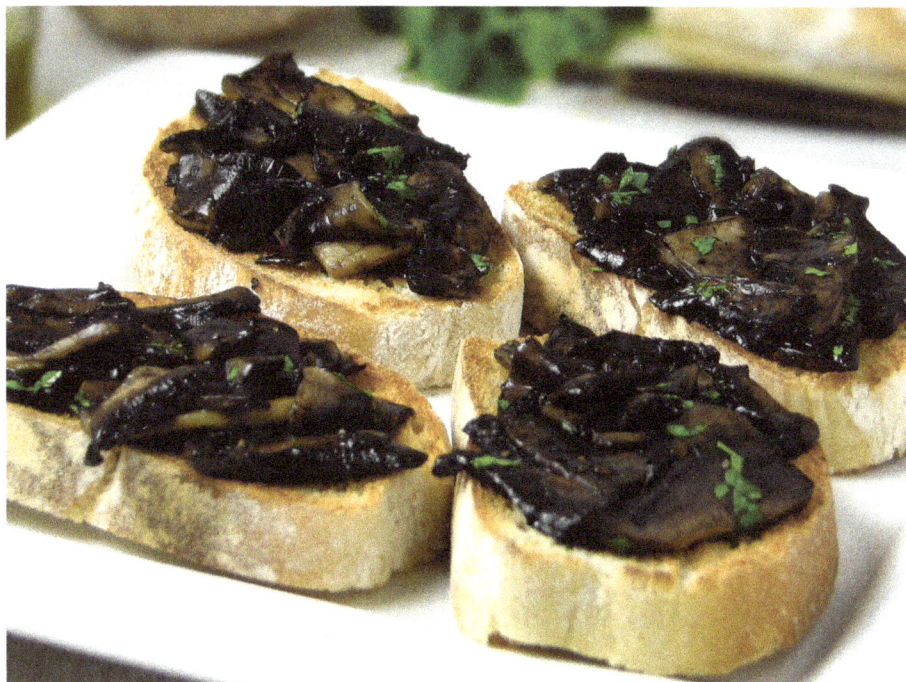

CHAPTER 21

SOUPS

Pho Bo

SERVES 4

Pho bo is a Vietnamese beef and noodle soup that is often eaten for breakfast, but also makes a satisfying lunch or light dinner. The boiling stock, fragrant with spices and sauces, is poured over the noodles, bean sprouts, and scallions, and it poaches the paper-thin slices of raw beef just before serving.

4 oz (115g) dried rice stick noodles

8 cups beef stock

1 onion, finely chopped

4 tablespoons hoisin sauce

2 tablespoons fish sauce

2 teaspoons finely grated fresh ginger

1 teaspoon ground black pepper

1 teaspoon five-spice powder

2 cups bean sprouts

2 scallions, thinly sliced

10 oz (280g) very thinly sliced bite-sized lean beef

2 tablespoons freshly squeezed lemon juice

Cilantro (fresh coriander) leaves, for garnish

Strips of fresh red chili, for garnish

SOAK the noodles in a bowl of boiling water for 10 minutes. PLACE the stock, onion, hoisin sauce, fish sauce, ginger, pepper, and five-spice powder in a saucepan. BRING to a boil, cover, and simmer over a medium heat for 10 minutes. DRAIN the noodles and place equal amounts into soup bowls. PLACE equal amounts of the sprouts, scallions, and beef slices on top of the noodles. POUR over the boiling stock to cover and allow to stand for 1 minute to poach, ensuring the beef is immersed. SERVE the soup drizzled with lemon juice and garnished with cilantro leaves and chili strips on top.

Variation: Use thinly sliced firm tofu or smoked salmon instead of beef.

Tip: To help cut the beef into paper-thin slices, place the meat in the freezer for about 30 minutes to firm up before slicing with a very sharp knife.

Soupe au Pistou

SERVES 4

A hearty, fiber-rich Provençal soup chock full of protein-packed beans and chunky vegetables.

2 tablespoons extra virgin olive oil

1 onion, diced

1 carrot, halved lengthwise and sliced into half-rounds

1 zucchini, halved lengthwise and sliced into half-rounds

1 potato, peeled and cut into small cubes

16 green beans, cut into 1-inch pieces

6 cups vegetable or chicken stock

1 teaspoon salt

½ teaspoon freshly ground black pepper

14 oz (400g) canned cannellini beans, rinsed and drained

¼ cup pesto (store-bought or homemade)

HEAT the oil in a large saucepan over a medium heat. COOK the onion for 4 minutes. ADD the carrot and cook for 2 minutes, then add the zucchini, potato and green beans and cook for 2 minutes more, stirring occasionally. ADD the stock, salt and pepper, bring to the boil, then cover the pot, reduce the heat and simmer for 15 minutes. ADD the white beans and pesto and cook for 1 minute.

Spanish Broccoli & Almond Soup

SERVES 4

The combination of ground almonds and broccoli makes a deliciously creamy yet creamless soup with a rich, green color.

5 cups vegetable stock

4 cups broccoli florets

1 red onion, roughly chopped

1 medium-sized potato, peeled and cut into small cubes

½ cup ground almonds

1 clove garlic, roughly chopped

1 teaspoon salt

½ teaspoon freshly ground black pepper

1 tablespoon extra virgin olive oil

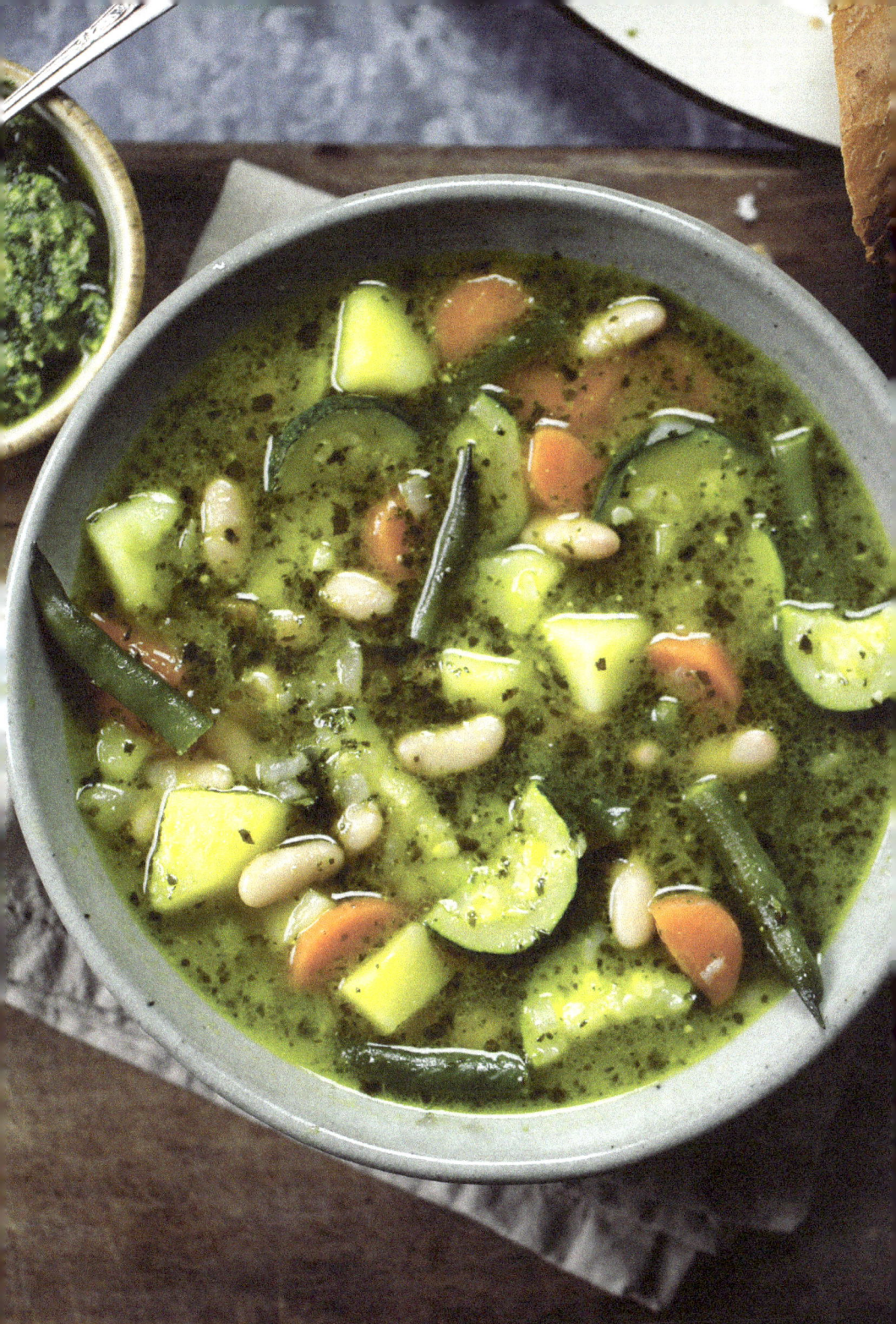

Soupe au Pistou

PLACE the stock, broccoli, onion, potato, almonds, garlic, salt, and pepper in a large saucepan and bring to a boil. COVER the pot, reduce the heat to medium, and simmer for 15 minutes. TRANSFER the soup to a blender and process until smooth, then return to the saucepan. STIR in the olive oil and heat thoroughly before serving.

Serving Idea: You can also chill this soup and serve it cold as a light summer meal with bread.

Miso Soup with Tofu & Mushroom

SERVES 4

This nourishing Japanese soup takes only minutes to prepare and can be served for breakfast, lunch, or as part of a main meal. Miso—fermented soy bean paste—adds a rich flavor and is highly valued in Japan for its health-giving properties.

6 cups dashi stock (dashi stock powder is available at Asian food stores)

4 thinly sliced fresh mushrooms (shiitake or white button)

3 tablespoons shiro (white) miso paste

2 tablespoons Japanese soy sauce

3 oz (85g) silken tofu, cut into cubes

1 scallion, green parts only, thinly sliced on the diagonal

BRING the stock to a gentle boil in a saucepan, add the mushrooms, reduce the heat and simmer for 3 minutes. MIX together the miso and soy sauce in a small bowl, then add to the hot stock. ADD the tofu. HEAT the soup and, just before it comes to a boil, remove from the heat. POUR the soup into bowls and garnish with the sliced scallions on top to serve.

Variation: You can add various other ingredients to make a more substantial soup, such as cooked shrimp, snow pea sprouts, cooked rice noodles, or paper-thin slices of fresh ginger.

Tuscan White Bean & Garlic Soup

SERVES 4

The garlic used in this recipe becomes surprisingly sweet and soft as it cooks, and makes this heart-warming soup extra heart-healthy.

3 tablespoons extra virgin olive oil

1 onion, chopped

14 oz (400g) canned cannellini beans, rinsed and drained

1 potato, peeled and cut into bite-sized cubes

4 cloves unpeeled garlic

½ teaspoon dried rosemary

5 cups chicken or vegetable stock

1 teaspoon sea salt

½ teaspoon freshly ground black pepper

HEAT 2 tablespoons of the olive oil in a large saucepan over medium heat. ADD the onions and cook, stirring, until softened, about 8 minutes. ADD the beans, potatoes, and rosemary and cook for a minute, stirring to combine. ADD the stock, unpeeled garlic cloves, salt, and pepper, bring to a boil, and cover with a lid. REDUCE the heat to medium-low and simmer gently for 20 minutes, stirring once or twice. REMOVE the garlic cloves and rinse them briefly under cold water. SQUEEZE the soft cooked garlic from each clove into a blender or food processor. POUR in half the soup and blend for about 15 seconds until smooth. RETURN the puree to the soup, stir in the reserved oil, and heat through before serving.

Minestrone Soup

SERVES 4

This classic Italian minestrone soup is packed with flavor and nutrients.

4 tablespoons extra virgin olive oil

2 slices lean bacon, finely chopped

1 red onion, diced

1 carrot, peeled and diced

1 stick celery, diced

2 cloves garlic, minced

6 cups vegetable stock

2 cups canned chopped tomatoes

1 teaspoon salt

½ teaspoon freshly ground black pepper

½ cup small pasta, such as macaroni or orzo

½ cup frozen green peas, thawed

1 zucchini (courgette), cut in half lengthways and thinly sliced into half-moons

1 cup canned white beans (like cannellini), rinsed and drained

2 tablespoons finely chopped flat-leaf parsley

Finely grated Parmesan cheese

HEAT 2 tablespoons of the oil in a large saucepan and cook the bacon, stirring occasionally, for 2 minutes. ADD the onion, carrot, and celery and cook, covered, for 3 minutes. STIR again and cook, covered, for another 3 minutes. ADD the garlic and cook, stirring regularly, for a minute. ADD the stock, tomatoes, salt, and pepper and stir to combine. BRING to a boil, cover, reduce the heat to medium, and simmer for 10 minutes. ADD the pasta, peas, zucchini, and beans, stir to combine, increase the heat to medium-high and cook, covered, until pasta is tender, about 8 minutes. REMOVE from the heat and stir in the parsley and the reserved 2 tablespoons of olive oil. SERVE in bowls sprinkled with a little grated Parmesan cheese.

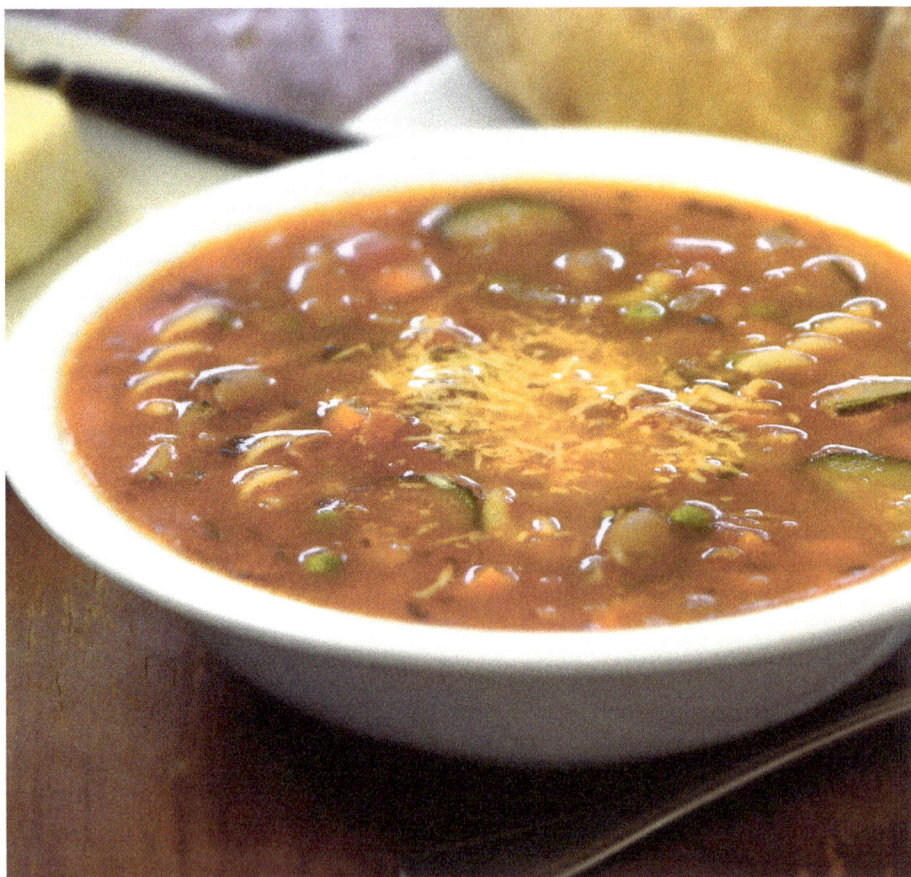

Thai-Spiced Sweet Potato Soup

SERVES 6

A velvety-smooth soup accented with Thai seasonings. The sweet potato adds not only texture and a vivid color to the soup, but also a healthy dose of beta-carotene and dietary fiber.

1 tablespoon peanut oil

1 onion, chopped

3 cloves garlic, chopped

2 tablespoons Thai red curry paste

6 cups chicken or vegetable stock

1 cup coconut milk

3 tablespoons fish sauce

2 pounds (900g) orange sweet potatoes, peeled and roughly chopped

1 cup red lentils

2 teaspoons brown sugar

2 tablespoons freshly squeezed lemon juice

Cilantro (fresh coriander) leaves, for garnish

HEAT the oil in a large saucepan over a medium heat. ADD the onion and cook, stirring occasionally, until softened, about 5 minutes. ADD the garlic and red curry paste and cook, stirring constantly, for 1 minute. ADD the stock, coconut milk, fish sauce, sweet potatoes, red lentils, and brown sugar, stir to combine, and bring to a boil. REDUCE the heat to medium and simmer, covered, for 20 minutes. REMOVE from the heat and allow to cool a little. PUREE the soup in two batches in a blender or food processor until smooth. RETURN to the saucepan to reheat and stir in the lemon juice. SERVE in bowls garnished with cilantro.

Variations: Replace the sweet potatoes with butternut squash (or pumpkin). Substitute lime juice for the lemon juice.

Thai Chicken Soup with Basil

SERVES 4

A warming and delicately spiced Thai chicken soup accented with fresh basil and lime juice.

2 tablespoons peanut oil

2 tablespoons Thai red curry paste

4 garlic cloves, finely chopped

6 cups chicken stock

2 cups coconut milk

4 tablespoons fish sauce

4 teaspoons brown sugar

20 green beans, cut into ½-inch pieces

2 cups bean sprouts

2 scallions, thinly sliced on the diagonal (reserve some green scallion to garnish)

2 cups shredded rotisserie chicken

3 tablespoons finely chopped fresh basil (plus some whole basil leaves to garnish)

3 tablespoons lime juice

2 red chilies, thinly sliced into rounds, to garnish (optional)

HEAT the oil in a large saucepan over a medium heat. ADD the curry paste and garlic and cook for 1 minute, stirring. ADD the stock, coconut milk, fish sauce and brown sugar and bring to the boil. ADD the green beans, then reduce heat to medium-high and simmer for 3 minutes, uncovered. ADD the bean sprouts, chicken and scallion and simmer for 2 minutes, uncovered. REMOVE from the heat and stir in the basil and lime juice. SPOON into bowls, garnish with extra basil leaves, scallion and sliced red chili (if using).

Variations: To turn this soup into a complete meal you can add cooked rice noodles. It can also be varied in many different ways: for a seafood version, add shrimp, squid, scallops, fish or mussels; for a vegetarian version, use tofu or tempeh in place of chicken; use different combinations of fresh vegetables such as mushrooms, snow peas, or thinly sliced zucchini; add some canned Asian veggies like sliced bamboo shoots, water chestnuts or baby corn; replace the lime juice with lemon juice; or use cilantro (fresh coriander) instead of basil.

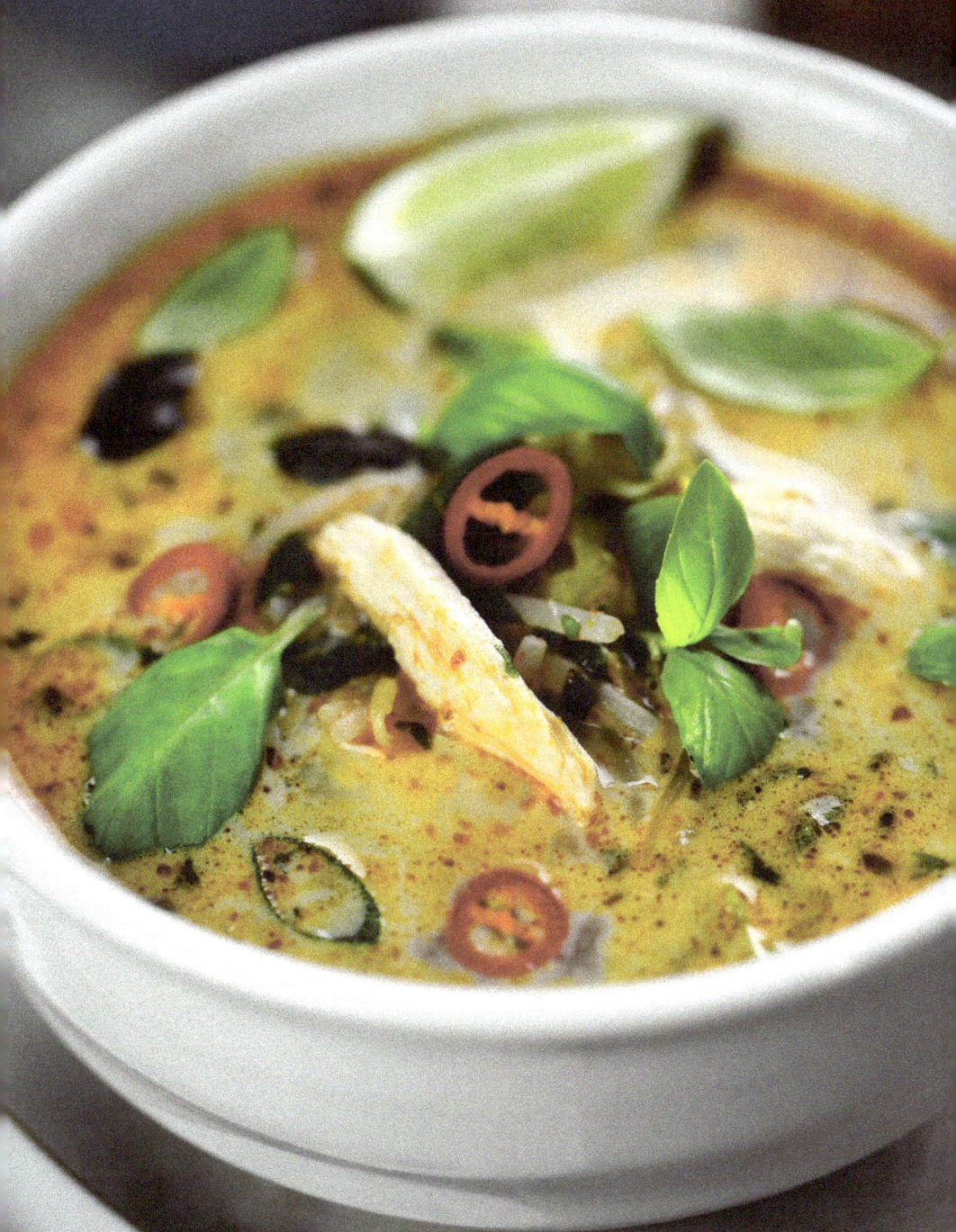

Tunisian Chickpea & Vegetable Soup

SERVES 4

This hearty chickpea and vegetable soup is flavored with warm spices including saffron, cumin, cinnamon, ground ginger and turmeric. The addition of cilantro, parsley, and lemon juice toward the end of cooking adds a fresh herby-citrus taste, while the pasta adds body and texture.

2 tablespoons extra virgin olive oil

1 onion, finely chopped

1 stick celery, finely chopped

1 teaspoon salt

½ teaspoon turmeric

½ teaspoon ground ginger

½ teaspoon cinnamon

½ teaspoon ground cumin

½ teaspoon ground black pepper`

1 zucchini (courgette), sliced into thin rounds

14 oz (400g) canned chopped tomatoes

½ cup red lentils

6 cups vegetable stock

¼ teaspoon saffron strands, soaked in ½ cup boiling water

1 cup canned chickpeas, rinsed and drained

1 oz capellini (angel-hair) pasta, broken into pieces

2 tablespoons chopped cilantro (fresh coriander)

2 tablespoons chopped fresh flat-leaf parsley

2 tablespoons freshly squeezed lemon juice

HEAT the oil in a large saucepan over a medium heat. ADD the onion and celery and cook, stirring occasionally, until softened, about 5 minutes. ADD the salt, turmeric, ginger, cinnamon, cumin, and pepper and cook, stirring, for 1 minute. ADD the zucchini, tomatoes, and lentils and stir to combine. ADD the stock and saffron liquid and bring to a boil. COVER the pot, reduce the heat to medium, and simmer for 15 minutes. ADD the chickpeas, pasta, cilantro, parsley, and lemon juice and stir to combine. COOK, covered, for 5 minutes and serve.

Greek Spinach & White Bean Soup

SERVES 4

A delicately seasoned Greek soup with white beans and a range of vegetables including spinach, carrots, onion, celery, and potato.

3 tablespoons extra virgin olive oil

1 onion, diced

1 carrot, peeled and diced

1 stick celery, diced

1 potato, peeled and diced

1 clove garlic, finely chopped

6 cups vegetable stock

2 tablespoons finely chopped fresh flat-leaf parsley

14 oz (400g) canned white beans (like cannelini), rinsed and drained

8 oz (230g) pack frozen spinach, defrosted and drained

½ cup frozen green peas, thawed

1 teaspoon salt

½ teaspoon freshly ground black pepper

HEAT 2 tablespoons of the oil in a large saucepan and cook the onion, carrot, and celery, stirring occasionally, until softened, about 7 minutes. ADD the potato and garlic and cook, stirring, for 1 minute. Add the stock and parsley, bring to a boil, then reduce the heat to medium and simmer for 15 minutes. ADD the white beans, spinach, peas, salt, and pepper, return to a simmer, and cook for another 5 minutes. REMOVE from the heat, stir in the remaining oil, and serve.

Gazpacho

SERVES 4

There are about as many gazpacho recipes as there are Spanish cooks. This is our quick version, which requires little effort but produces an authentic result. This cold soup is delicious and refreshing—a perfect summertime meal served with bread.

6 cups tomato juice

2 cups peeled, deseeded and chopped cucumber

1 small red onion, deseeded and chopped

1 red bell pepper, deseeded and chopped

1 green bell pepper, chopped

1 clove garlic, chopped

2 tablespoons extra virgin olive oil

2 teaspoons white wine vinegar

1 teaspoon salt

½ teaspoon ground black pepper

PLACE all ingredients in a food processor or blender and process until smooth. CHILL in the fridge until you're ready to serve.

Tip: The flavors of gazpacho develop over time, so allow the soup to chill in the fridge for at least 20 minutes, and up to a day ahead.

CHAPTER 22

SALADS

Insalata di Riso (Italian Rice Salad)

SERVES 4

A hearty Italian rice salad packed with tasty and healthful ingredients including tuna, tomatoes, toasted pine nuts, mushrooms, peas, cubed mozzarella cheese, artichoke hearts, and diced green bell pepper. This salad can be served as a side dish or eaten in larger quantities as a light meal.

1 cup long-grain white rice, cooked and left to cool (or use leftover rice)

2 artichoke hearts (jarred or canned), roughly chopped

6 oz (170g) canned light meat tuna in olive oil, drained and broken into chunks

⅓ cup frozen peas, cooked and cooled

1 large tomato, diced

¼ cup cubed mozzarella cheese

¼ green bell pepper, diced

2 white button mushrooms, thinly sliced

2 tablespoons pine nuts, lightly toasted

2 tablespoons finely chopped fresh flat-leaf parsley

4 tablespoons extra virgin olive oil

1½ tablespoons freshly squeezed lemon juice

1 clove garlic, finely chopped

1 teaspoon salt

½ teaspoon freshly ground black pepper

MIX together the rice, artichoke hearts, tuna, peas, tomato, cheese, bell pepper, mushrooms, pine nuts, and parsley in a bowl. MIX together the oil, lemon juice, garlic, salt, and pepper in a small bowl until well combined (or shake together in a screw-top jar). POUR the dressing over the rice mixture, mix together gently to combine thoroughly, and serve.

Variation: You can vary this salad endlessly—add black or green olives, sun-dried tomatoes, capers or use red bell peppers instead of green or finely chopped basil instead of parsley.

Greek Salad

SERVES 4

Greek salad, or *horiatiki salata*, is a rough country salad of juicy tomatoes, crisp cucumber, sliced red onion, green bell pepper, crumbly feta cheese, and plump kalamata olives. Serve this delightful combination as a side dish or as a light meal with some crusty bread.

3 tablespoons extra virgin olive oil

1½ tablespoons freshly squeezed lemon juice

1 clove garlic, minced

½ teaspoon dried oregano

¼ teaspoon salt

¼ teaspoon freshly ground black pepper, and extra for garnish

3 tomatoes, cut into wedges

¼ red onion, sliced into rings

½ cucumber, sliced lengthwise, then cut into thick half-moons

½ green bell pepper, cut into thin strips

16 pitted kalamata olives

4 oz (115g) feta cheese, cut into small cubes

PLACE the olive oil, lemon juice, garlic, oregano, salt, and pepper in a small jar with a screw-top lid and shake to combine. PLACE the tomatoes, onion, cucumber, bell pepper, olives, and cheese in a large bowl. POUR the dressing over the salad and toss gently to combine, just before serving. GARNISH with a little freshly ground black pepper.

Japanese Soba Noodle Salad

SERVES 4

Soba noodles combined with creamy avocado, a selection of crisp vegetables, and a Japanese soy-ginger dressing.

5 oz (140g) dried soba noodles

5 tablespoons Japanese soy sauce

3 tablespoons Japanese rice vinegar

1½ tablespoons finely grated fresh ginger

1 teaspoon sugar

20 thinly sliced rounds of cucumber, cut into halves

15 snow peas, ends trimmed and cut in half on the diagonal

1 carrot, peeled and grated

1 scallion, thinly sliced on the diagonal

1 avocado, peeled and cut into small cubes

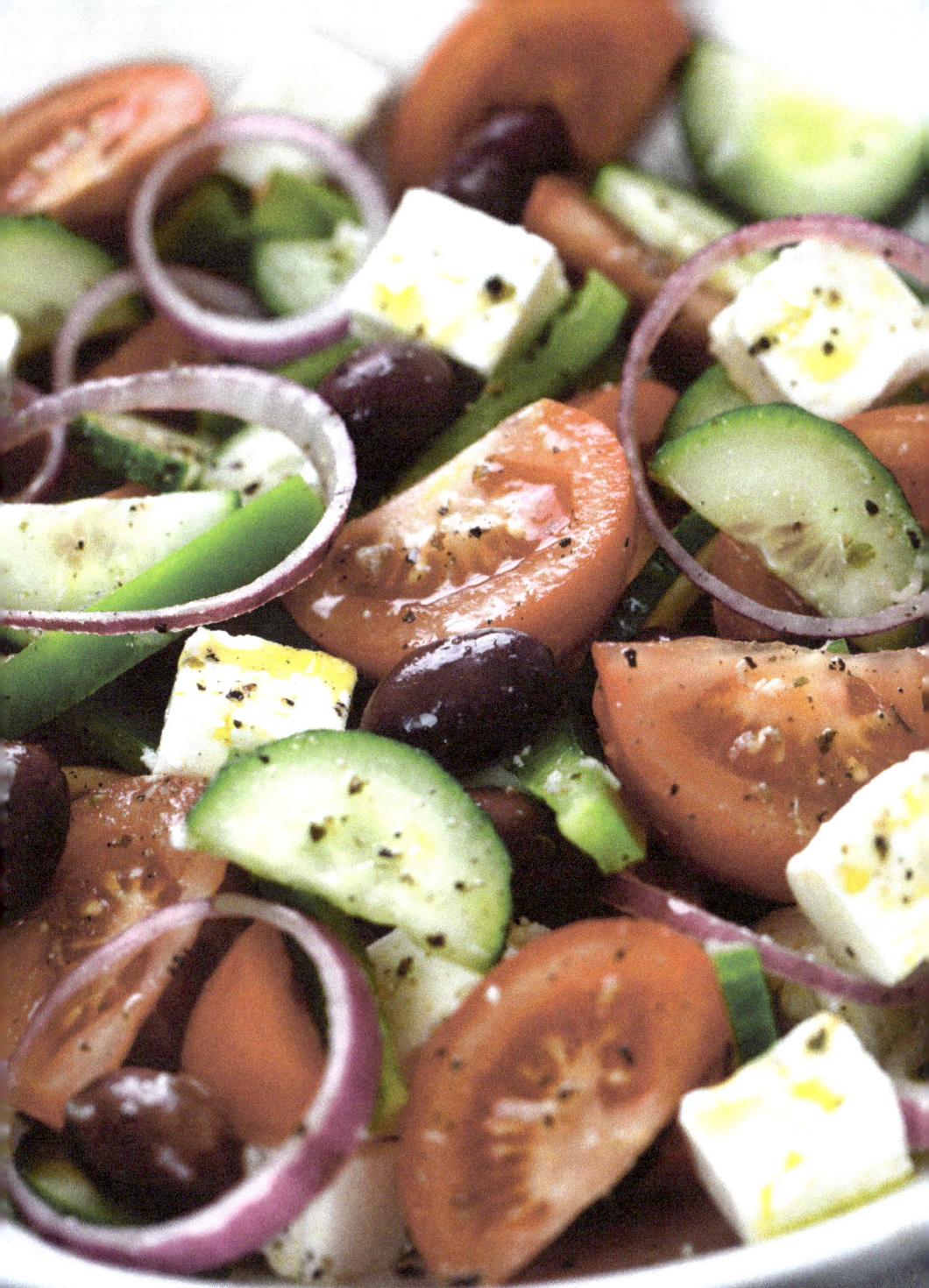

Greek Salad

COOK the noodles in boiling water for 5 minutes, rinse under cold water, drain, and set aside. MIX together the soy sauce, rice vinegar, ginger, and sugar in a small bowl. PLACE the noodles in the bottom of a large mixing bowl. ADD the cucumber, snow peas, carrot, scallion, and avocado. DRIZZLE with the soy dressing, toss gently to combine, and serve.

Variations: Add strips of smoked salmon to this salad for a more opulent version. For added bite, mix 1 teaspoon of wasabi into the dressing.

Pesto Pasta Salad with White Beans, Cherry Tomatoes & Artichoke Hearts

SERVES 4

Traditional pesto made with basil and pine nuts is ideal for this tasty pasta salad.

8 oz (230g) pasta of your choice (shells or spirals are ideal)	1 cup canned cannellini beans, rinsed and drained
¾ cup of pesto, homemade (page 285) or store-bought	1 cup jarred quartered artichoke hearts
8 oz (230g) cherry tomatoes, cut in half	2 tablespoons finely diced red onion

COOK the pasta in a large pot of boiling water according to package directions. DRAIN the cooked pasta, and refresh under cold water. TOSS the pasta with the pesto, cherry tomatoes, cannellini beans, artichoke hearts, and red onion until well combined.

Variation: Replace the cannellini beans with 1 cup of shredded cooked chicken breast. Add some sliced black olives.

Turkish Tomato, Cucumber & Olive Salad

SERVES 4

A simple combination of fresh tomatoes, cucumber, and black olives tossed with a tangy dressing made with lemon juice, vinegar, and olive oil.

4 tablespoons extra virgin olive oil

4 teaspoons freshly squeezed lemon juice

2 teaspoons white wine vinegar

2 teaspoons finely chopped fresh flat-leaf parsley

¼ teaspoon salt

¼ teaspoon freshly ground black pepper

4 tomatoes, sliced

24 thinly sliced rounds of cucumber

12 pitted black olives, sliced

MIX together the oil, lemon juice, vinegar, parsley, salt, and pepper in a bowl until well combined. PLACE the tomatoes, cucumber, and olives in a salad bowl. POUR the dressing over the salad and toss gently to combine just before serving.

Panzanella (Tuscan Bread Salad)

SERVES 4

This Tuscan summer dish uses day-old bread that is torn into pieces, softened with water, then mixed with tomatoes, fresh basil, red onion, and a simple olive oil vinaigrette.

4 cups cubed day-old Italian ciabatta bread

4 tomatoes, diced

4 tablespoons finely chopped red onion

16 basil leaves, roughly torn

6 tablespoons extra virgin olive oil

4 tablespoons red wine vinegar

1 clove garlic, minced

1 teaspoon salt

½ teaspoon freshly ground black pepper

PLACE the bread in a bowl, cover with water, and soak for 5 minutes until softened. REMOVE handfuls of the bread at a time and squeeze dry. PLACE the bread in a bowl with the tomatoes, red onion, and basil. MIX together the oil, vinegar, garlic, salt, and pepper in a small bowl until well combined. POUR the dressing over the salad, toss gently to combine, and serve.

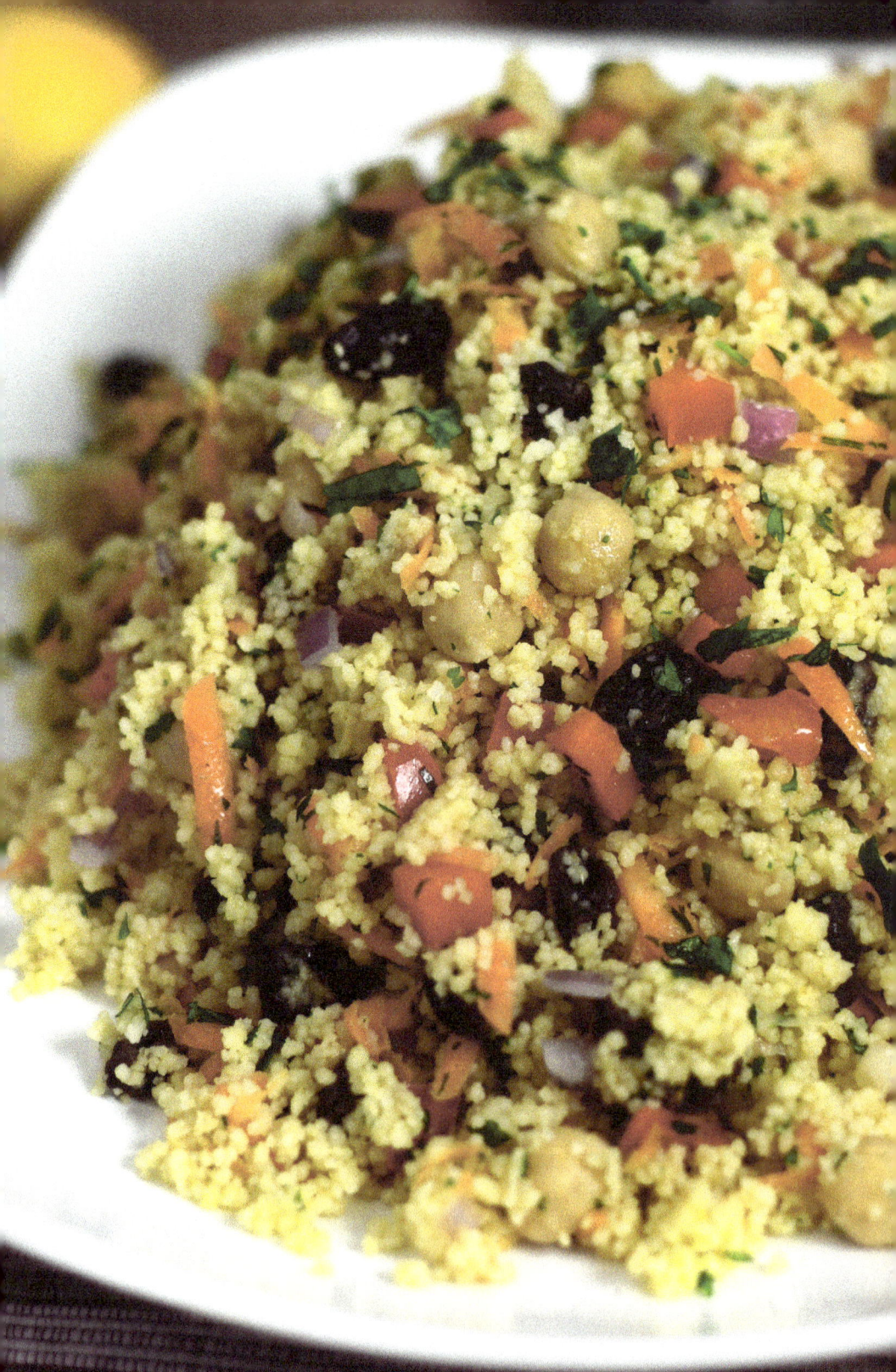

Moroccan Chickpea & Couscous Salad

Moroccan Chickpea & Couscous Salad

SERVES 4

An exotic Moroccan couscous salad with chickpeas, raisins and colorful vegetables coated in a delicately spiced olive oil and lemon dressing. Chickpeas not only add a wonderful flavor and texture to this Moroccan salad, they're a good source of vegetable protein and a number of important vitamins and minerals including calcium and folate. They're also a great source of dietary fiber, which helps lower cholesterol levels and regulate blood sugar levels.

1 cup quick-cooking couscous

¼ cup raisins

1¼ cups boiling chicken or vegetable stock

3 tablespoons extra virgin olive oil

2 tablespoons lemon juice

1 garlic clove, minced

1 teaspoon ground cumin

1 teaspoon ground coriander

½ teaspoon ground ginger

1 teaspoon salt

1 carrot, peeled and grated

½ red pepper, diced

¼ red onion, finely diced

1 cup canned chickpeas, rinsed and drained

2 tablespoons finely chopped fresh flat-leaf parsley

MIX the couscous with the raisins in a bowl and pour over the boiling stock. COVER with a dish towel, plate or plastic wrap to seal in the steam and let sit for 5 minutes. PLACE the oil, lemon juice, garlic, spices, and salt in a jar with a screw-top lid and shake to mix. FLUFF the couscous with a fork to separate the grains and stir through the carrot, red pepper, onion, chickpeas and parsley. POUR over the dressing and toss together until well combined.

Gado Gado

SERVES 4

Gado gado is a classic Indonesian salad made with green beans, potatoes, carrots, cabbage, and bean sprouts garnished with sliced boiled eggs and drizzled with a luscious peanut sauce. Gado gado is such a hearty and filling salad that it can easily be eaten as a complete meal.

- 2 cups Indonesian Peanut Sauce (page 284)
- 2 potatoes, peeled and cubed
- 2 carrots, peeled and cut into rounds
- 20 green beans, ends trimmed
- ¼ head cauliflower, broken into small florets
- 2 cups shredded cabbage
- 2 cups bean sprouts
- 4 large eggs, hard-boiled, shelled, and cut into quarters

WHILE the peanut sauce is simmering, bring a large saucepan of lightly salted water to a boil. ADD the potatoes and cook for 3 minutes. ADD the carrots, green beans, and cauliflower and boil for another 4 minutes. ADD the cabbage and bean sprouts and boil for 2 minutes. DRAIN the vegetables and rinse under cold water to refresh. ARRANGE equal amounts of each vegetable on plates, garnish with egg quarters, and drizzle with peanut sauce to serve.

Thai Chicken Salad

SERVES 4

Strips of chicken breast and a selection of colorful vegetables served with a lemon juice and sweet chili dressing.

- 8 handfuls of green mignonette or butter lettuce, washed and dried
- 28 thinly sliced rounds of peeled cucumber
- ½ red bell pepper, cut into very thin strips
- 1 carrot, peeled and grated
- 12 oz (340g) precooked chicken breast, skin removed and flesh torn into strips
- 4 tablespoons fish sauce
- 2 tablespoons sweet chili sauce
- 2 tablespoons freshly squeezed lemon juice
- 2 teaspoons sesame oil
- 1 clove garlic, minced
- 2 tablespoons finely chopped fresh mint

ARRANGE the lettuce, cucumber, bell pepper, carrot, and chicken on a serving platter. MIX together the fish sauce, chili sauce, lemon juice, sesame oil, and garlic in a small bowl until well combined. DRIZZLE the dressing over the salad and garnish with mint to serve.

Tabbouleh

SERVES 4

A traditional Middle Eastern salad made with chopped fresh herbs (mainly flat-leaf parsley, but also mint), bulgur, diced tomato, and scallion, and dressed with extra virgin olive oil and lemon juice.

½ cup bulgur

1½ cups finely chopped flat-leaf parsley

2 tomatoes, diced

1½ tablespoons finely chopped fresh mint

2 scallions, thinly sliced

¼ cup extra virgin olive oil

3 tablespoons freshly squeezed lemon juice

1 teaspoon salt

¼ teaspoon ground black pepper

MIX the bulgur with ¾ cup of water in a saucepan. BRING to a boil, cover, then turn the heat on very low and cook for 15 minutes. FLUFF with a fork to separate the grains, then allow to cool while preparing the other ingredients. PLACE the bulgur in a salad bowl with the parsley, tomatoes, mint, scallions, oil, lemon juice, salt, and pepper. TOSS well to combine and serve.

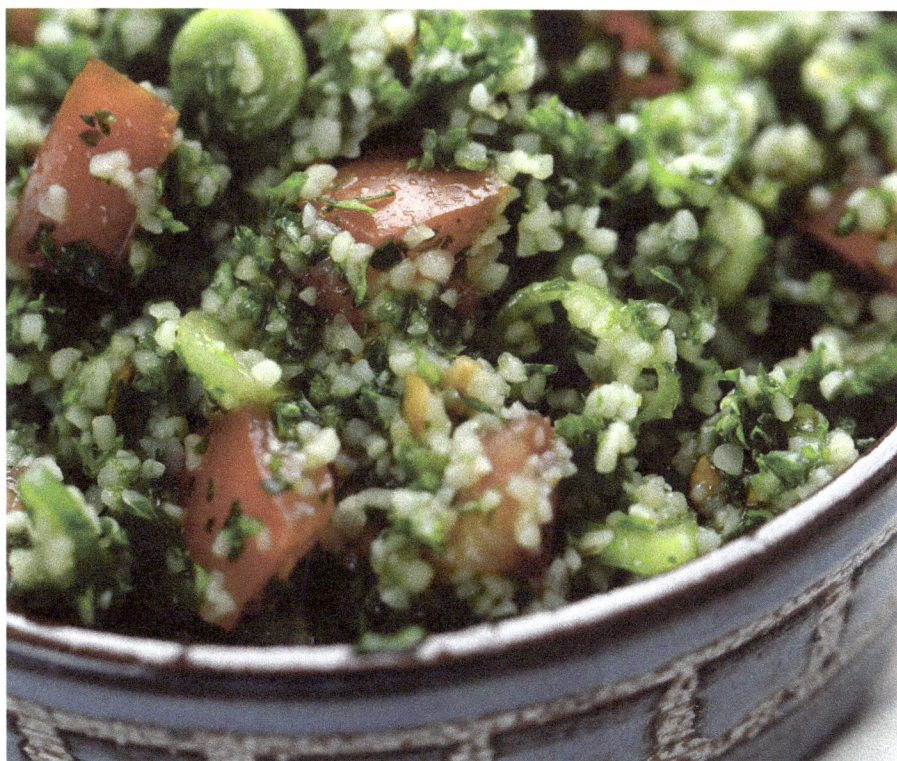

Salade Niçoise

SERVES 4

A mouthwatering and colorful salad from the Provence region of southern France which is a powerhouse of valuable nutrients. The tuna and anchovies provide protein and are a rich source of omega-3s, the olives and olive oil supply heart-healthy monounsaturated fat, the eggs provide protein and vitamins, the potatoes provide energy-giving carbohydrates, as well as plenty of potassium and fiber, and the salad vegetables add more fiber as well as a healthy dose of phytochemicals and antioxidants. Talk about good food that's good for you!

2 small potatoes, peeled and cut into bite-size cubes

20 green beans, ends trimmed and halved

4 anchovy fillets

4 tablespoons extra virgin olive oil

2 tablespoons white wine vinegar

1 garlic clove, minced

1 teaspoon Dijon mustard

½ teaspoon salt

½ teaspoon freshly ground black pepper

3 large eggs, hard-boiled, peeled and quartered

10 romaine (cos) lettuce leaves, washed and dried

14 oz (400g) canned tuna in olive oil, drained and broken into chunks

3 tomatoes, cut into wedges

¼ red onion, thinly sliced and separated into rings

16 black olives (Niçoise are ideal)

COOK the potatoes in a large pot of boiling water for 10 minutes, adding the beans for the final 5 minutes of cooking, then set aside to cool. FINELY chop the anchovies, then use the side of a knife blade to mash into a paste. SCRAPE the anchovies into a screw-top jar, then add the olive oil, vinegar, garlic, Dijon mustard, salt and pepper and shake to combine. ARRANGE the lettuce, potatoes, beans, tuna, tomatoes, onion, eggs and olives on a serving platter. POUR the dressing evenly over the salad to serve.

Variation: For a more opulent version, you can poach or grill fresh fillets of salmon or tuna, allow to cool, and cut into cubes to replace the canned tuna.

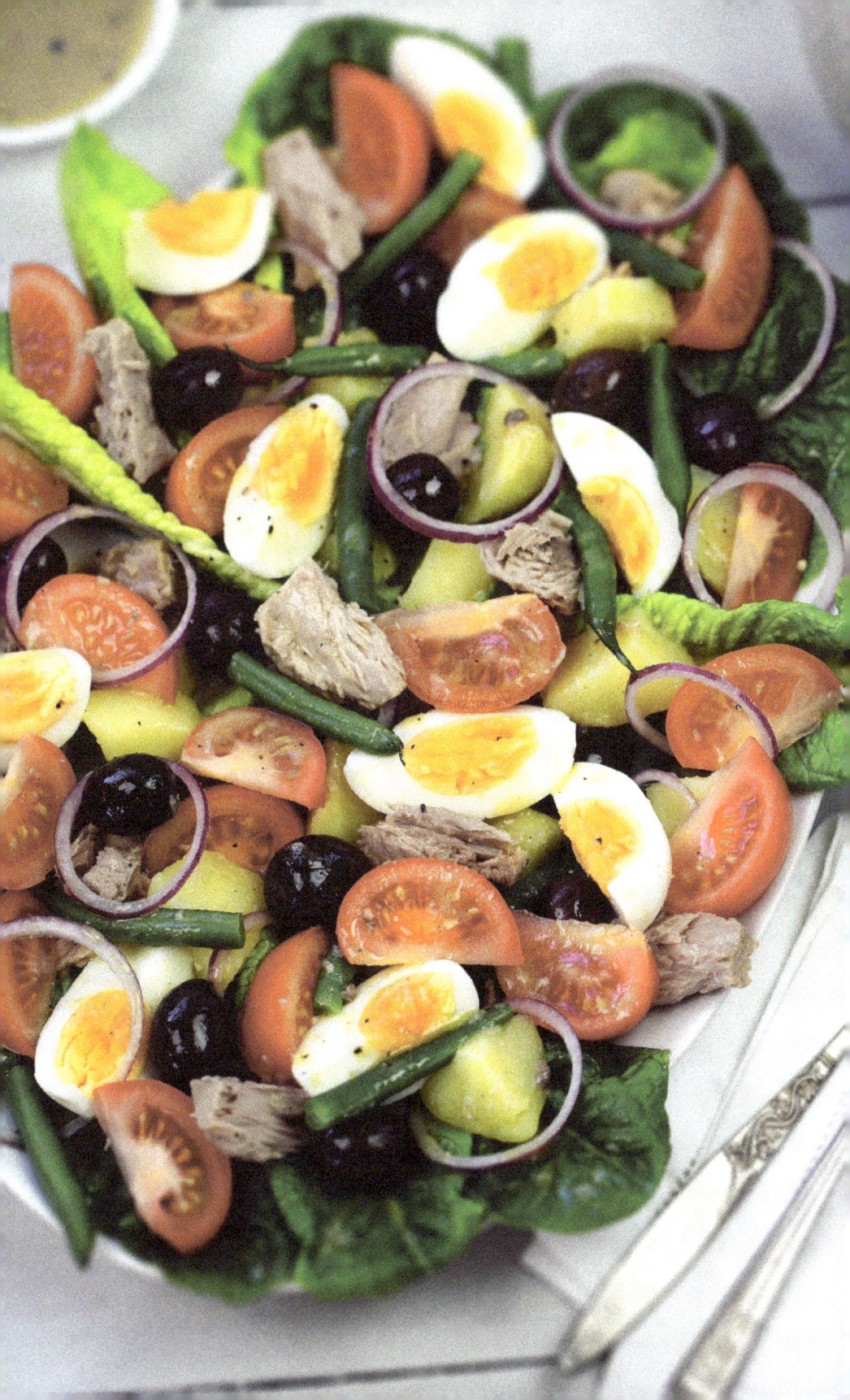

CHAPTER 23

BREAKFASTS

Chakchouka

SERVES 4

Also known as Shakshuka, this colorful and spicy Tunisian vegetable and egg dish makes a tasty and healthy breakfast or light lunch.

3 tablespoons extra virgin olive oil

1 red onion, diced

1 large red bell pepper, cut into thin strips

1 large green bell pepper, cut into thin strips

2 cloves garlic, finely chopped

1 small red chili, deseeded and finely chopped (or ½ teaspoon chili powder)

1 teaspoon cumin

1 teaspoon paprika

1 teaspoon salt

14 oz (400g) canned chopped tomatoes

4 large eggs

HEAT the oil in a large skillet over medium heat and cook the onion, stirring, for 2 minutes. ADD the bell peppers, garlic, and chili and cook, stirring regularly, for 10 minutes. ADD the cumin, paprika, salt, and tomatoes, mix well, and simmer gently until thickened, about 10 minutes. MAKE four indentations in the mixture with the back of a spoon, and crack one egg into each. COVER and simmer until the eggs are set, about 5 minutes. SERVE with crusty bread or lightly buttered whole grain toast on the side.

Smoked Salmon Bruschetta with Arugula & Lemon-Chive Ricotta

SERVES 4

This is a lighter, Italian version of the classic smoked salmon and cream cheese bagel. Instead of bagels it uses toasted slices of Italian ciabatta bread (or you could substitute sourdough), and instead of cream cheese it uses ricotta cheese (which has almost half the calories of cream cheese).

1½ cups ricotta cheese

1 tablespoon lemon juice

1 teaspoon finely chopped lemon zest

2 tablespoons finely chopped chives (plus extra to garnish)

1 teaspoon salt

½ teaspoon freshly ground black pepper

8 thick slices of crusty Italian bread (ciabatta is ideal)

8 teaspoons extra virgin olive oil

2 cups arugula (rocket)

7 oz (200g) thinly sliced smoked salmon

MIX together the ricotta cheese, lemon juice and zest, chives, salt and pepper in a bowl until well combined. TOAST the ciabatta on both sides then brush the top of each with 1 teaspoon of olive oil. SPREAD the ricotta mixture evenly on the bread slices, arrange the arugula over each, then place the salmon on top. GARNISH with extra chives and freshly ground black pepper.

Italian-Style Scrambled Eggs

SERVES 4

Soft, creamy scrambled eggs combined with a selection of Italian-style vegetables and Parmesan cheese.

8 large eggs

4 tablespoons milk

1 teaspoon salt

½ teaspoon freshly ground black pepper

2 tablespoons extra virgin olive oil

1 onion, finely chopped

½ red bell pepper, finely diced

1 zucchini (courgette), finely chopped

4 tablespoons grated Parmesan cheese

8 slices of lightly buttered whole grain toast, for serving

IN a bowl, whisk the eggs, milk, salt, and pepper together gently. HEAT the olive oil in a large skillet over medium heat until lightly sizzling. ADD the onion, bell pepper, and zucchini and cook, stirring occasionally, until the vegetables are softened, about 8 minutes. REDUCE the heat to medium-low, add the egg mixture, and cook, stirring continuously, until the eggs are barely set, about 2 minutes. STIR in the Parmesan cheese and cook until the eggs are creamy, about 30 seconds more. REMOVE from the heat and serve with slices of lightly buttered whole grain toast.

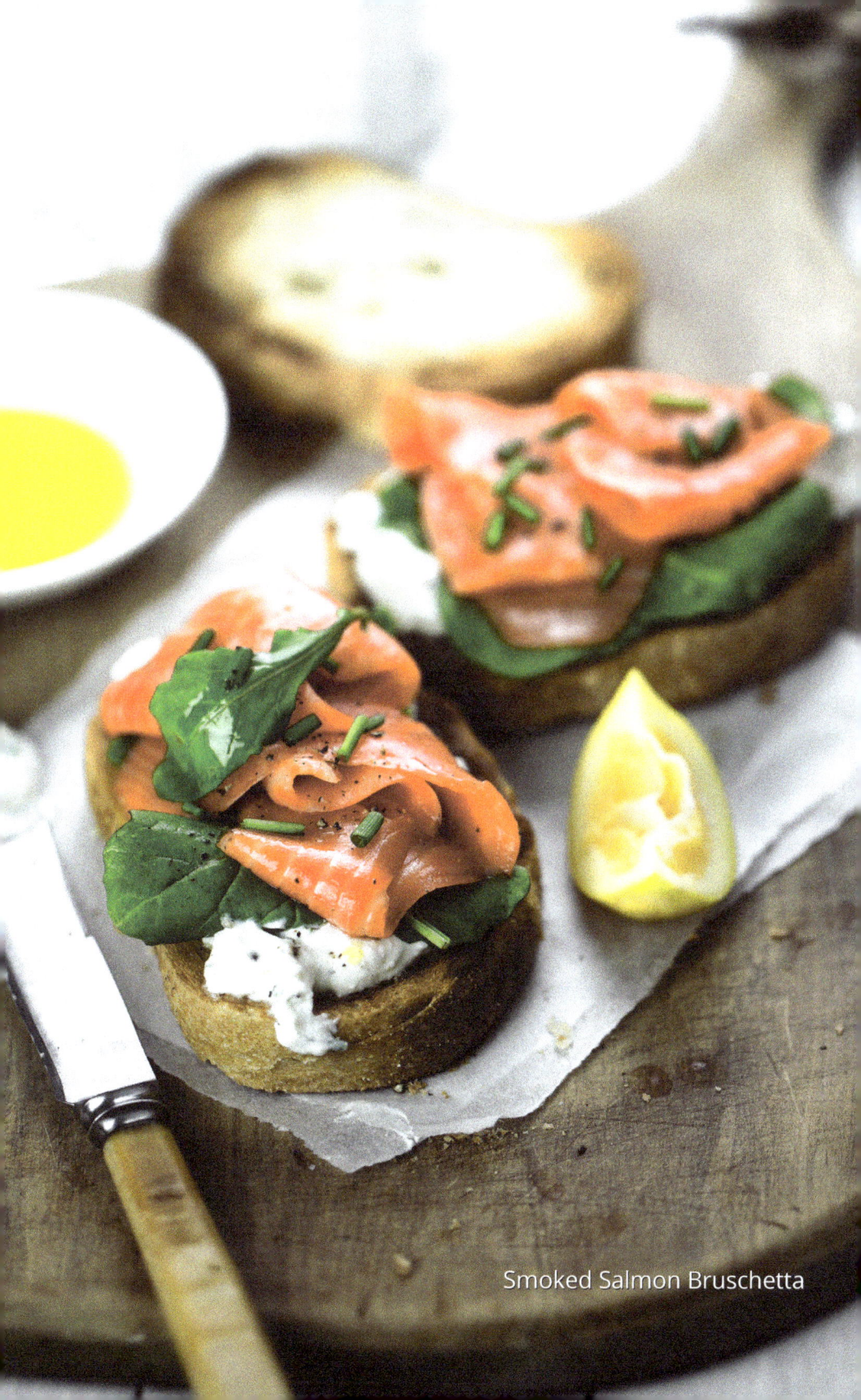
Smoked Salmon Bruschetta

Tuna, Pea & Corn Frittata

SERVES 4

Frittata is the Italian equivalent of an omelet. This specialty is very easy to prepare and is ideal either as a hearty breakfast served with slices of lightly buttered whole grain toast or plain bruschetta, or eaten as a delightful light dinner with a salad and some crusty bread.

2½ tablespoons extra virgin olive oil

1 onion, finely chopped

½ cup frozen green peas, thawed

½ cup corn kernels

1 clove garlic, minced

6 oz (170g) canned tuna in olive oil, drained and flaked

8 large eggs

1 tablespoon chopped fresh flat-leaf parsley

1 teaspoon salt

½ teaspoon freshly ground black pepper

½ cup grated Parmesan cheese

PREHEAT the oven broiler (griller). HEAT 2 tablespoons of the oil in a medium-size skillet over medium heat and cook the onion, stirring occasionally, for 5 minutes. ADD the peas, corn, and garlic and cook, stirring occasionally, for another 3 minutes. TRANSFER the mixture to a bowl, mix in the flaked tuna, and allow to cool slightly. WHISK the eggs in a bowl with the parsley, salt, and pepper, then mix together with the tuna and vegetable mixture. HEAT the remaining oil in the skillet over medium heat, then pour in the egg, tuna, and vegetable mixture. COOK the frittata gently over a low heat, covered, about 8 minutes. SPRINKLE the top with the cheese and cook under the preheated oven broiler for 1 minute. CUT the frittata into wedges and serve.

Variation: Use 2 thin slices of diced ham in place of the tuna.

Sardine Toast Topper

SERVES 4

Sardines are the perfect match with lemon juice and capers, and make a great breakfast spread on hot buttered toast (lightly buttered, of course).

8 oz (230g) canned sardines in water or oil, drained	1 teaspoon salt
	½ teaspoon freshly ground black pepper
4 teaspoons freshly squeezed lemon juice	8 slices of whole grain bread, toasted and lightly buttered
4 teaspoons capers, rinsed and drained	4 lemon wedges, for serving

MASH together the sardines, lemon juice, capers, salt, and pepper in a bowl until well combined. SPREAD equal amounts of the mixture over the pieces of lightly buttered toast and serve with lemon wedges for drizzling.

Tortilla de Patatas

SERVES 4

Tortilla de Patatas is a traditional Spanish egg dish similar to a French omelet and an Italian frittata. This version includes potatoes, red onion, and green bell peppers.

2 potatoes, peeled and cut into small cubes	8 large eggs
3 tablespoons extra virgin olive oil	2 tablespoons finely chopped fresh flat-leaf parsley
1 red onion, finely chopped	1 teaspoon salt
1 green bell pepper, deseeded and finely diced	½ teaspoon freshly ground black pepper

PREHEAT the oven broiler (griller). COOK the potato in a pot of boiling water for 6 minutes. HEAT the oil in a medium-size skillet over medium heat and cook the onion and bell pepper, stirring occasionally, until softened, about 5 minutes. ADD the potato and cook, stirring to combine, for another 2 minutes. WHISK the eggs together in a bowl with the parsley, salt, and pepper. POUR the eggs over the vegetables in the skillet, cover, and cook gently over low heat for 8 minutes. REMOVE the lid and place under the preheated broiler to cook for 1 minute or until the top is set. CUT into wedges to serve.

Serving Ideas: You can serve wedges of tortilla de patatas warm or cold (it keeps well, covered and chilled, for 1 to 2 days).

Fruity Couscous with Honey-Ginger Yogurt

SERVES 4

Apricot and raisin studded couscous served with a dollop of honey-ginger yogurt.

1¼ cups orange juice

1 cup quick-cooking couscous

½ cup dried apricots, cut into halves

¼ cup raisins

1 cup Greek yogurt

2 tablespoons liquid honey

2 teaspoons ground ginger

HEAT the orange juice in a small saucepan over a high heat and bring to a boil. PLACE the couscous, apricots and raisins in a heat-proof bowl, pour over the boiling orange juice, cover with a plate or clean dishcloth, and allow to steam for 5 minutes. WHILE the couscous steams, mix together the yogurt, honey and ginger in a small bowl. FLUFF up the couscous and dried fruit with a fork. SERVE the fruit couscous with the honey-ginger yogurt drizzled on top.

Creamy Fruit & Nut Oatmeal

SERVES 4

A bowl of this creamy oatmeal sprinkled with dried fruits and nuts makes a warming and sustaining breakfast.

5 cups cold water

2 cups rolled oats

½ teaspoon salt

½ teaspoon cinnamon

Cold milk, for serving

Brown sugar or honey, for serving

½ cup chopped dried fruit (such as raisins, figs, or apricots), for serving

4 tablespoons chopped nuts (such as walnuts, hazelnuts, or almonds)

COMBINE the water, oats, salt, and cinnamon in a saucepan. BRING to a boil over medium-high heat, stirring regularly to avoid lumps. REDUCE the heat to medium and simmer stirring occasionally, until thick and creamy (8-10 minutes). SERVE in bowls with milk, a little brown sugar or honey, and sprinkled with the fruit and nuts.

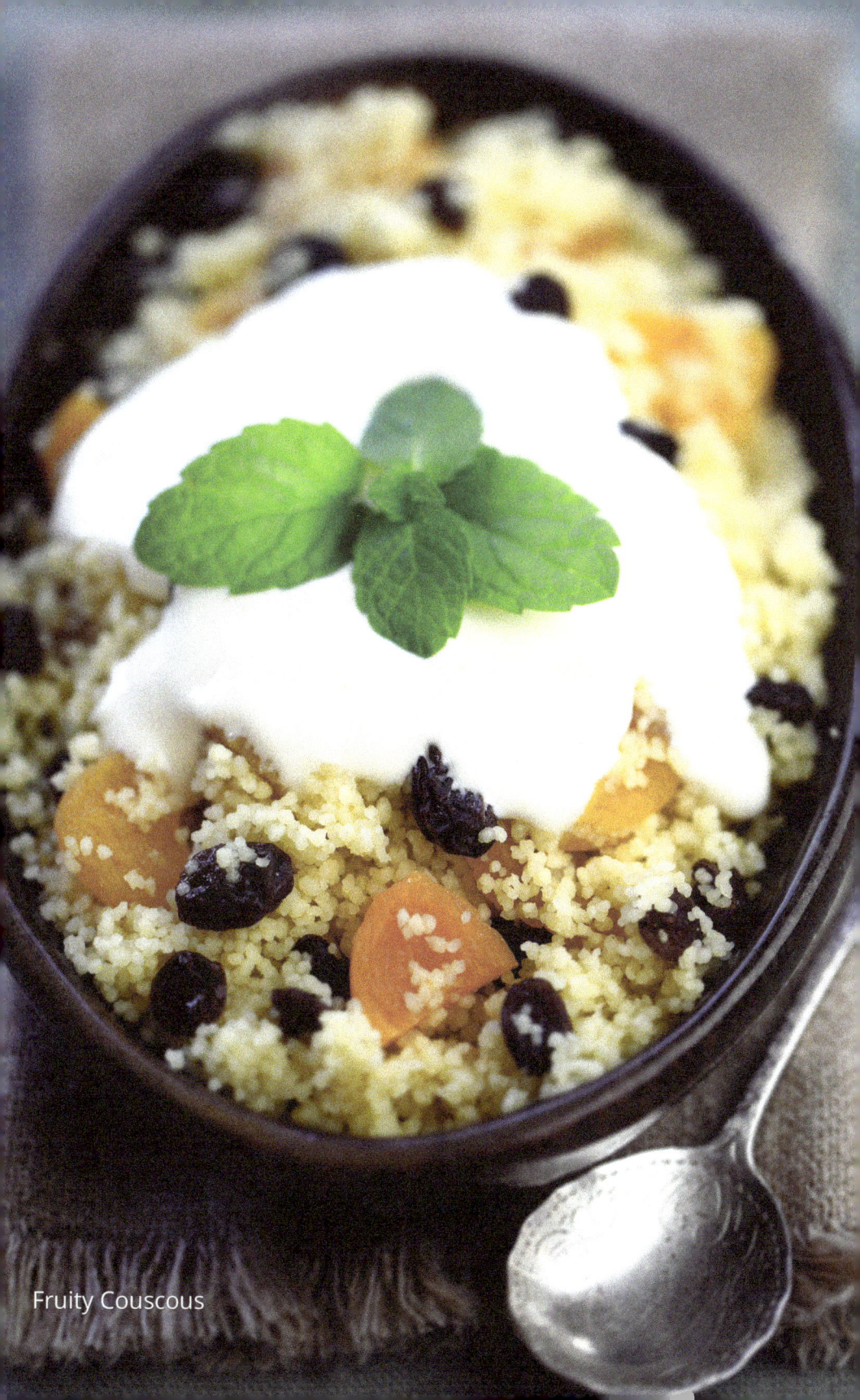

Fruity Couscous

Italian-Style Pan-Fried Sandwich

SERVES 4

A simple toasted sandwich with an Italian twist.

8 slices whole grain bread

4 thin slices ham

3 oz (85g) thinly sliced mozzarella cheese

2 tomatoes, thinly sliced

4 teaspoons finely chopped fresh basil

Salt and freshly ground black pepper to taste

8 teaspoons extra virgin olive oil

2 cloves garlic, peeled and cut in half

TOP four slices of bread evenly with ham, cheese, tomatoes, and basil, and season with salt and pepper. COVER with the other four bread slices and lightly brush the sandwiches on both sides with the oil. HEAT a large skillet over medium heat and place the sandwiches into the pan (wait until the pan is hot before you add the sandwiches or else they'll stick). COOK for 4 minutes on each side, or until golden brown. REMOVE from the skillet, rub one side of each sandwich with the cut side of the garlic, and cut in half to serve.

Variations: Add rings of thinly sliced onion or a few sliced olives. Replace the basil with a smear of pesto or use finely chopped sun-dried tomatoes instead of fresh.

Raisin, Apricot & Almond Muesli

MAKES 14 CUPS

One of the quickest and tastiest breakfasts is muesli. And because muesli typically contains a mixture of rolled oats (which are a whole grain), dried fruit, and nuts it also makes a healthy start to the day. This recipe makes the equivalent of a large box of breakfast cereal.

8 cups of Wheaties (also known as Weeties in some countries)

4 cups rolled oats

½ cup raisins

½ cup sliced almonds

½ cup chopped dried apricots

½ cup desiccated or shredded unsweetened coconut

IN a very large bowl combine the Wheaties, rolled oats, raisins, almonds, apricots, and coconut. MIX together thoroughly and store in an air-tight container.

CHAPTER 24

SAUCES, DIPS & SPREADS

Baba Ghanoush

MAKES 1 CUP

The smoky flavor and creamy texture of this Middle Eastern eggplant puree is truly unique and absolutely delectable. It's wonderful served as a dip or a spread.

1 large eggplant (aubergine), cut in half lengthways

2 tablespoons freshly squeezed lemon juice

2 tablespoons tahini (sesame paste)

2 tablespoons extra virgin olive oil

1 clove garlic, roughly chopped

1 teaspoon salt

½ teaspoon ground black pepper

PREHEAT an oven broiler (griller). Place the eggplant halves, skin side up, on a baking tray. COOK the eggplant directly under the heat source for 20 minutes. REMOVE the eggplant and let it cool to room temperature. SCOOP out the eggplant flesh from the skin with a spoon, and place in a food processor or blender with the lemon juice, tahini, oil, garlic, salt, and pepper; process until smooth. STORE in the refrigerator, covered, for up to 3 days, or in the freezer for up to 3 months.

Tapenade

MAKES ½ CUP

Tapenade is a luscious Provençal paste made with olives, olive oil, anchovies, capers, and garlic. Traditionally it's made using a mortar and pestle, but to save time and energy you can get similar results by using a food processor.

1 clove garlic, roughly chopped

1 tablespoon freshly squeezed lemon juice

2 tablespoons extra virgin olive oil

¾ cup pitted black olives

1 tablespoon capers

2 anchovy fillets

¼ teaspoon freshly ground black pepper

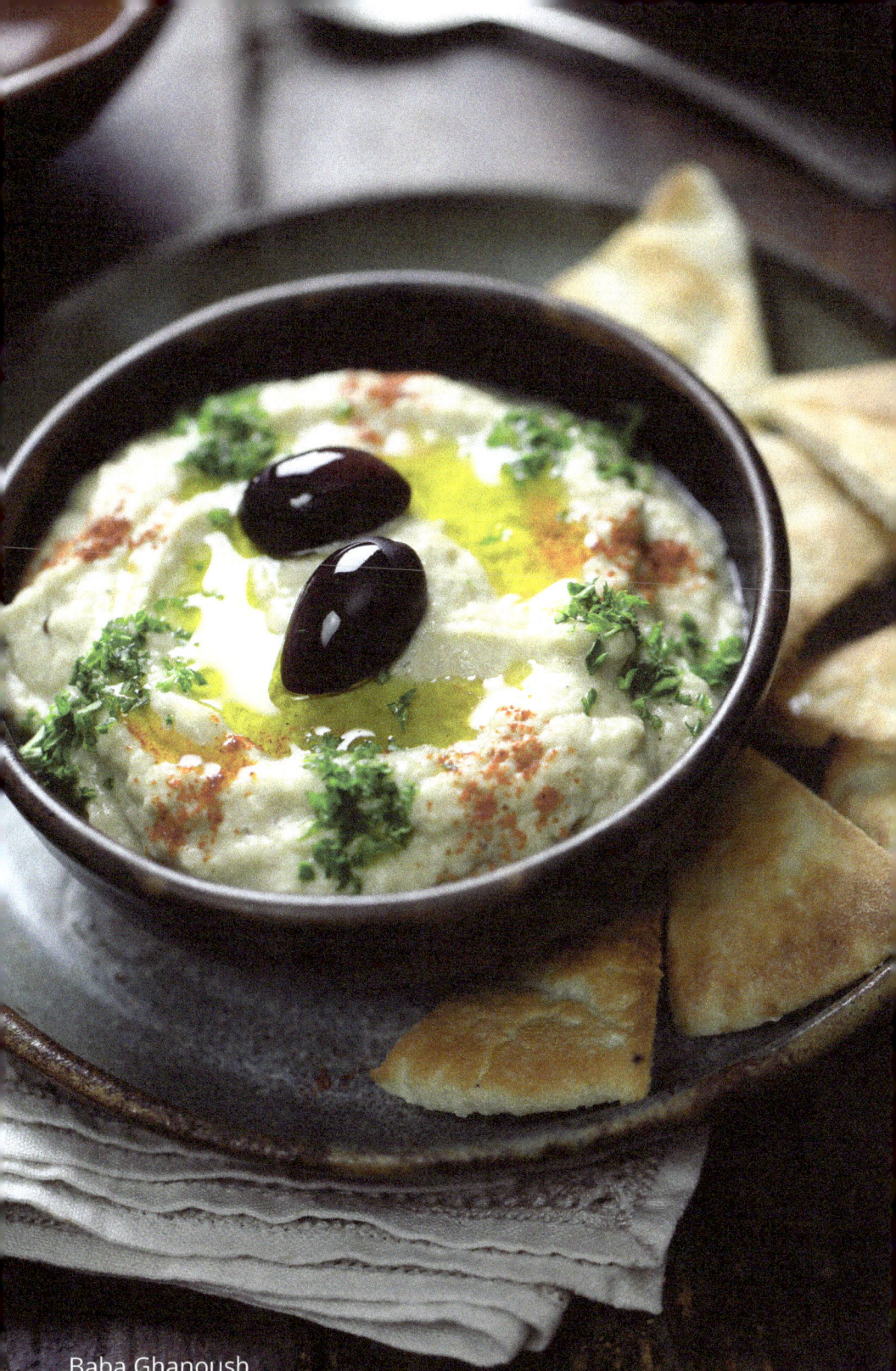

Baba Ghanoush

PLACE all ingredients in a food processor or blender and process until smooth. STORE in the refrigerator, covered, for up to 3 days, or in the freezer for up to 3 months.

Serving Ideas: Tapenade can be used to season grilled fish or chicken; it's delicious spread on sliced baguette and topped with chopped tomatoes; or simply serve it with crackers or crusty bread and vegetable crudités for dipping.

Romesco Sauce

MAKES 1 CUP

A robust Spanish sauce made from a pureed mix of grilled red peppers, toasted almonds, garlic, chili, red wine vinegar, and olive oil. This delicious and versatile sauce can be drizzled over grilled fish, chicken, seafood, or vegetables; used as a salad dressing, dip, or spread; stirred into stews to add richness and color; and it makes a wonderful pasta sauce.

1 red bell pepper, deseeded and quartered

½ cup sliced almonds

⅓ cup extra virgin olive oil

1½ tablespoons red wine vinegar

1 tablespoon water

1 clove garlic, roughly chopped

1 small red chili, deseeded and finely chopped (or ½ teaspoon chili powder)

½ teaspoon salt

¼ teaspoon freshly ground black pepper

PLACE the bell pepper (skin side up) directly under a hot oven broiler (griller) until the skin blackens all over, about 12 minutes. REMOVE and cover the charred pepper with a clean dishcloth or plastic wrap for 5 minutes to allow the steam to loosen the skin from the pepper flesh. WHILE the pepper cools, place the almonds in a frying pan and toast over a gentle heat, stirring regularly so they don't burn, until golden brown. PEEL off the blackened skin from the pepper and roughly cut the flesh into pieces. IN a blender or food processor, combine the roasted pepper, toasted almonds, oil, vinegar, water, garlic, chili, salt, and pepper and blend until smooth. STORE in the refrigerator, covered, for up to 3 days, or in the freezer for up to 3 months.

Raita

The combination of cucumber and yogurt makes a traditional cooling accompaniment to serve with spicy Indian dishes such as South Indian Shrimp and Chickpea Curry (page 179) or Fragrant Chicken Curry (page 182).

1 cup plain thick yogurt (Greek yogurt is best)

½ cup finely chopped cucumber, peeled and deseeded

½ clove garlic, minced

2 teaspoons freshly squeezed lemon juice

½ teaspoon salt

IN a small bowl, mix together the yogurt, cucumber, garlic, lemon juice, and salt until well combined. STORE in the refrigerator, covered, for up to 2 days.

Indonesian Peanut Sauce

MAKES 2 CUPS

This mouthwatering peanut sauce has a rich, nutty flavor and a delightful creamy texture. It makes an ideal dipping sauce for satay (marinated and grilled chicken, meat, or seafood skewers) and a pouring sauce for the classic Indonesian salad Gado Gado (page 266).

1 tablespoon peanut oil

2 cloves garlic, finely chopped

½ teaspoon shrimp paste (or 1 tablespoon fish sauce added at the same time as the coconut milk)

1 cup coconut milk

1 cup water

6 tablespoons natural peanut butter

4 tablespoons soy sauce

4 teaspoons brown sugar

½ teaspoon dried chili flakes

1 tablespoon freshly squeezed lemon juice

HEAT the oil in a skillet over medium heat. ADD the garlic and shrimp paste and cook, stirring constantly to dissolve the shrimp paste, for 1 minute. ADD the coconut milk, water, peanut butter, soy sauce, sugar, and dried chili flakes and bring to a boil. REDUCE the heat and simmer, stirring regularly, until the sauce reaches a creamy consistency, 10 to 12 minutes. ADD the lemon juice, and stir to combine. STORE in the refrigerator, covered, for up to 3 days, or in the freezer for up to 3 months.

Pesto Genoese

MAKES 1 CUP

This traditional pesto sauce combines fresh basil with pine nuts, garlic, Parmesan cheese and extra virgin olive oil. It originates in Genoa, the capital of Italy's Liguria region, where basil flourishes and is used extensively. Traditionally, pesto is made by grinding the ingredients together with a mortar and pestle; however, it's much quicker just to whip it up in a food processor or blender.

1 cup tightly packed fresh basil

⅓ cup freshly grated Parmesan cheese

⅓ cup pine nuts, lightly toasted

1 clove garlic, roughly chopped

2 tablespoons water

½ teaspoon salt

¼ teaspoon freshly ground black pepper

⅓ cup extra virgin olive oil

IN a food processor or blender, combine the basil, Parmesan, pine nuts, garlic, water, salt, and pepper. WHILE you process, slowly pour the olive oil into the mix until all the ingredients turn into a smooth paste (you may have to scrape the sides occasionally). STORE in the refrigerator, covered, for up to 3 days, or in the freezer for up to 3 months.

Serving Ideas: Pesto has a myriad of uses, such as tossed with hot pasta; spread over bruschetta, used as a pizza sauce, stirred into soups like minestrone just before serving, mixed with mayonnaise to dress salads and sandwiches, or served as a dip with vegetable crudités.

Variations: Walnuts, pistachios, macadamias, almonds, or cashews can be substituted for the pine nuts.

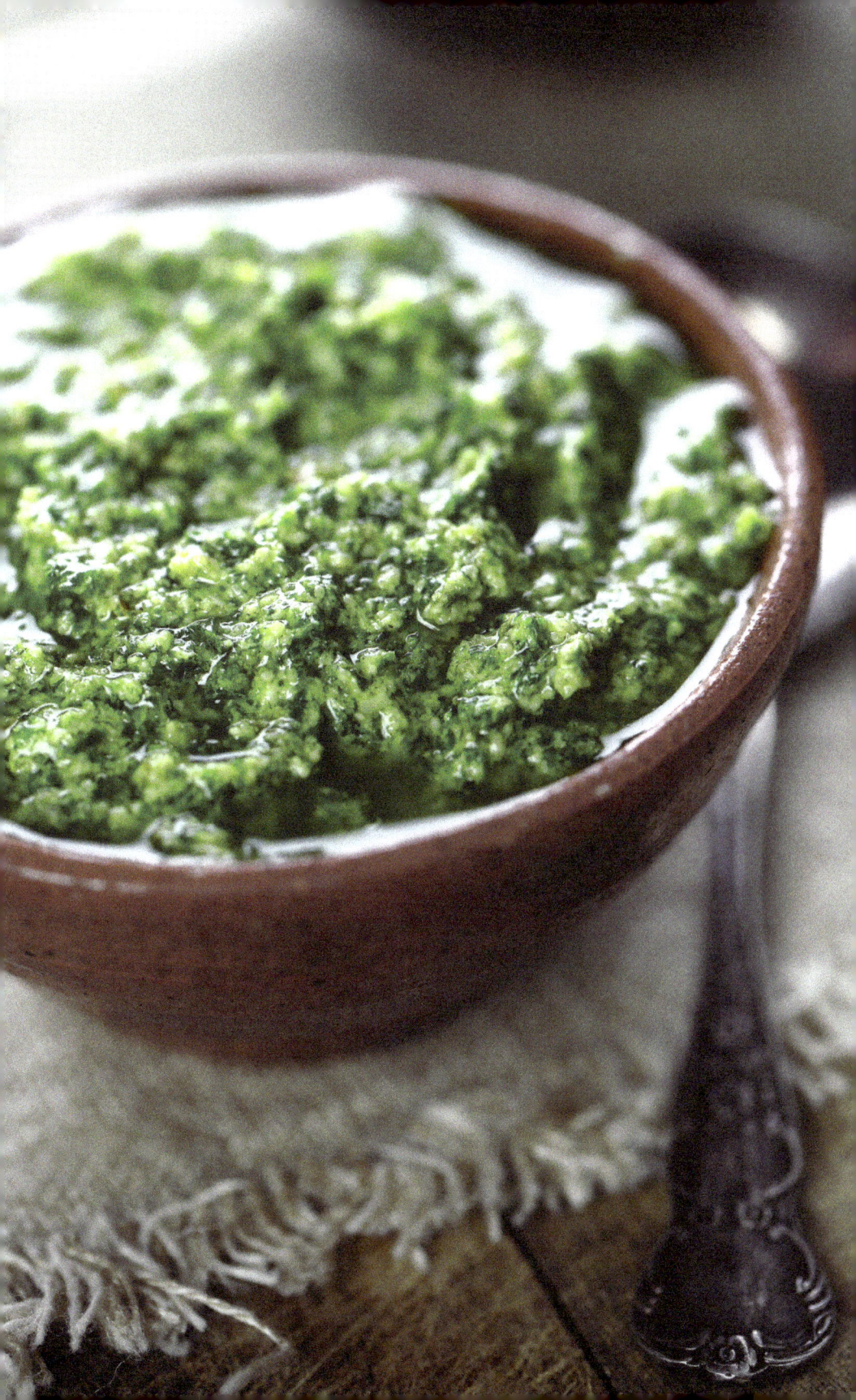

Sun-Dried Tomato & Walnut Pesto

MAKES 1 CUP

A deliciously different pesto made with walnuts and richly flavored sun-dried tomatoes. You can use this pesto tossed through pasta, as a dip or spread, you can stir it into soups to add richness and flavor.

1 cup tightly packed fresh basil

⅓ cup freshly grated Parmesan cheese

⅓ cup walnuts

6 oil-packed sun-dried tomatoes, roughly chopped

1 large clove garlic, roughly chopped

2 tablespoons water

½ teaspoon salt

¼ teaspoon freshly ground black pepper

⅓ cup extra virgin olive oil

IN a food processor, combine the basil, Parmesan, walnuts, sun-dried tomatoes, garlic, water, salt, and pepper. WHILE you process, slowly pour the olive oil into the mix until all the ingredients turn into a smooth paste (you may have to scrape the sides occasionally). STORE in the refrigerator, covered, for up to 3 days, or in the freezer for up to 3 months.

Asian Cilantro-Peanut Pesto

MAKES 1 CUP

This Asian-inspired pesto makes an enticing change from traditional pesto and is wonderful tossed through Asian noodles with vegetables and seafood or chicken.

1 cup tightly packed cilantro (fresh coriander)

⅓ cup unsalted roasted peanuts

1 small green chili, deseeded and roughly chopped

1 clove garlic, roughly chopped

1 teaspoon finely grated fresh ginger

2 tablespoons freshly squeezed lime juice

1 tablespoon fish sauce

½ tablespoon brown sugar

½ teaspoon salt

⅓ cup peanut oil

IN a food processor or blender, combine the cilantro, peanuts, chili, garlic, ginger, lime juice, fish sauce, sugar, and salt. WHILE you process, slowly pour the peanut oil into the mix until all the ingredients turn into a smooth paste (you may have to scrape the sides occasionally). STORE in the refrigerator, covered, for up to 3 days, or in the freezer for up to 3 months.

Hummus

MAKES 2 CUPS

Hummus is a creamy puree of chickpeas and tahini (sesame seed paste) seasoned with lemon juice and garlic, and is a popular spread and dip in Greece and throughout the Middle East. Hummus can be served as part of a meze platter; with bread or vegetable crudités for dipping; as a spread or filling for pita, lavash, or Turkish *pide* bread; or as a tasty, creamy alternative to butter in sandwiches.

14 oz (400g) canned chickpeas (garbanzo beans), rinsed and drained

½ cup tahini (sesame paste)

¼ cup freshly squeezed lemon juice

⅓ cup water

2 cloves garlic, roughly chopped

1 teaspoon salt

PLACE all ingredients in a food processor or blender and process until smooth, scraping the sides occasionally. STORE in the refrigerator, covered, for up to 1 week, or the freezer for up to 3 months.

Salsa Verde

MAKES ½ CUP

Made from a mixture of fresh herbs, capers, and anchovies, this piquant Italian green sauce can be served as a no-cook pasta sauce (such as Pasta with Salsa Verde and Smoked Salmon, page 152), with grilled fish or chicken, or tossed with potatoes for a Mediterranean-style potato salad.

4 anchovy fillets, finely chopped

4 tablespoons extra virgin olive oil

3 tablespoons finely chopped fresh flat-leaf parsley

3 tablespoons finely chopped fresh basil

2 tablespoons freshly squeezed lemon juice

1 scallion, finely chopped

1 tablespoon capers, rinsed, drained, and finely chopped

1 clove garlic, minced

½ teaspoon salt

¼ teaspoon freshly ground black pepper

MIX together all ingredients in a bowl until well combined. STORE in the refrigerator, covered, for up to 2 days.

Tzatziki

SERVES 4

A tangy and luxuriously textured Greek sauce that can be enjoyed as a dip or spread, served on souvlaki, in a gyro, pita sandwich, or with grilled fish, meat or vegetables.

1 cucumber, peeled and cut in half lengthways

2 cups Greek yogurt

2 garlic cloves, minced

1 tablespoon lemon juice

1½ tablespoons finely chopped fresh dill

1 tablespoon extra virgin olive oil

1 teaspoon salt

SCRAPE the seeds out of the cucumber halves using the pointy end of a teaspoon, and discard. GRATE the cucumber flesh into a bowl then squeeze out any excess moisture using your hands (a small handful at a time works best). PLACE the grated cucumber into a large bowl and add the yogurt, garlic, lemon juice, olive oil, dill, salt and pepper. STIR well to combine. PLACE the tzatziki in the refrigerator for at least 2 hours to let the flavors meld and intensify.

Variation: Use finely chopped fresh mint instead of dill.

Nuoc Cham Dipping Sauce

MAKES ½ CUP

This delicious, sweet and spicy Vietnamese dipping sauce is the perfect accompaniment to Vietnamese rice paper rolls or any Asian-style finger food.

2 tablespoons water

1 tablespoon sugar

2 tablespoons freshly squeezed lemon juice

2 tablespoons fish sauce

2 tablespoons rice vinegar

1 clove garlic, minced

1 red chili, deseeded and finely chopped

MIX together the water and sugar and water in a small bowl until dissolved. STIR in the lemon juice, fish sauce, vinegar, garlic, and chili until well combined. STORE in the refrigerator, covered, for up to 1 week.

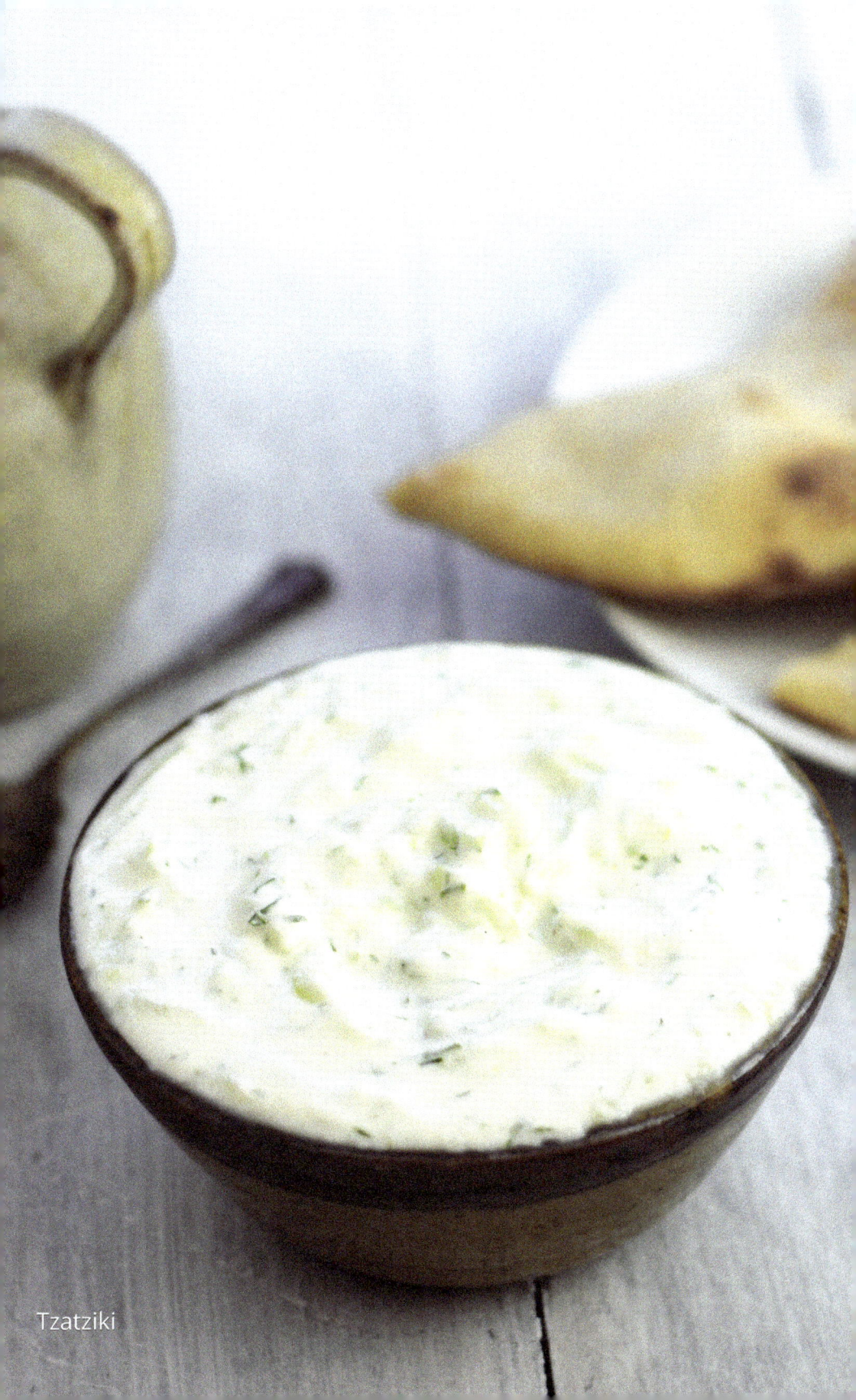

Tzatziki

Flavored Mayonnaise

Good-quality store-bought mayonnaise can be blended with different ingredients to create a range of flavorful sauces.

Aioli. Mix together 4 tablespoons mayonnaise with 1 clove minced garlic and 2 teaspoons extra virgin olive oil. This easy version of traditional Provençal garlic mayonnaise makes a delicious accompaniment with cooked fish and shellfish, roast chicken, or a selection of boiled eggs, potatoes, raw and cooked vegetables, and bread.

Dijon Mayonnaise. Mix together 4 tablespoons of mayonnaise with 2 teaspoons Dijon mustard.

Pesto Mayonnaise. Mix together 4 tablespoons mayonnaise with 2 tablespoons Pesto (page 285).

Wasabi Mayonnaise. Mix together 4 tablespoons mayonnaise with 2 teaspoons wasabi paste.

Lime Mayonnaise. Mix together 4 tablespoons mayonnaise with 1 tablespoon freshly squeezed lime juice and ½ teaspoon finely chopped lime zest.

Sweet Chili Mayonnaise. Mix together 4 tablespoons mayonnaise with 2 tablespoons sweet chili sauce.

Curry Mayonnaise. Mix together 4 tablespoons mayonnaise with 1 teaspoon curry powder.

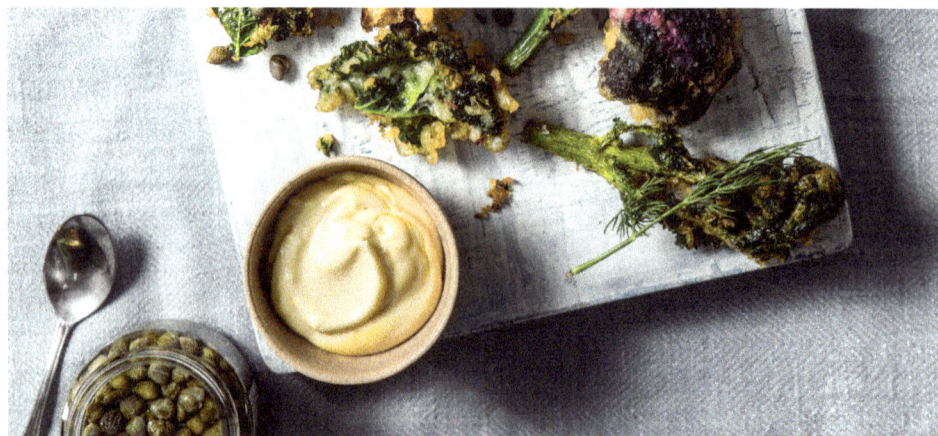

Chinese-Style Dipping Sauce

MAKES ¾ CUP

This is a good dipping sauce for Chinese-Style Chicken and Vegetable Rolls (page 225) and Asian-Style Corn Fritters (page 302).

½ cup chicken stock

2 tablespoons soy sauce

2 teaspoons Chinese rice wine

1 teaspoon sesame oil

1 teaspoon finely grated fresh ginger

½ clove garlic, crushed

1 teaspoon sugar

MIX together all ingredients in a small bowl until well combined. STORE in the refrigerator, covered, for up to 3 days.

Sesame-Hoisin Dipping Sauce

MAKES ⅓ CUP

The combination of thick, savory-sweet hoisin sauce with salty soy sauce, nutty sesame oil and a hint of garlic makes a heavenly dipping sauce to serve with rice paper rolls (page 222).

3 tablespoons hoisin sauce

3 tablespoons soy sauce

2 tablespoons water

2 teaspoons sesame oil

½ clove garlic, minced

MIX together all ingredients in a small bowl until well combined. STORE in the refrigerator, covered, for up to 3 days.

Savory Salmon Spread

MAKES 1 CUP

This easy-to-prepare omega-3-rich spread can be used as a sandwich or wrap filling, and also makes a tasty whole grain cracker topping.

14 oz (400g) canned Alaskan red salmon, bones removed

2 tablespoons mayonnaise

2 tablespoons extra virgin olive oil

½ teaspoon salt

½ teaspoon freshly ground black pepper

1½ tablespoons finely chopped red onion

1 tablespoon freshly squeezed lemon juice

1 tablespoon finely chopped fresh flat leaf parsley

1 teaspoon finely chopped capers

MASH the salmon in a bowl with the mayonnaise, olive oil, salt, and pepper. ADD the onion, lemon juice, parsley, and capers and mix thoroughly to combine.

Savory Tuna Spread

MAKES 1 CUP

This versatile spread can be used as a sandwich filling or toast topping (makes a delicious savory tuna melt), spread on whole grain crackers, served as part of a salad plate, or tossed through hot pasta.

14 oz (400g) canned tuna

2 tablespoons mayonnaise

2 tablespoons extra virgin olive oil

½ teaspoon salt

½ teaspoon freshly ground black pepper

2 tomatoes, diced

8 pitted black olives, finely chopped

1½ tablespoons finely chopped red onion

MASH the tuna a bowl with the mayonnaise, olive oil, salt, and pepper. ADD the tomatoes, olives, and onion and mix thoroughly to combine.

Italian Vinaigrette

MAKES ¼ CUP

A simple and flavorful all-purpose salad dressing.

2½ tablespoons extra virgin olive oil

1½ tablespoons balsamic vinegar

½ clove garlic, minced

¼ teaspoon salt

¼ teaspoon freshly ground black pepper

SHAKE all ingredients together in a screw-top jar until well combined.

CHAPTER 25

APPETIZERS

Thai Fish Cakes with Sweet Chili-Lime Dipping Sauce

SERVES 4

Fish cakes are a popular appetizer and snack in Thailand—and they're really easy to make at home. We not only love eating them as an appetizer, we also slice them and add them to stir-fries. The fish cake mixture can also be used in other ways. You can roll it into balls and add them to Southeast Asian soups and curries—they poach beautifully in hot broths and curry sauces. You can also shape the mixture into larger patties for Thai-style fish burgers with lettuce, cucumber, grated carrot, and sweet chili sauce mixed with mayo for the dressing.

20 oz (550g) roughly chopped firm white fish fillets

1 tablespoon Thai red curry paste

2 garlic cloves, minced

2 tablespoons plus 2 teaspoons fish sauce

2 tablespoons cornstarch

4 kaffir lime leaves, finely chopped (or 2 teaspoons finely chopped lime zest)

2 scallions, thinly sliced

4 tablespoons peanut or canola oil

½ cup sweet chili sauce

2 tablespoons lime juice

PLACE the chopped fish fillets in a food processor or blender and pulse until smooth. ADD the red curry paste, garlic, 2 tablespoons of fish sauce, and cornstarch and pulse until well combined. TRANSFER the fish mixture to a bowl, add the kaffir lime leaves and scallion, and stir to combine. DIVIDE the mixture into 12 equal portions and shape each with damp hands into patties. HEAT the oil in a large skillet over medium heat. COOK the fish cakes for 3 minutes each side. WHILE the fish cakes cook, mix together the sweet chili sauce, lime juice and 2 teaspoons of the fish sauce in a small bowl until well combined. SERVE the fish cakes warm or at room temperature with the sweet chili-lime sauce for dipping.

Variations: Use Thai green curry paste instead of red. Add 4 thinly sliced green beans to the fish cake mixture before shaping and frying.

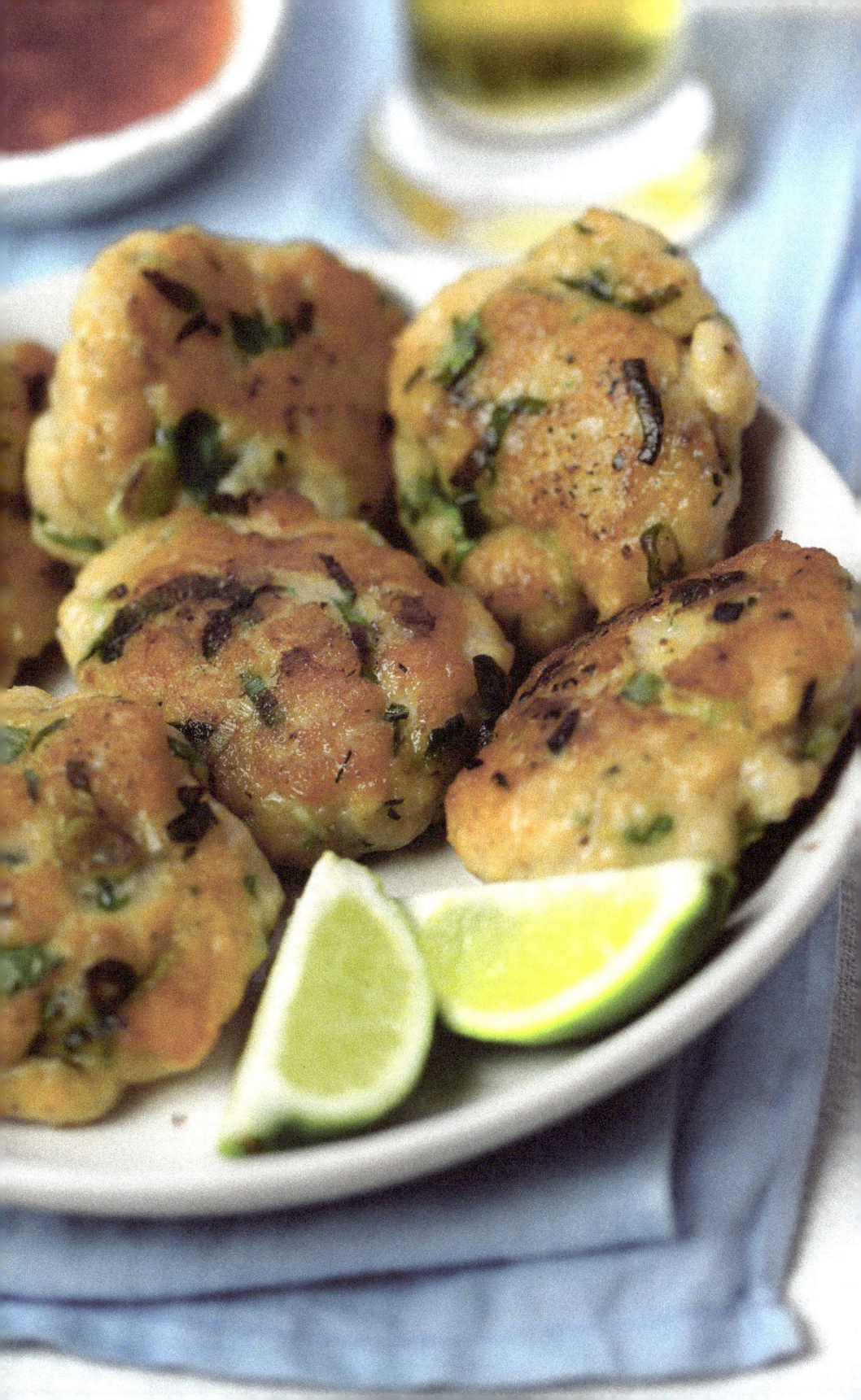

Garlic Shrimp

SERVES 4

A sizzling dish of shrimp flavored with fresh garlic, salt, and parsley and served with lemon wedges. Perfect as an appetizer on its own, or served as part of a selection of tapas.

4 tablespoons extra virgin olive oil

24 large uncooked shrimp (prawns), peeled and deveined with bottom of tail left intact

4 cloves garlic, finely chopped

1 teaspoon salt

2 teaspoons finely chopped fresh flat-leaf parsley

Lemon wedges, for serving

HEAT the oil in a large skillet over medium heat and add the shrimp, garlic, and salt. COOK, tossing regularly, about 3 minutes. SPRINKLE with parsley and serve with lemon wedges for squeezing.

Variation: To make Chili-Garlic Shrimp, add 2 small fresh red chilies, deseeded and finely chopped, with the garlic and shrimp.

Fava Bean Puree with Pita Wedges

SERVES 4

The vibrant green color and scrumptious flavor of the fava bean puree is a perfect combination with crisp baked pita wedges.

4 medium-size whole grain pita breads

4 cups frozen fava (broad) beans, cooked in boiling water for 5 minutes, rinsed under cold water, and skins removed

6 tablespoons extra virgin olive oil

2 tablespoons freshly squeezed lemon juice

2 cloves garlic, minced

1 teaspoon salt

½ teaspoon freshly ground black pepper

PREHEAT the oven to 450°F (230°C). CUT each pita bread into 8 wedges. PLACE on a baking tray and bake for 5 minutes. WHILE the pita wedges are baking, place the cooked fava beans, olive oil, lemon juice, garlic, salt, and pepper in a food processor or blender and process until smooth, scraping the sides occasionally. SPOON the puree into a bowl and serve with the pita wedges.

MediterrAsian Oysters

SERVES 4

A succulent combination of Mediterranean-seasoned and Asian-seasoned oysters on the half shell. This dish is very easy to whip up and can be enjoyed as an appetizer, or served as part of a seafood platter.

Crushed ice, for serving

24 very fresh raw oysters on the half shell

Mediterranean Dressing

2 tablespoons extra virgin olive oil

2 tablespoons freshly squeezed lemon juice

4 teaspoons finely chopped fresh flat-leaf parsley, plus sprigs for serving

2 teaspoons finely chopped red onion

Pinch of freshly ground black pepper

Asian Dressing

2 tablespoons fish sauce

2 tablespoons freshly squeezed lime juice

4 teaspoons finely chopped cilantro (fresh coriander), plus sprigs for serving

2 teaspoons finely chopped red chili

2 teaspoons finely chopped scallion

Place the crushed ice on a large serving plate and arrange the oysters evenly over the top. MIX together all the Mediterranean dressing ingredients in one bowl, and all the Asian dressing ingredients in another bowl. DRIZZLE half the oysters with the Mediterranean dressing and the other half with the Asian dressing. GARNISH with a sprig of parsley or cilantro and serve immediately.

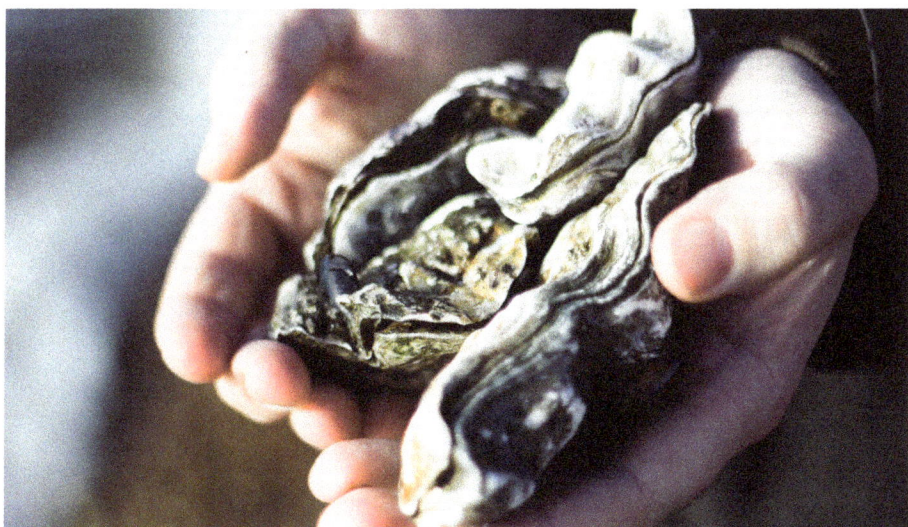

Phyllo Tartlets with Spinach, Pumpkin, Feta & Pine Nuts

SERVES 4

Roasted pumpkin, spinach and creamy feta cheese encased in delicate phyllo pastry, topped with pine nuts and baked until golden.

6 phyllo (filo) pastry sheets

2 cups peeled, diced pumpkin or winter squash

5 tablespoons extra virgin olive oil

1 onion, finely chopped

8 oz (230g) fresh spinach, stems removed and leaves roughly chopped

1 tablespoon finely chopped fresh dill

½ teaspoon salt

¼ teaspoon freshly ground black pepper

4 oz (115g) feta cheese, crumbled

1 tablespoon butter, melted

2 tablespoons pine nuts

PREHEAT oven to 350°F/180°C. TOSS the diced pumpkin with 1 tablespoon of olive oil, place in a single layer on a baking tray and cook for 15 minutes. WHILE the pumpkin bakes, heat 2 tablespoons of olive oil in a frying pan over a medium heat. COOK the onion for 6 minutes, then add the spinach and cook for 4 minutes, stirring regularly. STIR in the dill, salt and pepper and remove from the heat. STIR in the crumbled feta and baked pumpkin (keep the oven heated to 350°F/180°C) and set aside. COMBINE the remaining 2 tablespoons of olive oil with the melted butter in a small bowl. PLACE 2 phyllo sheets side-by-side on a work surface and brush each sheet evenly with the butter-oil mix. Place 2 more sheets on top and brush with butter-oil, then repeat once more. CUT each stack into six 5-inch (12.5 cm) squares, for a total of 12 stacks with 3 sheets each. LIGHTLY grease a standard 12-cup muffin pan with the butter-oil mix. PLACE each square phyllo stack into a muffin cup, pressing gently to mould the pastry into the bottom. SPOON ¼ cup of the spinach-pumpkin filling into each and fold the extra pastry back over the filling, roughly crumpling around the edges so that the filling is still exposed. BRUSH the edges with the remaining butter-oil mix. SPRINKLE pine nuts in the middle of each tart. BAKE for 22 minutes, then remove from the oven, and transfer the tarts from the muffin pan to a cooling rack. LET cool slightly then serve.

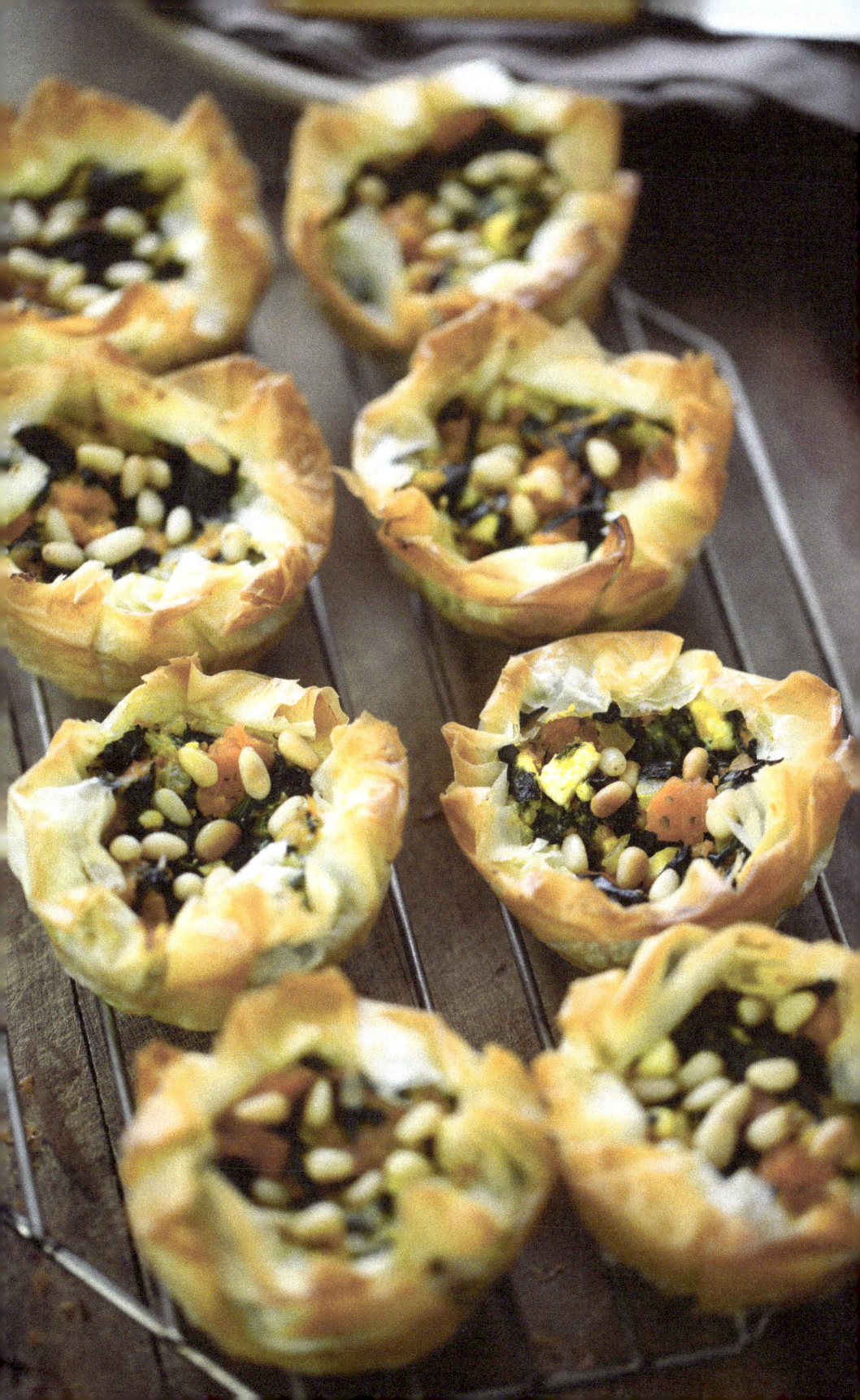

Lemongrass & Chili Mussels

SERVES 4

Steamed mussels infused with classic Thai-style seasonings.

1 cup coconut milk

2 scallions, thinly sliced on the diagonal

4 teaspoons finely chopped fresh lemongrass

4 teaspoons finely grated fresh ginger

2 small red chilies, deseeded and finely diced

2 cloves garlic, finely chopped

32 fresh mussels, cleaned and debearded

Cilantro (fresh coriander) leaves, for garnish

PLACE the coconut milk, scallions, lemongrass, ginger, chilies, and garlic in a large saucepan over high heat and bring to a boil. ADD the mussels, cover the pot, and steam over low heat, shaking the pan occasionally, until the mussels open, about 5 minutes. TRANSFER the mussels to serving bowls, reserving the liquid in the pan. HEAT the reserved liquid over high heat until reduced by half, about 3 minutes. POUR the liquid over the mussels and garnish with the cilantro leaves to serve.

Tip: Discard any mussels that haven't opened after cooking.

Asparagus with Garlic & Toasted Almonds

SERVES 4

Fresh asparagus spears are sautéed in olive oil, seasoned with white wine, garlic, salt and freshly ground pepper, then scattered with freshly toasted sliced almonds. Makes an appetizing side dish; can be served as an antipasto, meze or tapas dish; and can also be served cold as a salad.

½ cup sliced almonds

4 tablespoons extra virgin olive oil

1 red onion, finely diced

24 asparagus spears, woody ends removed

2 cloves garlic, minced

1 teaspoon salt

½ teaspoon freshly ground black pepper

4 tablespoons dry white wine

TOAST the almonds lightly in a skillet over medium heat until golden, 3 to 5 minutes. REMOVE and set aside. HEAT 3 tablespoons of the olive oil in the skillet over medium heat and cook the onion, stirring, for 3 minutes. ADD the asparagus, garlic, salt, and pepper and cook, stirring regularly, for 2 minutes. ADD the wine, cover the pan, and cook for 4 minutes. ADD the toasted almonds, mix thoroughly, and serve on a plate drizzled with the remaining half tablespoon of olive oil.

Asian-Style Corn Fritters

SERVES 4

These tasty fritters are delicious served with dipping sauces such as Nuoc Cham and Chinese-Style Dipping Sauce.

4 cups corn kernels, preferably fresh

2 cups self-rising flour

4 scallions, thinly sliced

2 large eggs, lightly beaten

4 tablespoons finely chopped cilantro (fresh coriander), plus sprigs for garnish

2 tablespoons fish sauce

2 teaspoons red curry paste mixed with 2 teaspoons boiling water

2 teaspoons salt

1 teaspoon ground black pepper

6 tablespoons peanut or canola oil

Thinly sliced cucumber, for garnish

Nuoc Cham Dipping Sauce (page 289), for serving

Chinese-Style Dipping Sauce (page 292), for serving

IN a bowl, mix together the corn, flour, scallions, eggs, cilantro, fish sauce, curry paste, salt, and pepper until well combined. SHAPE the mixture into fritters using wet hands to prevent sticking. HEAT a large skillet over medium heat, add half the oil, and swirl to coat the surface. COOK half the fritters for 3 minutes each side, then remove from the pan and keep warm. HEAT the remaining oil in the same pan and cook the other fritters. GARNISH the fritters with sliced cucumber and sprigs of fresh cilantro. SERVE with the dipping sauce of your choice.

Variation: To make shrimp fritters, replace the corn kernels with 2 cups of chopped cooked and peeled shrimp.

Fava Beans with Marinated Artichoke Hearts & Olives

SERVES 4

A tasty Greek meze (appetizer) dish with succulent kalamata olives, tender fava beans, and marinated artichoke hearts.

3 cups frozen fava beans (broad beans)

32 kalamata olives

4 jarred marinated artichoke hearts, quartered

4 tablespoons extra virgin olive oil

2 tablespoons freshly squeezed lemon juice

1 clove garlic, minced

1 teaspoon salt

4 teaspoons finely chopped fresh flat-leaf parsley

Freshly ground black pepper

COOK the fava beans in rapidly boiling water for 4 minutes, then rinse under cold water. REMOVE the leathery outer skin from the fava beans and discard. MIX together the shelled fava beans, olives, and artichoke hearts in a bowl. MIX together the olive oil, lemon juice, garlic, and salt in a small bowl. PLACE equal amounts of the fava bean mixture on serving plates. DRIZZLE with the dressing, and top with the parsley and a little freshly ground black pepper.

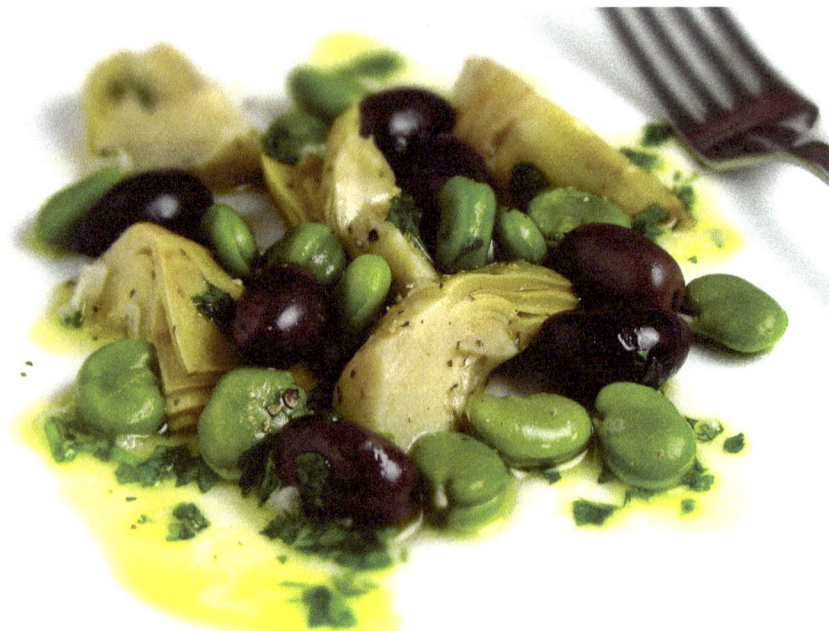

CHAPTER 26

DESSERTS

Fruit & Nut Salami

MAKES 2 LOGS

A scrumptious fruit 'salami' made from dried figs, dates, and apricots, and studded with chopped pistachio nuts. It's not only one of our favorite sweet treats, we also use it in a variety of delicious savory ways too, including as part of a cheese board (it goes perfectly with shaved Parmesan or Spanish manchego cheese).

12 oz (340g) dried figs, roughly chopped

¼ teaspoon ground cinnamon

¼ teaspoon vanilla extract

4 oz (115g) dried dates, finely chopped

4 oz (115g) dried apricots, finely chopped

3 oz (85g) lightly toasted unsalted pistachio nuts, finely chopped

PLACE the figs, cinnamon and vanilla extract in a food processor and process to a sticky paste. IN a large bowl, mix the fig paste with the chopped dates, apricots and pistachio nuts until thoroughly combined. DIVIDE the mixture in half and place each portion along the center of a sheet of baking paper in a log shape. TIGHTLY roll up each 'salami' in the baking paper to form a neatly packed cylinder (you can also use a sushi rolling mat to make this even easier). SQUEEZE firmly to make sure each roll is tightly packed, and secure the ends by twisting them. REFRIGERATE for 2 hours before slicing into rounds.

Mango with Lime Syrup & Toasted Coconut

SERVES 4

A sweet and simple Thai dessert, perfect for cooling the palate after a hot Thai curry.

½ cup water

4 tablespoons freshly squeezed lime juice

2 tablespoons sugar

2 teaspoons coarsely grated lime zest

4 tablespoons shredded dried coconut

4 mangoes, peeled, seeds removed, and flesh cut into cubes

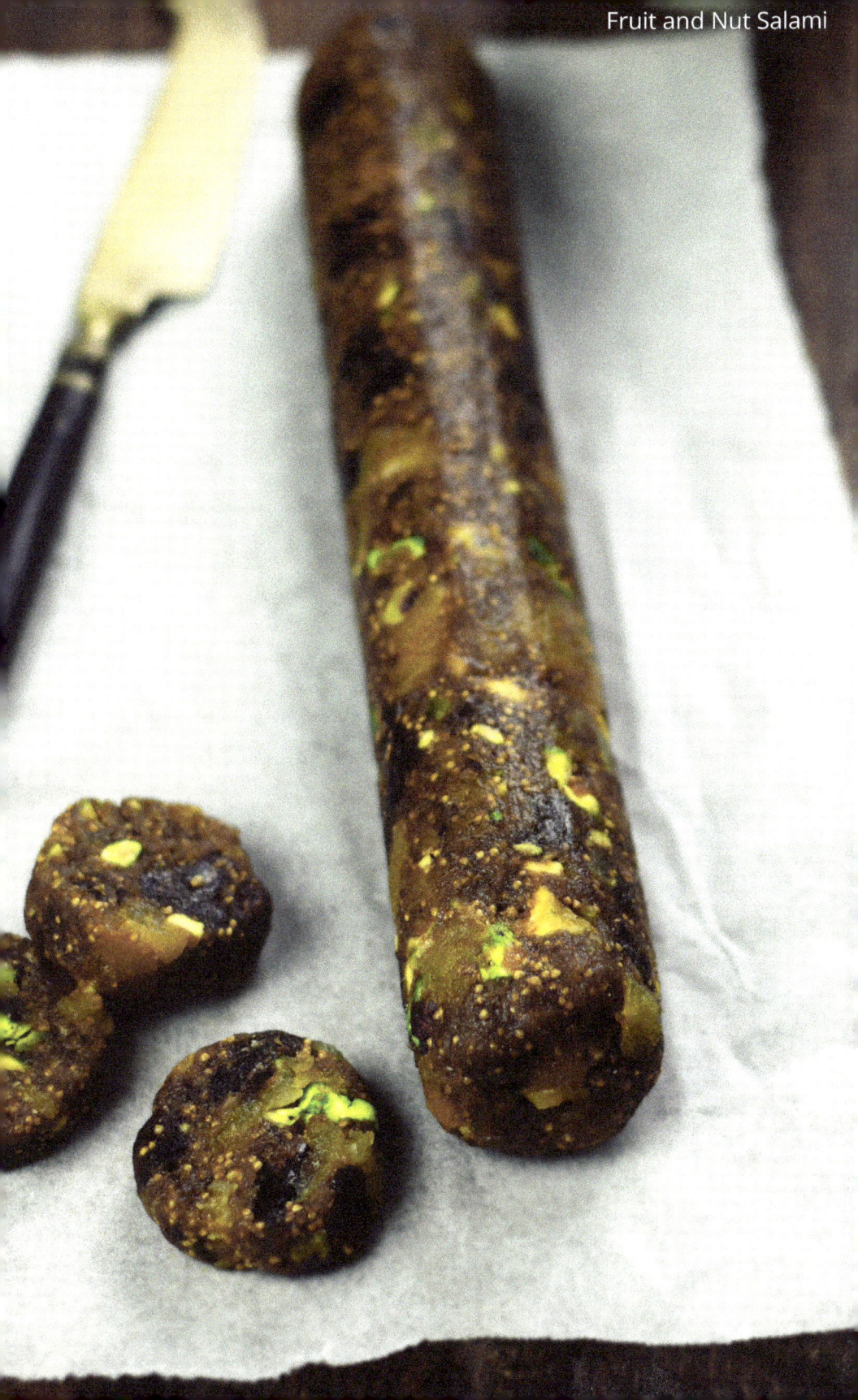
Fruit and Nut Salami

COMBINE the water, lime juice, sugar, and lime zest in a small saucepan, stir to combine, simmer gently for 5 minutes until reduced by about half, then strain to remove the zest. TOAST the coconut in a skillet over medium heat. ARRANGE the cubed mango on plates, drizzle with the lime syrup, and sprinkle with the toasted coconut to serve.

Provençal Apple & Walnut Pie

SERVES 4

This dessert tastes delicious served warm from the oven and topped with a scoop of good-quality vanilla ice cream.

2 large egg whites	½ cup all-purpose (plain) flour
½ cup sugar	1 cup peeled and diced apple
1 teaspoon vanilla extract	¼ cup chopped walnuts
1 teaspoon baking powder	Vanilla ice cream, for serving
½ teaspoon cinnamon	

PREHEAT the oven to 350°F/180°C and lightly grease a pie plate. BEAT the eggs, sugar, vanilla, baking powder, and cinnamon in a mixing bowl. MIX in the flour until well blended, then stir in the apples and walnuts. Pour the mixture into the prepared pie plate and bake for 30 minutes. SERVE cut in wedges and topped with a scoop of vanilla ice cream.

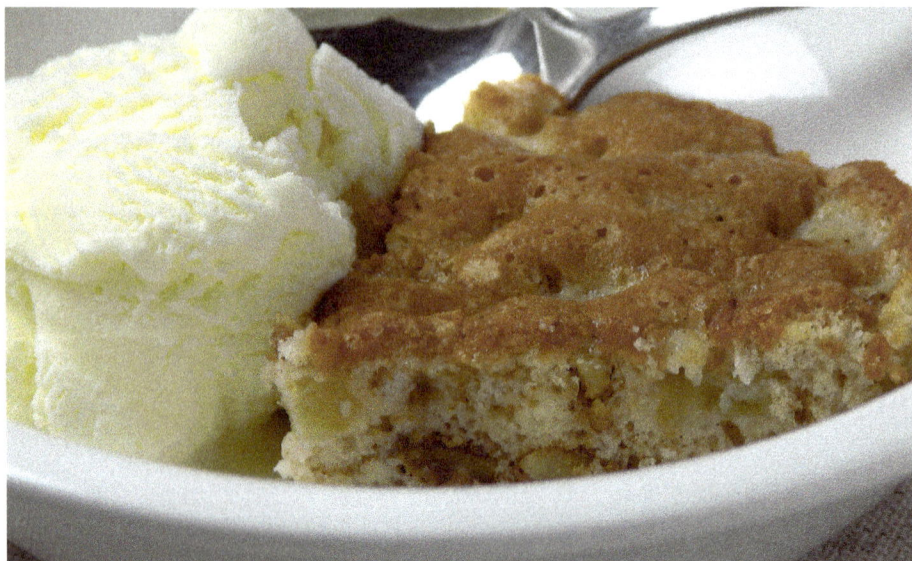

Pears with Peach Ricotta Whip & Almonds

SERVES 4

Ricotta cheese makes the perfect base for this creamy fruit dessert.

¾ cup ricotta cheese

¾ cup drained canned sliced peaches

1 tablespoon confectioners' (icing) sugar

12 canned pear halves

4 tablespoons sliced almonds

PLACE the ricotta cheese, peaches, and sugar in a food processor or blender and process for 1 minute. POUR the mixture into a bowl and chill, covered, in the refrigerator for 2 hours to firm (or in the freezer for 1 hour). PUT three pear halves in each serving bowl, pour over the peach ricotta whip, and sprinkle with the almonds.

Mango, Grape & Honeydew Melon Salad

SERVES 4

The luscious flesh of these fruits, which range in color from pale green to deep orange, makes a delicious fruit salad. Orange fruits are an excellent source of beta-carotene, a powerful antioxidant that converts in the body to vitamin A, which is important for healthy skin and good vision.

2 cups red or green seedless grapes

4 mangoes, peeled, seeds removed, and flesh cut into cubes

1 honeydew melon, peeled and flesh cut into cubes

2 tablespoons sugar

4 tablespoons water

Ice cream, fresh or frozen yogurt, or sorbet, for serving

COMBINE all the fruits in a serving dish. MIX the sugar and water until dissolved and toss gently with the fruit to coat. SERVE by itself or with a scoop of ice cream, fresh or frozen yogurt, or sorbet.

Tunisian Orange, Date, & Pistachio Salad

SERVES 4

Cinnamon adds an exotic touch to a plate of refreshing sliced oranges garnished with dates and pistachio nuts. Serve this simple dessert as is, or with a scoop of ice cream or yogurt.

8 oranges (6 oranges peeled and all the white pith removed with a sharp knife, and 2 oranges juiced)

2 teaspoons confectioners' (icing) sugar

½ teaspoon cinnamon

12 dried dates, finely chopped

20 pistachio nuts, peeled and chopped

SLICE the peeled oranges into rounds and arrange, overlapping, in a shallow serving bowl. COMBINE the orange juice with the sugar and cinnamon. DRIZZLE the juice over the orange rounds and garnish with the chopped dates and pistachio nuts.

Variation: Replace the pistachio nuts with toasted slivered almonds.

Strawberries & Mascarpone Cheese

SERVES 4

This dessert is simplicity itself.

1 cup mascarpone cheese

2 tablespoons confectioners' (icing) sugar

28 fresh, ripe strawberries, hulled

MIX together the mascarpone cheese and sugar in a small bowl until well combined. SERVE the strawberries with the sweetened mascarpone cheese for dipping.

Variations: Replace the mascarpone cheese with crème fraîche. As an alternative, you can macerate the strawberries to allow them to soften: Remove the stems and cut the strawberries lengthwise into quarters. Toss them in a bowl with a little superfine or confectioners' sugar and dash of fruit liqueur like Cointreau. Cover and allow to macerate in the refrigerator for at least 1 hour.

Mixed Berry Coulis

SERVES 4

Fresh strawberries and blueberries are folded through a berry sauce and served with vanilla-flavored Greek yogurt and almonds.

16 ounces (450g) strawberries, hulled

10 ounces (280g) blueberries

4 tablespoons confectioners' (icing) sugar

1 cup Greek yogurt

1 teaspoon vanilla extract

4 tablespoons sliced almonds (lightly toasted, if desired)

PUT half the strawberries and half the blueberries in a blender with 2 tablespoons of the sugar, and process until smooth. CUT the remaining strawberries into quarters, toss with the remaining blueberries, then fold into the berry sauce. MIX together the yogurt, vanilla, and remaining sugar in a small bowl until well combined. SPOON the berry coulis into four dessert bowls, top with the vanilla yogurt, and scatter each with a tablespoon of almonds.

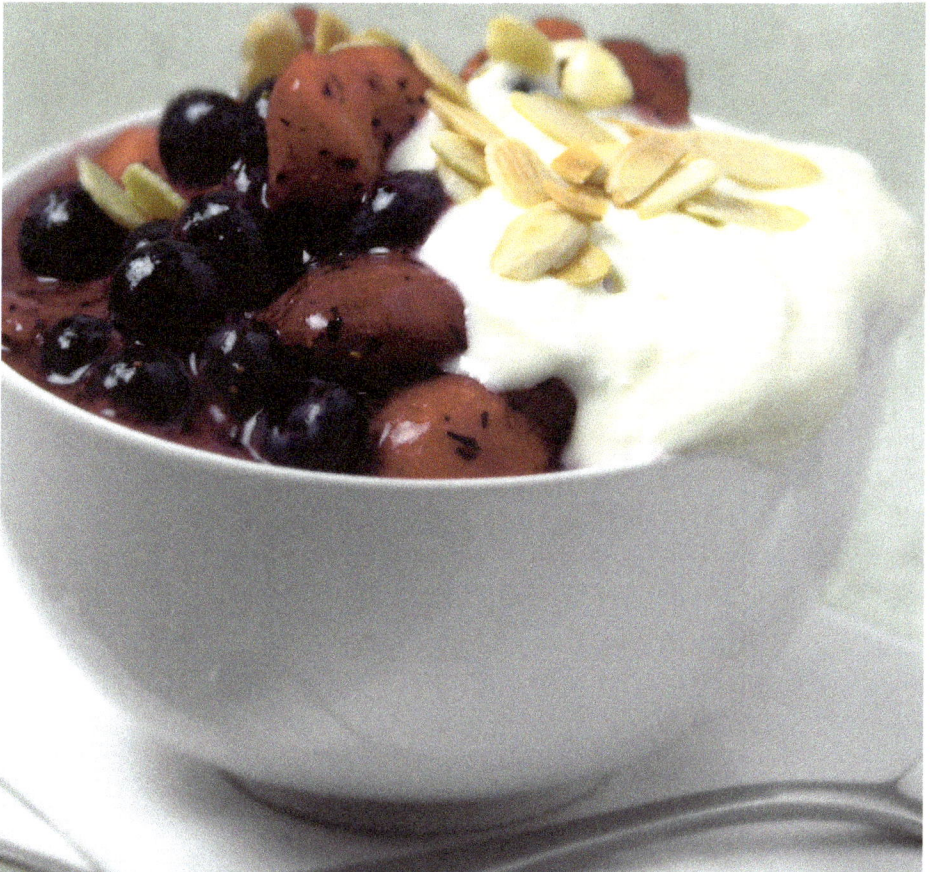

Asian-Style Fruit Salad

SERVES 4

This exotic salad of fresh and canned fruits provides the perfect ending to any Asian meal (or any meal, for that matter).

2 kiwi fruit, peeled and thinly sliced

2 mangoes, peeled, seeds removed, and flesh cut into cubes

2 mandarins, peeled and divided into segments

1 cup drained canned lychees

1 cup drained canned pineapple pieces

Ice cream, fresh or frozen yogurt, or sorbet, for serving

COMBINE all the fruits in a bowl and toss gently to mix. SERVE with a scoop of ice cream, fresh or frozen yogurt, or sorbet.

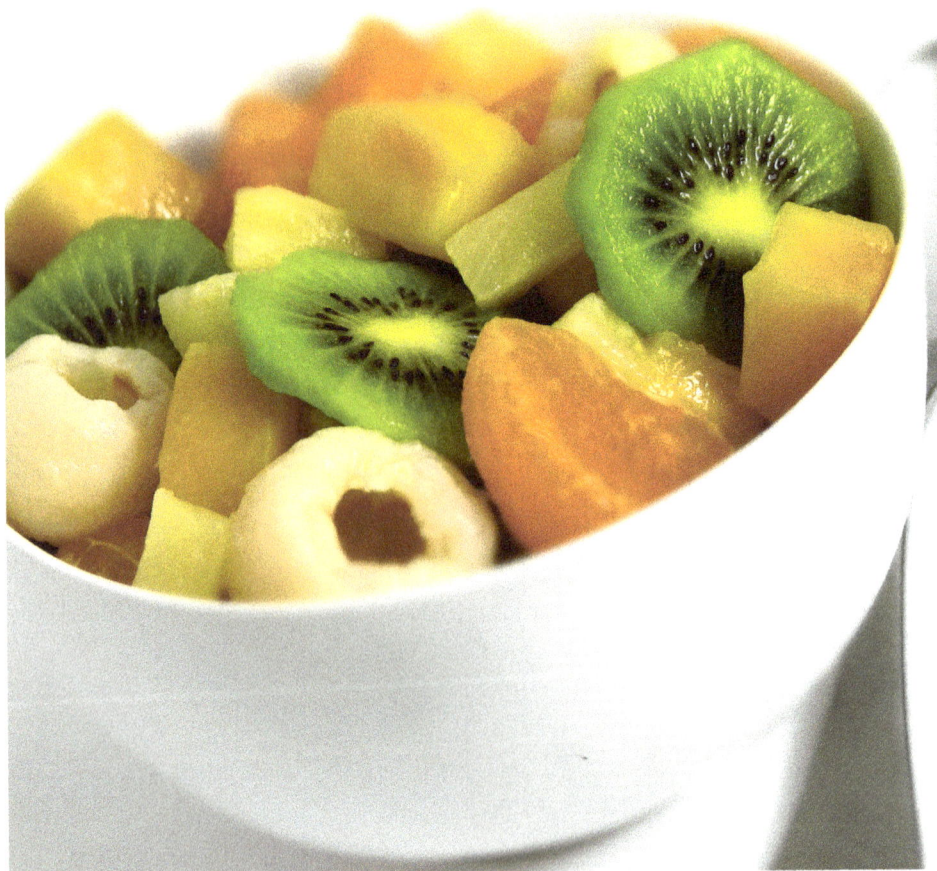

Middle Eastern Fruit & Nut Compote

SERVES 4

A simple but exotic Middle Eastern dessert in which dried fruits are simmered in a cinnamon-infused syrup until plump and tender.

1 cup orange juice

½ cup water

1 tablespoon brown sugar

½ teaspoon cinnamon

1 cup dried apricots

½ cup dried figs

½ cup raisins

Ice cream or fresh or frozen yogurt, for serving

4 tablespoons toasted sliced almonds

PLACE the orange juice, water, sugar, and cinnamon in a small saucepan, stir to combine, and bring to a boil. ADD the apricots, figs, and raisins, cover the pot, reduce the heat to medium-low, and simmer for 20 minutes. SERVE the fruit compote in bowls with a spoonful of ice cream or yogurt and sprinkled with the almonds.

Variation: Other dried fruits like prunes, apples, and peaches can also be used, and pistachio nuts or pine nuts can be substituted for the almonds.

INDEX

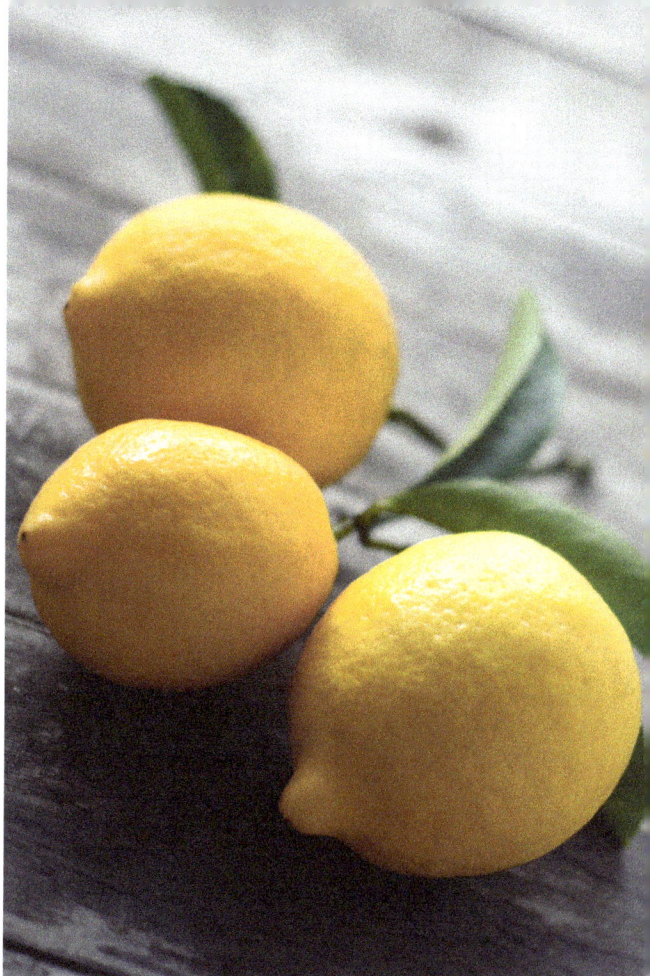

Lightning Source UK Ltd.
Milton Keynes UK
UKHW051339140319
339128UK00010B/119/P

9 780473 453763